D0763038

**This publication was supported by a grant from the
Mead Johnson Pediatric Nutrition Institute.**

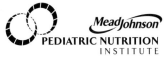

World Review of Nutrition and Dietetics

Vol. 110

Series Editor

Berthold Koletzko Munich

Nutritional Care of Preterm Infants

Scientific Basis and Practical Guidelines

Volume Editors

Berthold Koletzko Munich
Brenda Poindexter Indianapolis, Ind.
Ricardo Uauy Santiago de Chile

35 figures, 10 in color and 37 tables, 2014

KARGER Basel · Freiburg · Paris · London · New York · Chennai · New Delhi ·
Bangkok · Beijing · Shanghai · Tokyo · Kuala Lumpur · Singapore · Sydney

Berthold Koletzko
Div. Metabolic and Nutritional Medicine
Dr. von Hauner Children's Hospital
Univ. of Munich Medical Centre –
Klinikum d. Univ. München
München
Germany

Brenda Poindexter
Indiana University School of Medicine
Section of Neonatal-Perinatal Medicine
Riley Hospital for Children at Indiana University
Health
Indianapolis, Ind.
USA

Ricardo Uauy
Division of Neonatology Pontifical Catholic
University Medical School and Institute of
Nutrition INTA Universidad de Chile
Santiago de Chile
Chile

Bibliographic Indices. This publication is listed in bibliographic services, including Current Contents® and PubMed/MEDLINE.

© Copyright 2014 by S. Karger AG, P.O. Box, CH–4009 Basel (Switzerland)
www.karger.com
Printed in Germany on acid-free and non-aging paper (ISO 9706) by Kraft Druck, Ettlingen
ISSN 0084–2230
e-ISSN 1662–3975

Contents

List of Contributors

Laura D. Brown
Department of Pediatrics
Section of Neonatology
Perinatal Research Center
University of Colorado School of Medicine
13243 East 23rd Avenue
Aurora, CO 80045 (USA)

Femke de Groof
Department of Pediatrics
Medisch Centrum Alkmaar
Wilhelminalaan 12
NL–1815 JD Alkmaar (The Netherlands)

Scott C. Denne
Department of Pediatrics
University of Indiana School of Medicine
702 Barnhill Dr, Room 5900
Indianapolis, IN 46202 (USA)

Magnus Domellöf
Department of Clinical Sciences
Umea University
Pediatrics
SE–90185 Umea (Sweden)

Richard A. Ehrenkranz
Yale Pediatrics
Yale University School of Medicine
PO Box 208064
New Haven, CT 06520-8064 (USA)

Nicholas D. Embleton
Newcastle Neonatal Service
Ward 35 Royal Victoria Infirmary
Newcastle upon Tyne NE1 4LP (UK)

Christoph Fusch
Department of Pediatrics
McMaster University & Hamilton Health
Sciences
1280 Main Street west
Hamilton, Ont. L8S4K8 (Canada)

Michael K. Georgieff
Division of Neonatology
Department of Pediatrics
2450 Riverside Avenue
East Building MB-630
Minneapolis, MN 55454 (USA)

William W. Hay, Jr.
Department of Pediatrics
Section of Neonatology
Perinatal Research Center
University of Colorado School of Medicine
Anschutz Medical Campus F441
13243 East 23rd Avenue
Aurora, CO 80045 (USA)

Frank Jochum
Head of the Department of Pediatrics
Ev. Waldkrankenhaus Spandau
Stadtrandstr. 555
DE–13589 Berlin (Germany)

Gert Francois Kirsten
Head Neonatal Division
Tygerberg Children's Hospital and
University of Stellenbosch
PO Box 19063
Tygerberg
ZA–7505 Cape Town (South Africa)

Berthold Koletzko
Division of Metabolic and Nutritional Medicine
Dr. von Hauner Children's Hospital
University of Munich Medical Centre
Lindwurmstr. 4
DE–80337 Munich (Germany)

Zoe Lansdowne
National Institute for Health Research
Southampton Biomedical/ Pharmacy Research
Centre
Mailpoint 40
Southampton General Hospital
Tremona Road
Southampton SO16 6YD (UK)

Alexandre Lapillonne
Department of Neonatology
Necker-Enfants Malades Hospital
149 rue de Sevres
FR–75015 Paris (France)

Alison Leaf
National Institute for Health Research
Southampton Biomedical Research Centre
University of Southampton
Mailpoint 803
Child Health, Level F, South Block
Southampton General Hospital
Tremona Road
Southampton SO16 6YD (UK)

Ronit Lubetzky
Department of Pediatrics
Tel Aviv-Sourasky Medical Center
6 Weizman Street
IL–64239 Tel-Aviv (Israel)

Dror Mandel
Tel Aviv-Sourasky Medical Center
6 Weizman Street
IL–64239 Tel-Aviv (Israel)

Francis B. Mimouni
Department of Pediatrics
Tel Aviv Medical Center
6 Weizman Street
IL– 64239 Tel Aviv (Israel)

Fernando Moya
Director of Neonatology
Betty Cameron Women and Children's Hospital
2131 S. 17th Street
Wilmington, NC 28401 (USA)

Teresa Murguia-Peniche
Foege Fellow at Rollins School of Public Health
Hubert Department of Global Health
Emory University
1518 Clifton Road NE
Atlanta, GA 30322 (USA)

Josef Neu
Pediatrics/Neonatology
University of Florida
1600 SW Archer Road
Gainesville, FL 32610 (USA)

Brenda Poindexter
Indiana University School of Medicine
Section of Neonatal-Perinatal Medicine
Riley Hospital for Children at
Indiana University Health
699 Riley Hospital Dr. RR208
Indianapolis, IN 46202 (USA)

Sara E. Ramel
Division of Neonatology
University of Minnesota Amplatz Children's
Hospital
University of Minnesota School of Medicine
2450 Riverside Avenue
East Building MB-630
Minneapolis, MN 55454 (USA)

Thibault Senterre
University of Liège
Department of Neonatology
CHU de Liège
CHR de la Citadelle
Boulevard du XII de Ligne, 1
B–4000 Liège (Belgium)

Karen Simmer
Centre for Neonatal Research and Education
School of Paediatrics and Child Health
University of Western Australia (M550)
35 Stirling Highway
Crawley, W.A. 6009 (Australia)

Hania Szajewska
Department of Paediatrics
The Medical University of Warsaw
Dzialdowska 1
PL–01-184 Warsaw (Poland)

Reginald C. Tsang
3333 Burnet Ave
Cincinnati, OH 45229 (USA)

List of Contributors

Ricardo Uauy
Division of Neonatology Pontifical Catholic
University
Medical School and Institute of Nutrition INTA
Universidad de Chile
Macul 5540
11 Santiago de Chile (Chile)

Chris H. van den Akker
Department of Pediatrics
Sophia Children's Hospital
ErasmusMC
Postbus 2060
NL–3000 CB Rotterdam (The Netherlands)

Sophie R.D. van der Schoor
Department of Pediatrics
Onze Lieve Vrouwe Gasthuis
Oosterpark 9
NL–1091 AC Amsterdam (The Netherlands)

Johannes B. van Goudoever
Department of Pediatrics
Emma Children's Hospital
AMC, c/o Room H7-282
P.O. Box 22660
NL–1100 DD Amsterdam (The Netherlands)

Hester Vlaardingerbroek
Department of Pediatrics
Emma Children's Hospital
AMC, c/o Room H7-282
P.O. Box 22660
NL–1100 DD Amsterdam (The Netherlands)

Ekhard E. Ziegler
Department of Pediatrics
University of Iowa
2501 Crosspark Rd.
Coralville, IA 52241-8802 (USA)

Preface

Improved conditions of care for premature infants have led to markedly increased survival rates over the last few decades, particularly in infants with very low birth weight (<1,500 g) and extremely low birth weight (<1,000 g). Therefore, increased attention is now directed to improving long-term outcome, health and quality of life. Accumulating evidence demonstrates that nutritional care is a central cornerstone towards achieving this goal. Normal fetal growth in utero is extremely rapid, for example from 30 to 36 weeks of gestation fetal body weight doubles in only 6 weeks, along with remarkable tissue differentiation. It remains an enormous challenge to match this quantity and quality of growth and development in infants whose nutrient supply via the umbilical cord has been prematurely interrupted. Major progress has been achieved in our understanding of meeting their nutrient needs, but a surprising variability of neonatal nutritional support exists in clinical practice around the world, within countries, and even between different physicians working in one and the same neonatal unit. Current knowledge on nutrient requirements and the practice of nutritional care in premature infants is provided by this book, with a focus on very low birth weight infants. The most recent evidence and critical analyses were contributed by leading experts in the field from all five continents. The manuscripts have been shared among all authors and further reviewers who provided critical comments prior to a two-day authors' meeting held in Munich, Germany, in July 2013. The authors presented their chapters which were critically discussed, and agreement on conclusions and recommendations was sought. The manuscripts were then thoroughly revised to comprise these considerations and to include latest knowledge as guidance for clinical application.

The editors and authors wish to thank Prof. Reginald Tsang (Cincinnati, Ohio, USA) who inspired the creation of this volume by editing two previous landmark books on this topic [1, 2] and kindly served as senior editorial advisor in the current project. We are grateful to Dr. Colin Rudolph and colleagues at the Mead Johnson Pediatric Nutrition Institute who kindly provided financial support to Karger Publishers, Basel, Switzerland, to facilitate publication. We are indebted to the whole Karger team for their dedication and enthusiasm in producing this book.

Berthold Koletzko, Munich
Brenda Poindexter, Indianapolis, Ind.
Ricardo Uauy, Santiago de Chile

References

1 Tsang R, Lucas A, Uauy R, Zlotkin S (eds): Nutritional Needs of Preterm Infants. Scientific Basis and Practical Guidelines. Baltimore, Williams & Wilkins, 1993, pp 65–86.

2 Tsang R, Uauy R, Koletzko B, Zlotkin S (eds): Nutrition of the Preterm Infant. Scientific Basis and Practical Application, ed 2. Cincinnati, Digital Educ Publ, 2005, pp 97–139.

Koletzko B, Poindexter B, Uauy R (eds): Nutritional Care of Preterm Infants: Scientific Basis and Practical Guidelines.
World Rev Nutr Diet. Basel, Karger, 2014, vol 110, pp 1–3 (DOI: 10.1159/000358451)

Historical Perspective

Reginald C. Tsang

First, I want to warmly congratulate the editors and authors of this new volume of 'Nutritional Care of Premature Infants'. I was amused and privileged to be invited to attend the meeting of the authors in Munich, Germany, as the 'old man' to come to bless the event, on the invitation of esteemed Professors Koletzko and Uauy – wonderful editors who I have worked with on many occasions in the past.

The story of this book actually goes back to 1984 [1], when we first published 'Vitamin and Mineral Requirements in Preterm Infants', where my preface indicated the 'need to give tentative answers to "real-life situations" of the pre-term infant in the nursery'. The authors were instructed to concisely present their recommendations and provoke discussions with regard to the difficulties in arriving at these particular recommendations. Over the years, several books have also contributed directly and indirectly to the development and presentation of the present book. In sequence, they were, in 1988 'Nutrition during Infancy' [2]; in 1993 'Nutritional Needs of the Preterm Infant: Scientific Basis and Practical Guidelines' [3] wherein we stated: 'the book is meant to be practical and easily accessible so that in the "middle of the night" the practitioner would have information readily available for use in the management of preterm infants'; in 1997 'Nutrition during Infancy' [4], and the most recent book, in 2005, 'Nutrition of the Pre-Term Infant: Scientific Basis and Practical Guidelines' [5]. These books played important roles in developing our current thinking, in terms of content and how best to organize and present the information, particularly focusing on practical and useful information in the clinical setting.

What drove our relatively visionary effort was the feeling that most books in this field had been written for rather elite groups of investigators and neonatologists, who normally read the literature from original scientific articles, but were hard put to find a reference material that they could use for practical purposes. Thus developed the clear emphasis of bringing the theoretic considerations for determining nutrient requirements in preterm infants *into the practical world* of neonatology, and in particular for the developing preterm infant. It is particularly exciting *today*, in view of the rapid worldwide development of neonatology, that many more preterm infants are now surviving, and therefore their nutrition becomes of primary importance, rather than just the acute resuscitative efforts around the time of delivery or the first few days of life.

It was apparent throughout the various iterations that there was an enthusiastic team spirit during the key authors' meeting, with authors *encouraged to have* a major focus to provide coherence in recommendations and development of reasonable consensus. This focus has resulted in the book's now established practical utility for practicing neonatologists, nutritionists, and nurses in the newborn intensive care unit (NICU) all over the world.

Our rather unique involvement of industry was clearly a win-win situation for all concerned, because while NICU staff needed practical information to manage their infants, certainly many in the nutrition industry also needed accurate and scientific information to produce the best products possible for the infant. Indeed, their resources were extremely helpful in assembling the group of authors together, a rather novel approach at the time to produce a book, and they were particularly helpful in distributing books to various NICUs, often globally, so that the information arrived literally in the hands of NICU staff for immediate application.

Academicians like myself tend to not like to be 'pinned down' about the 'bottom line number' that is being recommended, and we tend to give 'academic answers' because of the lack of absolute certainty on many issues. However the practicing medical personnel need very practical conclusions to scientific deliberations; they face a baby that needs care, all theories aside. This interaction with industry basically also helped academicians to confront the realities of 'life in the real world'.

A few stories illustrate the progress over the years; one more interesting episode involved an investigator who required the editor to fly across the Atlantic to sit down for one whole day to finish a manuscript that was holding up the book; Alan Lucas' creative involvement of Princess Anne in one of the iterations provided some royal glamour (Princess Anne, Buckingham Palace, wrote: 'The whole process must be highly unusual, if not unique, in medical writing, was conducted with good grace and remarkably little acrimony; having meetings in exotic places like Captiva Island, FL, where authors were literally held *"captive"* on the premises, with no chance of enjoying the beautiful scenery because of the intensity of the work; the most recent book translated into Chinese [6], and even counterfeited – a sure sign of "recognition of its importance" apparently').

It is with great memories that I see the launch of the new book 'Nutritional Care of Premature Infants', and I wish all the authors and the readership to maximally utilize and 'dog-ear' this book from cover to cover, for the care of our precious charges.

References

1 Tsang RC (ed): Vitamin and Mineral Requirements in Preterm Infants. New York, Dekker, 1985.
2 Specker BL, Greer F, Tsang RC: Vitamin D; in Tsang RC, Nichols BL (eds): Nutrition during Infancy. Philadelphia, Hanley & Belfus, 1988, pp 264–276.
3 Tsang RC: Nutritional needs of the preterm Infant; in Tsang RC, Lucas A, Uauy R, Zlotkin S (eds): Scientific Basis and Practical Guidelines. Pawling/NY, Caduceus Medical Publishers, 1993.
4 Tsang RC, Nichols B, Zlotkin S, Hansen J: Nutrition during Infancy, p. v. Cincinnati, Digital Educational Publishing, Inc, 1997.
5 Tsang RC, Uauy R, Koletzko B, Zlotkin S (eds): Nutrition of the Pre-Term Infant: Scientific basis and practical guidelines, p. iii. Cincinnati, Digital Educational Publishing, Inc, 2005.

Reginald C. Tsang
3333 Burnet Ave
Cincinnati, OH 45229 (USA)
E-Mail rctsang@gmail.com

Koletzko B, Poindexter B, Uauy R (eds): Nutritional Care of Preterm Infants: Scientific Basis and Practical Guidelines.
World Rev Nutr Diet. Basel, Karger, 2014, vol 110, pp 4–10 (DOI: 10.1159/000358453)

Defining the Nutritional Needs of Preterm Infants

Ricardo Uauy[a] · Berthold Koletzko[b]

[a]Division of Neonatology, Pontifical Catholic University Medical School and Institute of Nutrition INTA Universidad de Chile, Santiago de Chile, Chile; [b]Dr. von Hauner Children's Hospital University of Munich Medical Centre, Munich, Germany

Reviewed by Hania Szajewska, Department of Paediatrics, The Medical University of Warsaw, Warsaw, Poland; Richard Ehrenkranz, Department of Pediatrics, Yale University School of Medicine, New Haven, Conn., USA

Abstract

Nutritional needs are defined as the amount and chemical form of a nutrient needed to support normal health, growth and development without disturbing the metabolism of other nutrients. Nutrient intake recommendations are based on the estimated average requirement (EAR) of a population group. Enteral and parenteral needs differ for many nutrients because of differences in bioavailability and utilization. Assuming a near-normal distribution of nutrient needs, the reference nutrient intake (RNI – also called population reference intake or recommended dietary allowance) is equal to the EAR plus two standard deviations of the distribution, with the exception of energy intake where the reference intake is equal to the EAR. The upper level (UL) is the highest level of intake where no untoward effects can be detected in virtually all individuals in a specific population group. The acceptable range of intakes (AR) is the range from the EAR to the UL that is considered safe, however preterm infants are not a homogeneous population thus intake often needs to be individualized based on clinical condition and developmental stage.   © 2014 S. Karger AG, Basel

Meeting the nutritional needs of preterm infants represents a continuing challenge facing neonatologists, gastroenterology and nutrition consultants, nutritionists and dieticians, nurses, as well as the infants' families [1]. Around the world, improvements of perinatal care have led to both increased survival and reduced long-term morbidity, such as chronic lung disease and neurodevelopmental impairment, in preterm infants, particularly in very low birth weight (VLBW) (birth weight <1,500 g) and extremely low birth weight (ELBW) infants (birth weight <1,000 g) [2–5]. These trends have led to a paradigm change with a shift of focus from securing survival to a concern with providing support optimal outcomes, development and quality of life in surviving infants. This paradigm change includes a markedly increased attention to nutritional care of preterm infants prompted by data that demonstrate a considerable importance

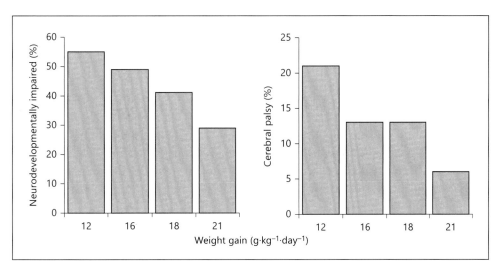

Fig. 1. In 490 ELBW infants, higher growth velocity on the neonatal intensive care unit similar to intrauterine growth rates predicts a better neurological outcome at 18–22 months' corrected age [drawn from 7].

of early nutrition and growth on long-term outcome [6]. For example, higher growth velocity on the neonatal intensive care unit that was similar to intrauterine growth rates predicts better neurological outcome at 18–22 months corrected age in 490 ELBW infants [7] (fig. 1). The early provision of human milk [8] and higher intakes of protein and energy in the first week of life [9] have been linked to improved neurodevelopmental outcomes. Evidence for a causal role of nutrition was provided by data from a randomized clinical trial in infants born with a birth weight <1,850 g. The trial results showed that provision of higher intakes of energy, protein and nutrients during an average 30 days after birth led to a significantly higher intelligence quotient at 7.5–8 years of age in boys, along with less cerebral palsy [10], and in the subgroup revisited in adolescents a persistent improvement of intelligence quotient associated with detectable differences in brain structure [11]. Benefits were also demonstrated for improved provision of specific nutrients. For example, a large randomized, double-blind controlled trial in 657 preterm infants born <33 gestational weeks showed that providing a higher DHA supply (1 vs. 0.3% of dietary fat) reduced severe neurodevelopmental impairment with a Bayley MDI <70 at 18 months by about one half [12].

These and other data support the importance of striving for optimal nutrition support in preterm infants and has placed a greater demand for: (a) knowledge on developmental biology, physiology and biochemistry as they provide the science base for the practices utilized in the nutritional care of low birth weight (LBW <2,500) infants, VLBW and ELBW, birth weight <1,000 g) infants; (b) the conduct of larger scale randomized controlled clinical trials to define safe, effective, and ultimately cost-effective feeding modalities required to establish evidence-based sound clinical practices. A new research agenda has been generated and partly answered over the past decades, yet much remains to be done. Moreover, knowledge on the consequences of early nutrition on later health and well-being has added a new dimension to the significance of early nutritional practices on life-long health. In addition to addressing the imperative of improving the survival of smaller and progressively more immature neonates, perinatal care must also consider the effects this might have on the long-term quality of life, performance, burden of disease and disability. Addressing the nutritional needs of small and preterm infants needs to generate guidance with a global scope that is oriented to all children independent of ethnic and socioeconomic condition.

Nutrition during early life is now recognized not only as a key determinant for immediate neonatal survival, growth and mental development during infancy, but also as a major conditioning factor for long-term health [13, 14]. The mechanisms for these effects are beginning to be unraveled, but still remain to be fully defined [15]. There are now convincing data for adequate nutrition as an important factor affecting the short- and long-term quality of life of those that survive the neonatal period. Nutrition not only contributes to recovery from neonatal disease and early discharge from the nursery, but also provides the substrates necessary for early brain growth and thus affects neurodevelopment in later life. In addition, the epigenetic programming of metabolic and other physiologic functions are marked by early life experiences. These effects include the effect of metabolic and nutritional deficits and excesses; these play an important role in defining later risk of adult chronic diseases (diabetes, hypertension, dyslipidemia and cardiovascular disease). The achievement of appropriate growth is not an easy task considering the special needs of the premature infants as a result of immaturity of the gastrointestinal tract, difficulties in metabolic adaptations, and the concomitant neonatal medical disease conditions. Defining what is 'normal' and or 'optimal' growth remains an elusive goal since in many cases the health outcomes are defined in part by our practices, including early nutrition. Thus, the only way to define 'optimal' in practice is by first establishing nutritional goals that will guide our nutritional prescription of high-risk neonates. These should be based on promoting survival with the lowest (early and late) burden of death and disability.

Definition of Key Concepts

Nutritional Needs: Nutrient requirements were defined by the Committee on Nutrition of the European Society for Paediatric Gastroenterology, Hepatology and Nutrition (ESPGHAN) as follows [16]: 'Physiological requirement is the amount and chemical form of a nutrient that is needed systematically to maintain normal health and development without disturbance of the metabolism of any other nutrient. The corresponding dietary requirement would be the intake sufficient to meet the physiological requirement. Ideally this should be achieved without extreme homeostatic processes and excessive depletion or surplus in bodily depots.' Nutrient intakes via the enteral or parenteral route meeting requirements will promote optimal growth and development, and prevent

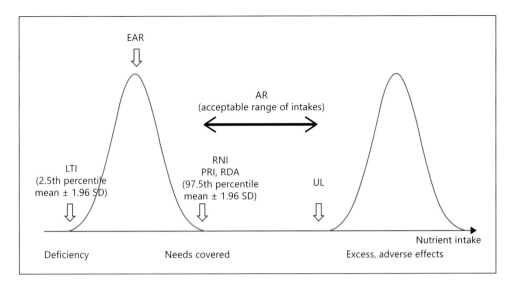

Fig. 2. Schematic depiction of the terms used for describing reference nutrient intakes. LTI = Lowest threshold intake; EAR = estimated average requirement; RNI = reference nutrient intake; PRI = population reference intake; RDA = recommended dietary allowance; UL = upper safe level of intake; AR = acceptable range of intakes (see text for details).

risks associated with nutritional deficiency or excess [17]. Most nutrient requirement estimates are intended for apparently 'healthy' individuals; healthy is defined by absence of disease, based on clinical signs and symptoms, and functional normalcy assessed by routine laboratory methods and physical evaluation [18]. Unfortunately, most VLBW and ELBW infants are sick, and thus the definition of their nutritional requirements cannot be simply extrapolated from the needs of healthy infants. Moreover, the science base to adjust nutrient needs by specific disease categories in most cases is lacking.

Enteral Nutritional Needs: The same as above but delivery is exclusive to the enteral route.

Individual Nutritional Requirement: The given level of a nutrient that will meet specified criteria of nutritional adequacy, preventing adverse consequences associated with nutritional deficit or excess for a given individual. These criteria may encompass a range of biological effects related to given nutrient intakes, thus the requirement value is linked to the specific criteria used; thus the first step in defining requirements should be agreement on criteria for sufficiency.

Estimated Average Requirement (EAR): EAR (fig. 2) is the average requirement value obtained from or estimated for a group of individuals. The estimation of requirements starts by defining the criteria that will be used to define adequacy and establishing the necessary corrections for physiological and dietary factors. Once a mean value is obtained from a group of subjects, the recommended range value is adjusted for group variability.

Reference Nutrient Intake (RNI) – Population Reference Intake (PRI) or Recommended Daily Allowance (RDA): The daily intake that meets the nutrient requirements of almost all (97.5%) apparently 'healthy' individuals; in our case 'medically stable' for a specific gestational age and/or birth weight-specific population group is more appropriate. Unless there is specific data to the contrary, it is generally assumed that the distribution of requirements follows a gaussian distribution; that is the mean ± 2 SD is expected to cover 97.5% of the population. If the SD is not known a value of 10–15% of the mean is generally assumed. In general, this approach follows the WHO and US National Academy of Science/Food and Nutrition Board (NAS/FNB)/Dietary Recommended intakes (DRI) process. However, requirements for some nutrients are known not to follow a normal distribution. For example, iron needs are not normally distributed but are markedly influenced by blood losses including blood sampling, transfusion, erythropoietin treatment, and others. Similarly, the needs for long-chain polyunsaturated fatty acids (LC-PUFA) differ in the subgroups with fatty acid desaturase genotypes associated with slower or more rapid conversion of precursor essential fatty acids to LC-PUFA [19]. At this time, definition of RNI usually tries to encompass the needs of all sizeable population subgroups defined by genetic or other variables, rather than providing separate RNI for such population subgroups.

Daily intake corresponds to an average over a given period; it does not need to be fulfilled every day. However, since stores are limited and needs are high, small infants should receive their recommended intakes ideally within 3–5 days after birth.

The mean and range of requirements is measured in a given category defined by gestational age and/or birth weight. It is commonly described by the mean or median (central tendency) and the distribution by percentiles or SD units (if normally distributed). In the absence of birth weight and/or gestational age-specific information, population groups will be assumed to follow a gaussian 'normal' distribution, thus permitting the derivation of a risk function for deficiency and excess as the mean ± 2 SDs.

The range of biological effects starts with the most extreme consequence, the prevention of severe nutritional deficiency or excess leading to death or major disability. For most nutrients, data on prevention of clinical or subclinical pathological conditions identified by functional assays are used since true mortality risk-related intakes are not available for most nutrients. The next set of markers that can be used to define requirements includes measures of nutrient stores, critical tissue pools, or functional effects on relevant organ systems. Intakes to assure adequate body stores are particularly important when deficiency conditions are highly prevalent. Presently, approaches to define requirements of most nutrients for LBW and ELBW use several criteria in combination; functional assays related to subclinical deficit or excess are considered the most relevant. Ideal biomarkers should be sensitive to changes in nutritional state, while at the same time remaining nutrient-specific. Criteria used to define requirements are important since recommendations vary widely depending on what has been used to define adequacy. The information base to scientifically support the definition of nutritional needs of small neonates, especially ELBW neonates, is extremely limited for most nutrients. Where relevant, requirement estimates should include allowance for variations in bioavailability and utilization by the enteral as compared to parenteral route (in the latter case absorption or bioavailability need not be considered).

Lowest Threshold Intake (LTI): The daily nutrient intake below which almost all individuals will be unable to meet their nutrient needs and to maintain metabolic integrity based on the criteria chosen for the respective nutrient.

Upper Safe Level of Intake (UL): For some nutrients a UL is defined if adverse effects have been identified. Intakes up to the UL are unlikely to pose a risk of adverse health effects in almost all (97.5%) medically stable individuals in a specific population group. ULs should be based on long-term exposure to the nutrient from all sources, combining enteral and parenteral routes. The special situation of ELBW and VLBW infants, where parenteral vitamins and minerals may be added to the enteral macronutrient intake leading to potential excess, should be specifically addressed. This may include carefully monitoring intake of critical nutrients with potential toxicity and avoiding exceeding the UL. The case of aluminum, contained in parenteral solution, is an example of this potential problem.

Acceptable Range of Intakes (AR): Based on the above limitations, the authors of this book have agreed to the use of clinically acceptable intake range (AR) for LBW and ELBW – defined as the range of intake derived from observational studies or evaluated under controlled conditions that appear to sustain adequate nutrition, based on absence of abnormal clinical signs/symptoms, or evidence that these levels preserve biochemical and functional normalcy. The lower value of the AR will be the EAR if one has been established for the given birth weight-specific group. The upper value will generally be lower than the UL if one has been established for the specific population group; if no UL can be derived, the upper value of the range will be defined based on intakes considered safe from available data from 'clinically stable' neonates. Thus the AR for most nutrients should be considered the best *'guesstimate'* from expert opinion, plus careful analysis of the available data. Under some conditions, such as parenteral nutrition, subgroups of infants receive substantially less or substantially more than their computed needs, as in the case for calcium and riboflavin respectively. The AR should be applied as a range of intake for individuals within a group that is homogeneous in terms of age, birth weight, and other characteristics believed to affect nutrient requirement. Moreover, since postnatal adaptations are critical in defining nutrient needs, we first must consider guidance for the initial feeding, then the transitional phase, and finally define goals that should be reached for optimal growth and development of small neonates.

Recommendations are presented wherever possible, as range of intakes for a given category rather than a single exact number for an individual subject. However, ELBW, VLBW, and LBW infants can hardly, if ever, be considered homogeneous because of concurrent medical conditions and variability in physiological development. Thus, health professionals caring for these special groups should attempt to individualize nutritional care based on tolerance to feedings and adjust nutrient delivery according to restrictions imposed by disease conditions and requirement as they relate to developmental stage and actual degree of depletion for the specific nutrient.

References

1 Tsang R, Uauy R, Koletzko B, Zlotkin S: Nutrition of the Preterm Infant. Scientific Basis and Practical Application, ed 2. Cincinnati, Digital Educational Publishing, 2005.

2 Botet F, Figueras-Aloy J, Miracle-Echegoyen X, Rodriguez-Miguelez JM, Salvia-Roiges MD, Carbonell-Estrany X: Trends in survival among extremely-low-birth-weight infants (less than 1,000 g) without significant bronchopulmonary dysplasia. BMC Pediatr 2012;12:63.

3 Jonsdottir GM, Georgsdottir I, Haraldsson A, Hardardottir H, Thorkelsson T, Dagbjartsson A: Survival and neurodevelopmental outcome of ELBW children at 5 years of age: comparison of two cohorts born 10 years apart. Acta Paediatr 2012;101:714–718.

4 Ruegger C, Hegglin M, Adams M, Bucher HU: Population-based trends in mortality, morbidity and treatment for very preterm- and very low birth weight infants over 12 years. BMC Pediatr 2012;12:17.

5 Hahn WH, Chang JY, Chang YS, Shim KS, Bae CW: Recent trends in neonatal mortality in very low birth weight Korean infants: in comparison with Japan and the USA. J Korean Med Sci 2011;26:467–473.

6 Koletzko B, Brands B, Poston L, Godfrey K, Demmelmair H: Early programming of long-term health. Proc Nutr Soc 2012;71:371–378.

7 Ehrenkranz RA, Dusick AM, Vohr BR, Wright LL, Wrage LA, Poole WK: Growth in the neonatal intensive care unit influences neurodevelopmental and growth outcomes of extremely low birth weight infants. Pediatrics 2006;117:1253–1261.

8 Corpeleijn WE, Kouwenhoven SM, Paap MC, van Vliet I, Scheerder I, Muizer Y, et al: Intake of own mother's milk during the first days of life is associated with decreased morbidity and mortality in very low birth weight infants during the first 60 days of life. Neonatology 2012;102:276–281.

9 Stephens BE, Walden RV, Gargus RA, Tucker R, McKinley L, Mance M, et al: First-week protein and energy intakes are associated with 18-month developmental outcomes in extremely low birth weight infants. Pediatrics 2009;123:1337–1343.

10 Lucas A, Morley R, Cole TJ: Randomised trial of early diet in preterm babies and later intelligence quotient. BMJ 1998;317:1481–1487.

11 Isaacs EB, Gadian DG, Sabatini S, Chong WK, Quinn BT, Fischl BR, et al: The effect of early human diet on caudate volumes and IQ. Pediatr Res 2008;63:308–314.

12 Makrides M, Gibson RA, McPhee AJ, Collins CT, Davis PG, Doyle LW, et al: Neurodevelopmental outcomes of preterm infants fed high-dose docosahexaenoic acid: a randomized controlled trial. JAMA 2009;301:175–182.

13 Symonds ME, Mendez MA, Meltzer HM, Koletzko B, Godfrey K, Forsyth S, et al: Early life nutritional programming of obesity: mother-child cohort studies. Ann Nutr Metab 2013;62:137–145.

14 Koletzko B, Decsi T, Molnar D, de la Hunty A (eds): Early Nutrition Programming and Health Outcomes in Later Life: Obesity and Beyond. New York, Springer, 2009.

15 Koletzko B, Symonds ME, Olsen SF: Programming research: where are we and where do we go from here? Am J Clin Nutr 2011;94:2036S–2043S.

16 Aggett PJ, Bresson J, Haschke F, Hernell O, Koletzko B, Lafeber HN, et al: Recommended dietary allowances (RDAs), recommended dietary intakes (RDIs), recommended nutrient intakes (RNIs), and population reference intakes (PRIs) are not 'recommended intakes'. J Pediatr Gastroenterol Nutr 1997;25:236–241.

17 Hermoso M, Tabacchi G, Iglesia-Altaba I, Bel-Serrat S, Moreno-Aznar LA, Garcia-Santos Y, et al: The nutritional requirements of infants. Towards EU alignment of reference values: the EURRECA network. Matern Child Nutr 2010;6(suppl 2):55–83.

18 Iglesia I, Doets EL, Bel-Serrat S, Roman B, Hermoso M, Pena Quintana L, et al: Physiological and public health basis for assessing micronutrient requirements in children and adolescents. The EURRECA network. Matern Child Nutr 2010;6(suppl 2):84–99.

19 Lattka E, Klopp N, Demmelmair H, Klingler M, Heinrich J, Koletzko B: Genetic variations in polyunsaturated fatty acid metabolism – implications for child health? Ann Nutr Metab 2012;60(suppl 3):8–17.

Ricardo Uauy, MD, PhD
Instituto de Nutrición y Tecnologia de los Alimentos
University of Chile, PO Box 138-11
Macul/Santiago de Chile 5540 (Chile)
E-Mail druauy@gmail.com

Koletzko B, Poindexter B, Uauy R (eds): Nutritional Care of Preterm Infants: Scientific Basis and Practical Guidelines.
World Rev Nutr Diet. Basel, Karger, 2014, vol 110, pp 11–26 (DOI: 10.1159/000358455)

Nutrition, Growth and Clinical Outcomes

Richard A. Ehrenkranz

Yale University School of Medicine, New Haven, Conn., USA

Reviewed by Brenda Poindexter, Indiana University School of Medicine, Indianapolis, Ind., USA; William Hay Jr.,
Department of Pediatrics, University of Colorado School of Medicine, Aurora, Colo., USA

Abstract

Recommendations about the nutritional management of preterm infants, especially of extremely
low gestational age (or extremely low birth weight) neonates, have been published by a number of
pediatric and nutritional organizations. The objectives of these recommendations are to provide
nutrients to approximate the rate of growth and composition of weight gain for a normal fetus of
the same postmenstrual age, to maintain normal concentrations of blood and tissue nutrients, and
to achieve a satisfactory functional development. Achieving these goals requires an understanding
of the intrauterine growth rate to be targeted and of the nutrient requirements of preterm infants.
Birth weight-based intrauterine curves should be used to monitor postnatal growth of preterm infants in neonatal intensive care units. Although primarily provided by observational studies or historic control studies, data demonstrate that growth and neurodevelopmental outcomes correlate
with nutritional intake. The implementation of standardized feeding guidelines reduces nutritional
practice variation and facilitates postnatal growth and improved clinical outcomes.

© 2014 S. Karger AG, Basel

Recommendations about the nutritional management of preterm infants, especially
of extremely low gestational age (or extremely low birth weight – ELBW) neonates,
have been published by such organizations as the American Academy of Pediatrics
[1], the Canadian Paediatric Society [2], the European Society of Paediatric Gastroenterology, Hepatology and Nutrition [3, 4], and the Life Science Research Office [5].
The guiding principles of these recommendations are similar: to provide nutrients to
approximate the rate of growth and composition of weight gain for a normal fetus of
the same postmenstrual age (PMA), to maintain normal concentrations of blood and
tissue nutrients, and to achieve a satisfactory functional development. However,
achieving these goals requires an understanding of the intrauterine (IU) growth rate
to be targeted and of the nutrient requirements of preterm infants. Unfortunately, the
composition of the optimal diet is unknown and, as displayed in figure 1, extrauterine

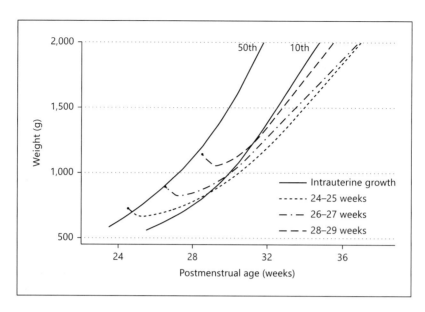

Fig. 1. NICHD Growth Observational Study, 1999. Average body weight versus PMA in weeks for infants 24–29 weeks' GA plotted with smoothed 10th and 50th percentile reference IU growth curves. The infants are stratified by GA weeks 24–25, 26–27, and 28–29. Reproduced with permission from Pediatrics [6, p. 287]; Copyright 1999 by the AAP.

growth restriction (EUGR) remains all too common [6, 7], having been facilitated by nutritional practices in which parenteral and enteral support permit the development of energy, protein and mineral deficits [8].

This chapter will review and discuss the manner in which the postnatal growth of preterm infants is monitored in neonatal intensive care units (NICUs) and data that demonstrate that growth and neurodevelopmental outcomes are associated with the adequacy of postnatal nutrient intake. Since achievement of nutritional and growth milestones is facilitated by the reduction of practice variation, the implementation of standardized feeding guidelines will be recommended.

Monitoring Postnatal Growth in the Neonatal Intensive Care Unit

Birth Weight-Derived Intrauterine Growth Curves
In several papers published between 1963 and 1967, Lubchenco and her colleagues [9–11] were the first to describe IU growth using percentile curves. In the initial publication [9], data on the birth weights of 5,635 live-born Caucasian infants 24–42 weeks of gestation delivered near Denver, Colorado, between July 1948 and January 1961, were analyzed. Gestational age (GA) was determined from the onset of the mother's last normal menstrual period. The data were presented in figures and tables that displayed smoothed 10th, 25th, 50th, 75th and 90th weight percentiles for males

and females together and separately at each GA. Smooth percentiles for IU length and head circumference (HC) between 26 and 44 weeks' GA were reported in a subsequent publication [10] on over 4,700 live-born infants included in this cohort. The authors acknowledged several limitations to their analysis, including: 'The sample has an undeterminable bias because premature birth itself is probably related to unphysiological states of variable duration in either mother or fetus. Since the weight of fetuses who remain in utero cannot be measured, the curves presented herein are submitted with these reservations as estimates of intrauterine growth' [9]. A third paper [11] introduced the terms small for gestational age (SGA), appropriate for gestational age (AGA), and large for gestational age (LGA) into our vocabulary; weights between the 10th and 90th percentiles were referred to as AGA, those less than the 10th percentile as SGA, and those greater than the 90th percentile as LGA. Lubchenco et al. [9] correctly predicted that these curves would be useful at birth, providing information about the infant's IU environment and revealing whether he/she was large or small for his/her GA, and useful after birth to monitor and compare postnatal growth to IU growth.

Following publication of the Lubchenco curves [9–11], birth weight (BW) by gestational curves that described IU growth for various populations, ethnic groups, and geographic locations around the world have been reported. As part of a recent project to revise preterm growth charts published in 2003 [12], Fenton and Kim [13] performed a systematic review and meta-analysis of population-based preterm growth studies from developed countries. Their inclusion criteria sought to identify reports with (a) corrected GAs through fetal ultrasound and/or infant assessment and/or statistical correction; (b) data percentiles at 24 weeks' GA or lower; (c) a sample size of at least 25,000 infants, with more than 500 <30 weeks' GA; (d) separate data on females and males; (e) data that had been published numerically or which was available from the investigators, and (f) data collected between 1987 and 2012. From almost 2,500 records identified via database searching, 75 full-text papers were evaluated in detail, and 6 were included in the meta-analysis [13] used to revise Fenton's 2003 preterm infant growth charts [12]. These revised preterm growth charts will be discussed below. In addition to the concerns noted above about the normalcy of prematurely born infants, the influence of an inaccurately determined GA on BW means, standard deviations, and percentile values must be acknowledged [14]. Nonetheless, curves and tables describing IU growth have been used widely by clinicians and researchers to assess fetal growth, and, if indicated, to evaluate or screen for problems associated with being SGA or LGA.

Following its publication in 2003, the Fenton [12] Fetal-Infant Growth Chart for Preterm infants had become one of the most widely used curves to monitor growth of preterm infants from 22 to 50 completed weeks of gestation. Smoothed 3rd, 10th, 50th, 90th, and 97th percentile curves were constructed from 3 IU growth datasets; BW for gestation data on about 676,000 Canadian infants from 22 to 40 weeks' gestation and length and HC data from 376,000 Swedish infants from 28 to 40 weeks' ges-

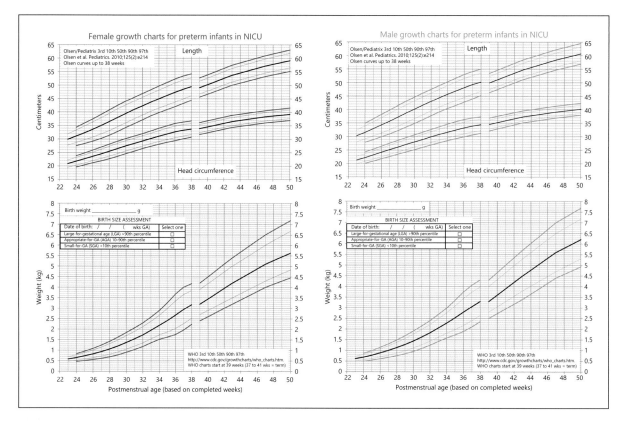

Fig. 2. Olsen IU growth curves combined with the WHO-CDC growth charts can be can be used to monitor postnatal growth of preterm infants from 23 to 50 weeks' GA Reproduced with the permission of Pediatrix Medical Group. Available at http://www.pediatrix.com/workfiles/NICUGrowthCurves7.30.pdf.

tation and from about 27,000 Australian infants from 22 to 40 weeks' gestation. Those data were combined with post-term data from the Center for Disease Control and Prevention (CDC)-2000 growth charts [15].

In 2010, Olsen et al. [16] described IU growth curves that were constructed and validated from an administrative dataset of anthropometric measurements collected on over 250,000 infants at 22–41 weeks' gestation delivered at 248 United States hospitals in 33 states between 1998 and 2006. Smoothed 3rd, 10th, 25th, 50th, 75th, 90th, and 97th percentile gender-specific data for BW, length and HC were presented in figures and tables. Updated growth curves (fig. 2) that combine these IU growth charts with the WHO-CDC 2010 charts [17] are now available online at http://www.pediatrix.com/workfiles/NICUGrowthCurves7.30.pdf, and can be used to monitor growth until 50 weeks' PMA.

As noted above, Fenton and Kim [13] revised the 2003 Fenton preterm infant growth charts [12] after performing a systematic review and meta-analysis. The revised curves combine data from 6 large population-based studies that include anthro-

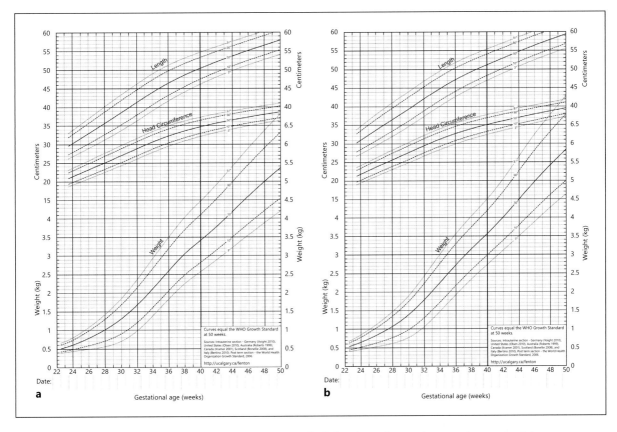

Fig. 3. Fenton preterm infant growth charts (**a** girls, **b** boys) can be used to monitor postnatal growth of preterm infants from 22 weeks' GA to 10 weeks post-term Reproduced with permission from Fenton and Kim [13]; Copyright licensee BioMed Central Ltd. This is an Open Access article distributed under the terms of the Creative Commons Attribution License (http://creativecommons.org/licenses/by/2.0) which permits unrestricted use, distribution, and reproduction in any medium, provided the original work is properly cited. Available at http://www.biomedcentral.com/1471-2431/13/59.

pometric measurements from almost 4 million infants at birth (almost 35,000 of these infants were <30 weeks' GA) with data until 50 weeks' PMA from the WHO 2006 multicenter growth study [18]. Infants were born between 1991 and 2007 in Germany, USA, Italy, Australia, Scotland, and Canada. Birth length values were available in 151,500 infants and birth HC values were available in about 173,600 infants. Smoothed 3rd, 10th, 50th, 90th, and 97th percentile gender-specific growth curves were developed for BW, length and HC (fig. 3). Since these curves are available for unrestricted use online, it is likely that they will become widely used and replace Fenton's 2003 curves [12] in clinical settings. Furthermore, exact z-scores have been made available online for download (http://ucalgary.ca/fenton).

Estimated Fetal Weight-Derived Intrauterine Growth Curves

Since the mid-1980s, sonographic techniques, including computational strategies to estimate fetal weight, have been developed and improved. By studying women in whom the menstrual history is well known and/or corroborated in the first trimester by ultrasound or clinical evaluation, several investigators have described fetal growth models based upon longitudinal studies in which serial ultrasound measurements of a fetus were made during pregnancy [19, 20] or with cross-sectional data in which a fetus was only measured once during a pregnancy [21]. Individualized or customized estimated fetal weight (EFW) curves have also been prepared [22]. Since EFW-based curves might be more representative of 'normal' fetal growth, reflecting growth of the larger population of infants delivered at term, growth along the 50th percentile line of an EFW-based curve might represent the most appropriate rate of IU growth and the rate that postnatal nutrition should target. However, determination of an EFW is limited by the ability to accurately obtain the sonographic measurements included within the formula used to calculate EFW. Furthermore, accurate knowledge of the GA is essential to assess the adequacy of fetal growth and to determine if fetal growth has been restricted. Therefore, BW-derived IU curves have continued to be widely used because the inherent errors associated with the construction of EFW-derived growth curves are similar to those associated with BW-derived growth curves.

The results of the INTERGROWTH-21st Project [23] should change the practice of using BW-derived growth curves to monitor the growth of preterm infants. This project is a multicenter, multiethnic, population-based study of growth, health and nutrition from early pregnancy to infancy and is being conducted in 8 geographical areas (Brazil, China, India, Italy, Kenya, Oman, UK, and USA). Similar to the WHO 2006 multicenter study [18] which developed prescriptive child growth standards that have also been adopted by the CDC [17], the INTERGROWTH-21st Project aims to produce prescriptive growth standards from early pregnancy to infancy. Therefore, the populations included in this project and used to construct the growth standards were required to live in environments with no socioeconomic constraints on growth and to receive up-to-date, evidence-based, medical care and appropriate nutrition. The goal was to recruit about 56,000 (about 7,000 at each site) mostly low- to medium-risk pregnant women prior to 14^{+0} weeks' of a singleton gestation. Each pregnancy will be followed prospectively; in addition to an ultrasound performed at the first prenatal visit for GA confirmation, scans will be performed at 5- ± 1-week intervals. Preterm infants will be followed after delivery to evaluate postnatal growth. The objectives are to construct new international standards that will describe (a) fetal growth assessed by clinical and ultrasound measurements, (b) postnatal growth of term and preterm infants up to 2 years of age, and (c) describe the relationship between BW, length and HC, GA and perinatal outcomes. Results should be available in late 2014. Since they should be prescriptive growth standards and describe how all fetuses and newborns should grow, they should become the preferred way for monitoring the postnatal growth of preterm infants and evaluating the relationship between nutrition, growth and long-term outcomes.

Postnatal Growth Curves

Postnatal growth curves for preterm infants have also been constructed from anthropometric measurements collected during the NICU stay [6, 24–27]. The smoothed curves displayed in these reports have usually represented infants within selected BW ranges and demonstrate initial weight loss after birth followed by steady weight gain, with BW being regained by about 14 days of age in extremely preterm (EPT) infants. Growth velocity (g/kg/day) has been estimated from these data; but for very low birth weight (VLBW) infants, the exponential model described by Patel et al. [28, 29] offers an easy and accurate method to estimate growth velocity and to compare the response to nutritional interventions. These reports have shown that compared to preterm infants who do not experience major morbidities, growth velocity is slower among preterm infants who experience such neonatal morbidities as necrotizing enterocolitis, bronchopulmonary dysplasia, and late-onset sepsis. Furthermore, as displayed in figure 1, when postnatal growth curves are plotted with BW-based IU growth curves, EUGR is evident for most preterm infants, especially EPT infants [6, 7]. Since two of the goals of the nutritional management of preterm infants are to approximate the rate of growth and composition of weight gain for a normal fetus of the same PMA, this observation emphasizes the need to use an IU growth chart to monitor growth in the NICU. Unfortunately, techniques such as dual energy x-ray absorptiometry or air displacement plethysmography to assess body composition, including bone mineral content, fat mass, and lean body mass, have not become incorporated into routine clinical practice.

Growth and Neurodevelopmental Outcomes Are Associated with Nutrient Intake

One of the other major goals of the nutritional management of preterm infants is to achieve a satisfactory functional development. Unfortunately the published literature about the relationship between nutritional support provided to hospitalized preterm infants and growth and neurodevelopmental outcomes is not replete with randomized control trials that demonstrate clear cause and effect relationships. In fact, most reports describe observational studies or historical control studies in which the impacts of nutritional practice changes are delineated. Table 1 lists a number of clinical investigations that illustrate one or more of the following statements: (a) better nutritional support is associated with improved growth and less EUGR; (b) improved growth is associated with improved neurodevelopmental outcomes, and (c) better nutritional support is associated with improved neurodevelopmental outcomes. These papers will be briefly reviewed in an effort to demonstrate that growth and outcomes are associated with the adequacy of postnatal nutrition provided to preterm infants.

Of the six reports listed in table 1 which support the statement that better nutritional support is associated with improved growth and less EUGR, only one was a

Table 1. Findings in clinical investigations in extremely preterm infants

Reference (first author)	Better nutritional support associated with improved growth and less EUGR	Improved growth is associated with improved neurodevelopmental outcomes	Better nutritional support is associated with improved neurodevelopmental outcomes
Wilson, 1997 [30]	X		
Pauls, 1998 [27]	X		
Dinerstein, 2006 [31]	X		
Maggio, 2007 [32]	X		
Cormack, 2013 [33]	X		
Shan, 2009 [34]	X		
Ehrenkranz, 2006 [35]		X	
Poindexter, 2013 [36]		X	
Belfort, 2011 [37]		X	
Poindexter, 2006 [39]	X		+ (effect suggested)
Stephens, 2009 [40]	+		X
Eleni dit Trolli, 2012 [41]	+		X
Tan, 2008 [43, 44]	X	X	X
Franz, 2009 [45]	X	X	X

randomized clinical trial. That trial, performed between 1990 and 1992 by Wilson et al. [30], randomized sick VLBW infants to an aggressive nutritional intervention or their standard nutritional or control practice. The report by Pauls et al. [27] was an observational study and three were historical control studies [31–33]. These five studies each described the response to nutritional regimes of early parenteral and enteral nutritional support; improved growth during the NICU hospitalization, without an increased risk of adverse clinical outcomes, was reported. As part of the early nutritional intervention, parenteral protein (0.5–3.0 g/kg/day) was initiated on the first day of life, often within hours of birth; lipid emulsion (0.5–1 g/kg/day) was initiated by day 2 of life, and minimal enteral feeding (human milk if possible; about 10–20 ml/kg/day) was mostly started on day 1 of life. In contrast, in the control patients, parenteral nutrition tended to be initiated on day 3 of life and enteral nutrition when the infants were considered stable by the clinicians [27, 30–32]; the study by Cormack and Bloomfield [33] compared a higher versus a lower protein intake. Dinerstein et al. [31] reported significant decreases in protein and energy deficits during the first month of life and significantly improved weight, length and HC were reported at hospital discharge [30–33]. The sixth study [34] was a multicenter, retrospective review of an administrative database which demonstrated that preterm infants managed by nutritional support teams were significantly less likely to develop EUGR.

Two of the three reports listed in table 1, which support the statement that improved growth is associated with improved neurodevelopmental outcomes, were derived from the Eunice Kennedy Shriver NICHD Neonatal Research Network (NRN)

VLBW registry; limited information about nutritional management was available for each analysis [35, 36]. The third report by Belfort et al. [37] was an observational analysis of data from the DHA for Improvement of Neurodevelopmental Outcome (DINO) trial in infants who were randomized to docosahexaenoic acid (DHA) supplementation [38].

Ehrenkranz et al. [35] described the relationship between in-hospital growth velocity and neurodevelopmental and growth outcomes at 18–22 months' corrected age in 495 infants 501–1,000 g BW whose growth was monitored in the NICHD NRN's Growth Observational Study performed from August 31, 1994 to August 9, 1995 [6] and who were evaluated at follow-up. The study cohort was divided into quartiles of in-hospital growth velocity rates, and as the rate of weight gain increased between quartile 1 and quartile 4, from 12.0 to 21.2 g/kg/day, the incidence of clinical morbidities and of neurodevelopmental impairment significantly decreased. Specifically, the incidence of any cerebral palsy or of a Bayley Scales of Infant Development (BSID) II-R Mental Developmental Index (MDI) <70 or a Psychomotor Developmental Index (PDI) <70 fell significantly as the rate of weight gain increased. In addition, significantly fewer infants in the highest quartile had anthropometric measurements at 18 months' corrected age below the 10th percentile values of the CDC-2000 growth curves [15]. Logistic regression analyses, controlled for potential demographic and clinical cofounders, and adjusted for center, suggested that in-hospital growth velocity rates exerted a significant, and possibly independent, effect on neurodevelopmental and growth outcomes at 18–22 months' corrected age.

Poindexter et al. [36] reviewed data on 2,463 infants $23^{0/7}$–$26^{6/7}$ weeks' gestation at born between 2008 and 2010 at NRN centers; 1,616 (65.6%) survived to discharge and 1,396 (86.4%) were seen at 18–22 months' corrected age. The objective of this report was to evaluate the association between in-hospital weight gain and growth and neurodevelopmental outcomes in this more contemporary population. Consistent with the findings reported by Ehrenkranz et al. [35], as the rate of weight gain increased from 12 to 18 g/kg/day between quartile 1 and quartile 4, the incidence of clinical morbidities and of profound/severe neurodevelopmental impairment decreased significantly. Specifically, the incidence of moderate/severe cerebral palsy or of a BSID-III Cognitive Score <70 or <85 fell significantly as the rate of weight gain increased. Also, significantly fewer infants in the highest quartile had anthropometric measurements at 18 months' corrected age below the 10th percentile values. Furthermore, adjusted logistic regression analyses again suggested that in-hospital growth was independently associated with neurodevelopmental outcomes.

Belfort et al. [37] examined the impact of growth before and after term on neurodevelopmental outcomes at 18 months' corrected age in 613 infants <33 weeks' gestation. Greater weight gain between 1 week of age and term was associated with higher BSID-II MDI and PDI scores, especially for infants weighing <1,250 g at birth. From term to 4 months' corrected age, greater weight gain and linear growth were associated with higher PDI scores. However, between 4 months' corrected age and 12 months' corrected age, none of the anthropometric measurements were associated with MDI or PDI scores.

The reports by Poindexter et al. [39], Stephens et al. [40], and Eleni dit Trolli et al. [41] support the statements that (a) better nutritional support is associated with improved growth and less EUGR and (b) better nutritional support is associated with improved neurodevelopmental outcomes (table 1). Poindexter's paper was a secondary analysis of the glutamine supplementation trial that was aimed at reducing late-onset sepsis [42] in infants ≤1,000 g BW; it cohorted infants by whether or not they received at least 3 g/kg/day of parenteral protein by the fifth day of life (early vs. late group, respectively). Significantly improved growth at 36 weeks' PMA was noted in the early group and males in the early group had significantly greater HCs at 18–22 months' corrected age. However, no significant differences between the groups were found on neurodevelopmental testing. In contrast, Stephens' report [40] was a single-center retrospective study in which adjusted, multiple logistic regression analyses found that higher protein intake during the first week of life was associated with significant increases in the BSID-II MDI and significantly associated with length growth at 18 months' corrected age. Energy intake during the first week of life was also significantly associated with increases in the MDI. It is likely that the greater variation in practices seen in 15 NRN centers compared to the practice variation seen at a single center contributed to the different neurodevelopmental outcome findings reported by these authors.

Eleni dit Trolli et al. [41] performed a retrospective analysis of prospectively collected data in a cohort of 48 infants <28 weeks' GA. They reported a significant univariate relationship between developmental outcomes at 1 year corrected age and the cumulative intake of energy and lipids at 14 days of age and with weight gain during the first 28 days of life. No correlation was found between 1-year outcomes and early protein or carbohydrate intake. However, protein intakes during the first week of life were higher and more consistent with current nutritional recommendations than protein intakes reported in studies which demonstrated an association between early protein intake and developmental outcomes. In multivariate analyses, only the association between 1-year outcomes and cumulative lipid intake at 14 days of life remained significant.

The final two reports listed in table 1 support each of the statements: (a) better nutritional support is associated with improved growth, better clinical outcomes and less EUGR; (b) improved growth is associated with improved neurodevelopmental outcomes, and (c) better nutritional support is associated with improved neurodevelopmental outcomes. Tan and co-workers [43, 44] performed a randomized controlled trial that tested a parenteral nutrition intervention in 142 infants <29 weeks' gestation; the primary outcome was HC growth and developmental outcome. The parenteral nutrition intervention provided protein (4 g/kg/day), glucose (16.3 g/kg/day) and fat

(4 g/kg/day) intakes above the standard recommendations; however, practices related to the initiation and advancement of enteral nutrition were similar for both groups, and parenteral nutrition was discontinued once infants received >50% of their total daily fluid intake enterally. Therefore, although the intervention significantly reduced the energy and protein deficit at 4 weeks' of age compared to the control group, 80% of the infants in the intervention group and 97% of the infants in the control group were in overall energy and protein deficit after 4 weeks. Nonetheless, when the groups were pooled, significant correlations existed between (a) energy intake and energy deficit during the first 4 weeks and total brain (MRI) volume at 40 weeks' PMA and with MDI and PDI at 3 months, but not at 9 months corrected age; (b) anthropometrics at 36 weeks' PMA and total brain (MRI) and cortical brain (MRI) volume at 40 weeks' PMA, and (c) body weight at 36 week's PMA and both mental and motor outcomes during the first year of life.

Franz et al. [45] evaluated the association of IU, early neonatal, and post-discharge growth with neurodevelopmental outcomes at about 5.4 years of age in 219 surviving VLBW children who were born between July 1996 and June 1999. All infants received intensive early nutritional support that included initiation of parenteral protein (2 g/kg/day) on day 1 and enteral feeds (about 16 ml/kg/day) on day 1; parenteral protein was increased to 3 g/kg/day; enteral feeds by about 16 ml/kg/day. Developmental assessments were performed at about 5 years of age and included a standardized neurologic examination, the Gross Motor Function Classification Scale, and the Kaufmann Assessment Battery for Children (KABC). Increased in-hospital growth was associated with a reduction in the risk of an abnormal neurological examination and higher mental processing composite score on the KABC (the mental processing composite score is similar to an IQ score). Post-discharge growth was not found to have a significant impact on neurodevelopmental outcomes. Overall, although only about 3% of the variability of the mental processing composite score was explained by in-hospital growth, its contribution to neurodevelopmental outcome was only exceeded by severe intraventricular hemorrhage and prolonged mechanical ventilation, which accounted for 21 and 13%, respectively. Therefore, they concluded that while improving early neonatal growth with additional nutritional efforts might improve long-term developmental outcomes, the effects might be small.

Benefits from Standardized Feeding Guidelines

The influence of nutritional practice variation, within and between NICUs, on nutritional and growth outcomes has been described [46, 47]. For example, a retrospective study conducted in 6 NICUs between 1994 and 1996 reported that variation in nutritional practices, especially related to the mean caloric and protein intake, accounted for the largest difference in growth among the 6 centers [48]. A quality improvement project performed between 1999 and 2001 in 51 NICUs demonstrated that the identification and implementation of potentially better nutritional practices observed at high-weight-gain centers by low-weight-gain centers could lead to significant increases in discharge weight and HC [49]. Furthermore, a recent report [50] that also utilized the prospective data collected in the NICHD NRN glutamine supplementation trial [42] demonstrated that practice decisions about the provision of early nutritional support to ELBW infants seemed to be related to the perceived severity of illness, as reflected by ventilation status on day 7 of life. Compared with more critically ill infants, less critically infants received significantly more total nutritional support during each of the first 3 weeks of life, had significantly faster growth velocities, less significant morbidities, fewer deaths, shorter lengths of hospital stay, and better neurodevelopmental outcomes at 18–22 months' corrected age. Adjusted analyses that included a formal mediation framework found that the influence of critical illness on the risk of adverse outcomes was mediated by total daily energy intake during the first week of life.

Evidence-based standardized feeding guidelines have often been developed from a consensus of discussions by the NICU medical and nursing staffs as part of a quality improvement project [51, 52]. Implementation of such guidelines has been found to reduce practice variation within a center. Standardized feeding guidelines commonly include early parenteral and enteral nutritional support, specify when trophic feedings should be initiated and how long they should be continued before the volume is increased, specify if initial feedings should be a mother's own milk, pooled, pasteurized donor human milk, or preterm formula, outline a strategy to evaluate and manage 'feeding intolerance', and aim to maintain a steady rate of postnatal growth by adjusting nutritional support if growth parameters are not met [53]. Benefits following implementation of a standardized feeding guideline have included improvements in achieving nutritional milestones such as a reduction in the time to reach full enteral feedings, a decrease in the duration of parenteral nutrition, and a more rapid growth velocity. Furthermore, several reports [54, 55] published within the last few years have suggested that the use of standardized feeding guidelines, regardless of the specifics of feeding volumes and rates of advancement, offer the best protection against necrotizing enterocolitis.

Finally, the value of active involvement of neonatal nutritionists in monitoring compliance with standardized feeding guidelines or in directing nutritional management cannot be overstated. They ensure that early, intense nutritional support is initiated and individualized to the infant, facilitate the smooth transition from parenteral to enteral nutrition, closely monitor growth on growth charts, and suggest adjustments to nutritional support aimed at maintaining steady growth. Although infants are often weighed daily, due to commonly observed fluctuations in daily measurements, weight change should be assessed over 5- to 7-day periods, and weight, length, and HC should be plotted weekly on preterm infant growth charts.

Summary and Conclusions

- Nutritional management of preterm infants, especially EPT infants, should:
- Provide nutrients to approximate the rate of growth and composition of weight gain for a normal fetus of the same PMA
- Maintain normal concentrations of blood and tissue nutrients
- Achieve a satisfactory functional development
- Achieving these goals requires an understanding of the:
- IU growth rate to be targeted
- Nutrient requirements of preterm infants
- Monitor postnatal growth of preterm infants in NICUs
- BW-derived IU curves should be used currently [13, 16]
- EFW-derived IU curves should be used once the results of the INTERGROWTH-21st Project are available in late 2014 [23]
- EUGR may be unavoidable in some infants, but growth and outcomes reflect nutritional support
- Implementation of standardized feeding guidelines facilitates postnatal growth and improved clinical outcomes.

Research Opportunities

- Most EPT infants can be managed successfully with standardized feeding guidelines. However, research needs to be performed to identify and address the specific nutritional needs (e.g. protein and energy) of critically ill EPT infants and of such selected populations as IUGR infants.
- Nutrition, growth and outcomes are intricately related. However, much work still needs to be done to understand the contribution of specific nutrients toward the promotion of optimal metabolism and development.
- Clinically-friendly techniques need to be developed to assess the relationship between nutrient intake and body composition, specifically fat and lean body mass and bone mineralization. These techniques will supplement routine anthropometric measurements performed during and after NICU hospitalizations and can be used to direct nutritional management.
- The prescriptive fetal and infant growth curves constructed by the INTERGROWTH-21st Project need to be validated with larger cohorts of EPT infants. Specifically, studies will need to be performed to demonstrate that the INTERGROWTH data facilitate monitoring of postnatal growth of EPT infants, identify infants who need adjustments in their nutritional support to maintain steady growth, and identify infants at risk of metabolic syndrome.

References

1 American Academy of Pediatrics, Committee on Nutrition: Nutritional needs of the preterm infant; in Kleinman RE (ed): Pediatrc Nutrition Handbook, ed 6. Elk Grove Village/IL, American Academy of Pediatrics, 2009, pp 79–112.

2 Canadian Paediatric Society (CPS), Nutrition Committee: Nutrient needs and feeding of premature infants. CMAJ 1995;152:1765–1785.

3 Agostoni C, Buonocore G, Carnielli VP, DeCurtis M, Darmaun D, Decsi T, Domellöf M, Embleton ND, Fusch C, Genzel-Boroviczeny O, Goulet O, Kalhan SC, Kolacek S, Koletzko B, Lapillonne A, Mihatsch W, Moreno L, Neu J, Poindexter B, Puntis J, Putet G, Rigo J, Riskin A, Salle B, Sauer P, Shamir R, Szajewska H, Thureen P, Turck D, van Goudoever JB, Ziegler EE, for the ESPGHAN Committee on Nutrition: Enteral nutrient supply for preterm infants: Commentary from the European Society for Paediatric Gastroenterology, Hepatology, and Nutrition Committee on Nutrition. J Pediatr Gastroenterol Nutr 2010;50:85–91.

4 Koletzko B, Goulet O, Hunt J, Krohn K, Shamir R, for the Parenteral Nutrition Guidelines Working Group: Guidelines on Paediatric Parenteral Nutrition of the European Society of Paediatric Gastroenterology, Hepatology, and Nutrition (ESPGHAN) and the European Society for Clinical Nutrition and Metabolism (ESPEN), Supported by the European Society of Paediatric Research (ESPR). J Pediatr Gastroenterol Nutr 2005;41:S1–S87.

5 Klein CJ, Heird WC: Summary and Comparison of Recommendations for Nutrient Contents of Low-Birth-Weight Infant Formulas. Bethesda, Life Sciences Research Office, Inc, 2005.

6 Ehrenkranz RA, Younes N, Lemons JA, Fanaroff AA, Donovan EF, Wright LL, Katsikiotis V, Tyson JE, Oh W, Shankaran S, Bauer CR, Korones SB, Stoll BJ, Stevenson DK, Papile LA: Longitudinal growth of hospitalized very low birth weight infants. Pediatrics 1999;104:280–289.

7 Cole TJ, Statnikov Y, Santhakumaran S, Pan H, Modi N, on behalf of the Neonatal Data Analysis Unit and the Preterm Growth Investigator Group: Birth weight and longitudinal growth in infants below 32 weeks' gestation: a UK population study. Arch Dis Child Fetal Neonatal Ed 2014;99:F34–F40.

8 Embleton NE, Pang N, Cooke RJ: Postnatal malnutrition and growth retardation: an inevitable consequence of current recommendations in preterm infants? Pediatrics 2001;107:270–273.

9 Lubchenco LO, Hansman C, Dressler M, Boyd E: Intrauterine growth as estimated from liveborn birth weight data at 24 to 42 weeks of gestation. Pediatrics 1963;32:793–800.

10 Lubchenco LO, Hansman C, Boyd E: Intrauterine growth in length and head circumference as estimated from live births at gestational ages from 26 to 42 weeks. Pediatrics 1966;37:403–408.

11 Battaglia FC, Lubchenco LO: A practical classification of newborn infants by weight and gestational age. J Pediatr 1967;71:159–163.

12 Fenton TR: A new growth chart for preterm babies: Babson and Benda's chart updated with recent data and a new format. BMC Pediatr 2003;3:13–22.

13 Fenton TR, Kim JH: A systematic review and meta-analysis to revise the Fenton growth chart for preterm infants. BMC Pediatr 2013;13:59.

14 Platt RW: The effect of gestational age errors and their correction in interpreting population trends in fetal growth and gestational age-specific mortality. Semin Perinatol 2002;26:306–311.

15 Ogden CL, Kuczmarski RJ, Flegal KM, Mei Z, Guo S, Wei R, Grummer-Strawn LM, Curtin LR, Roche AF, Johnson CL: Centers for Disease Control and Prevention 2000 growth charts for the United States: Improvements to the 1977 National Center for Health Statistics version. Pediatrics 2002;109:45–60.

16 Olsen IE, Groveman SA, Lawson ML, Clark RH, Zemel BS: New intrauterine growth curves based on United States data. Pediatrics 2010;125:e214–e224.

17 Grummer-Strawn LM, Reinold C, Krebs NF: Use of World Health Organization and CDC growth charts for children aged 0–59 months in the United States. MMWR 2010;59(RR-9):1–15.

18 World Health Organization: WHO Child Growth Standards: Length/Height-for-Age, Weight-for-Age, Weight-for-Height and Body Mass Index-for-Age: Methods and Development. Geneva, WHO, 2006.

19 Persson P-H, Weldner B-M: Intrauterine curves obtained by ultrasound. Acta Obstet Gynecol Scand 1986;65:169–173.

20 Maršál K, Persson P-H, Larsen T, Lilja H, Selbing A, Sultan B: Intrauterine growth curves based on ultrasonically estimated foetal weights. Acta Pædiatr 1996;85:843–848.

21 Hadlock FP, Harrist RB, Martinez-Poyer J: In utero analysis of fetal growth: a sonographic weight standard. Radiology 1991;181:129–133.

22 Gardosi J: Customised assessment of fetal growth potential: implications for perinatal care. Arch Dis Child Fetal Neonatal Ed, 2012;97:F314–F317.

23 Villar J, Altman D, Purwar M, Noble J, Knight H, Ruyan P, Cheikh Ismail L, Barros FC, Lambert A, Papageorghiou AT, Carvalho M, Jaffer YA, Bertino E, Gravett MG, Bhutta ZA, Kennedy SH, for the International Fetal and Newborn Growth Consortium for the 21st Century (INTERGROWTH-21st): The objectives, design and implementation of the INTERGROWTH-21st Project. BJOG 2013; 120(suppl 2):9–26.

24 Dancis J, O'Connell JR, Holt LE: A grid for recording the weight of premature infants. J Pediatrics 1948;33: 570–572.

25 Shaffer SG, Quimiro CL, Anderson JV, Hall RT: Postnatal weight changes in low birth weight infants. Pediatrics 1987;79:702–705.

26 Wright K, Dawson JP, Fallis D, Vogt E, Lorch V: New postnatal growth grids for very low birth weight infants. Pediatrics 1993;91:922–926.

27 Pauls J, Bauer K, Versmold H: Postnatal body weight curves for infants below 1,000 g birth weight receiving early enteral and parenteral nutrition. Eur J Pediatr 1998;157:416–421.

28 Patel AL, Engstrom JL, Meier PP, Kimura RE: Accuracy of methods for calculating postnatal growth velocity for extremely low birth weight infants. Pediatrics 2005;116:1466–1473.

29 Patel AL, Engstrom JL, Meier PP, Jegier BJ, Kimura RE: Calculating postnatal growth velocity in very low birth weight premature infants. J Perinatol 2009;29: 618–622.

30 Wilson DC, Cairns P, Halliday HL, Reid M, McClure G, Dodge JA: Randomised controlled trial of an aggressive nutritional regimen in sick very low birthweight infants. Arch Dis Child 1997;77:4–11.

31 Dinerstein A, Neito RM, Solana CL, Perez GP, Otheguy LE, Larguia AM: Early and aggressive nutritional strategy (parenteral and enteral) decreases postnatal growth failure in very low birth weight infants. J Perinatol 2006;26:436–442.

32 Maggio L, Cota F, Gallini F, Lauriola V, Zecca C, Romagnoli C: Effects of high versus standard early protein intake on growth of extremely low birth weight infants. J Pediatr Gastroenterol Nutr 2007;44:124–129.

33 Cormack BE, Bloomfield FH: Increased protein intake decreases postnatal growth faltering in ELBW babies. Arch Dis Child Fetal Neonatal Ed 2013;98: F399–F404.

34 Shan HM, Cai W, Cao Y, Fang BH, Feng Y: Extrauterine growth retardation in premature infants in Shanghai: a multicenter retrospective review. Eur J Pediatr 2009;168:1055–1059.

35 Ehrenkranz RA, Dusick AM, Vohr BR, Wright LL, Wrage LA, Poole WK, for the National Institutes of Child Health and Human Development Neonatal Research Network: Growth in the Neonatal Intensive Care Unit Influences Neurodevelopmental and Growth Outcomes of Extremely Low Birth Weight Infants. Pediatrics 2006;117:1253–1261.

36 Poindexter B, Hintz S, Langer J, Ehrenkranz R: Have we caught up? Growth and neurodevelopmental outcomes in extremely preterm infants. E-PAS 2013: 1395.2.

37 Belfort MB, Rifas-Shiman SL, Sullivan T, Collins CT, McPhee AJ, Ryan P, Kleinman KP, Gillman MW, Gibson RA, Makrides M: Infant growth before and after term: effects on neurodevelopment in preterm infants. Pediatrics 2011;128:e899–e906.

38 Makrides M, Gibson RA, McPhee AJ, Collins CT, Davis PG, Doyle LW, Simmer K, Colditz PB, Morris S, Smithers LG, Wilson K, Ryan P: Neurodevelopmental outcomes of preterm infants fed high-dose docosahexaenoic acid. JAMA 2009;301:175–182.

39 Poindexter BB, Langer JC, Dusick AM, Ehrenkranz RA, for the NICHD Neonatal Research Network: Early provision of parenteral amino acids in extremely low birth weight infants: relation to growth and neurodevelopmental outcome. J Pediatr 2006; 148:300–305.

40 Stephens BE, Walden RV, Gargus RA, Tucker R, McKinley L, Mance M, Nye J, Vohr BR: First-week of protein and energy intakes are associated with 18-month developmental outcomes in extremely low birth weight infants. Pediatrics 2009;123:1337–1343.

41 Eleni dit Trolli S, Kermorvant-Duchemin E, Huon C, Bremond-Gignac D, Lapillone A: Early lipid supply and neurological development at one year in very low birth weight preterm infants. Early Hum Dev 2012;88:S25–S29.

42 Poindexter BB, Ehrenkranz RA, Stoll BJ, Wright LL, Poole WK, Oh W, Bauer CR, Papile LA, Tyson JE, Carlo WA, Laptook AR, Narendran V, Stevenson DK, Fanaroff AA, Korones SB, Shankaran S, Finer NN, Lemons JA, for the NICHD Neonatal Research Network: Parenteral glutamine supplementation does not reduce the risk of mortality or late-onset sepsis in extremely low birth weight infants. Pediatrics 2004;113:1209–1215.

43 Tan MJ, Cooke RW: Improving head growth in very preterm infants – a randomized controlled trial I: neonatal outcomes. Arch Dis Child Fetal Neonatal Ed 2008;93:F337–F341.

44 Tan MJ, Cooke RW: Improving head growth in very preterm infants – a randomized controlled trial II: MRI and developmental outcomes in the first year. Arch Dis Child Fetal Neonatal Ed 2008;93:F342–F346.

45 Franz AR, Pohlandt F, Bode H, Mihatsch WA, Sander S, Kron M, Steinmacher J: Intrauterine, early neonatal, and postdischarge growth and neurodevelopmental outcome at 5.4 years in extremely preterm infants after intensive neonatal nutritional support. Pediatrics 2009;123:e101–e109.

46 Ehrenkranz RA: Early, Aggressive nutritional management for very low birth weight infants: what is the evidence? Semin Perinatol 2007;31:48–55.

47 Uhing MR, Das UG: Optimizing growth in the preterm infant. Clin Perinatol 2009;36:165–176.

48 Olsen IE, Richardson DK, Schmid CH, Ausman LM, Dwyer JT: Intersite differences in weight growth velocity of extremely premature infants. Pediatrics 2002;110:1125–1132.

49 Bloom BT, Mulligan J, Arnold C, Ellis S, Moffitt S, Rivera A, Kunamneni S, Thomas P, Clark RH, Peabody J: Improving growth of very low birth weight infants in the first 29 days. Pediatrics 2003;112:8–14.

50 Ehrenkranz RA, Das A, Wrage LA, Poindexter BB, Higgins R, Stoll BJ, Oh W, for the Eunice Kennedy Shriver National Institute of Child Health Human Development Neonatal Research Network: Early nutrition mediates the influence of severity of illness on extremely low birth weight infants. Pediatr Res 2011; 69:522–529.

51 McCallie KR, Lee HC, Mayer O, Cohen RS, Hintz SR, Rhine WD: Improved outcomes with a standardized feeding protocol for very low birth weight infants. J Perinatol 2011;31:S61–S67.

52 Rochow N, Fusch G, Mühlinghaus A, Niesytto C, Straube S, Utzig N, Fusch C: A nutritional program to improve outcome of very low birth weight infants. Clin Nutr 2012;31:124–131.

53 Ehrenkranz RA: Ongoing issues in the intensive care for the periviable infant-nutritional management and prevention of bronchopulmonary dysplasia and nosocomial infections. Semin Perinatol 2014;38:25–30.

54 Patole SK, de Klerk N: Impact of standardized feeding regimens on incidence of neonatal necrotizing enterocolitis: a systematic review and meta-analysis of observational studies. Arch Dis Child Fetal Neonatal Ed 2005;90:F147–F151.

55 Gephart SM, Hanson CK: Preventing necrotizing enterocolitis with standardized feeding protocols. Adv Neonatal Care 2013;13:48–54.

Prof. Richard A. Ehrenkranz, MD
Pediatrics and Obstetrics, Gynecology & Reproductive Sciences
Yale University School of Medicine, PO Box 208064
New Haven, CT 06520-8064 (USA)
E-Mail richard.ehrenkranz@yale.edu

Koletzko B, Poindexter B, Uauy R (eds): Nutritional Care of Preterm Infants: Scientific Basis and Practical Guidelines.
World Rev Nutr Diet. Basel, Karger, 2014, vol 110, pp 27–48 (DOI: 10.1159/000358457)

Assessing the Evidence from Neonatal Nutrition Research

Hania Szajewska[a] · Berthold Koletzko[b] · Francis B. Mimouni[c] ·
Ricardo Uauy[d]

[a]Department of Paediatrics, The Medical University of Warsaw, Warsaw, Poland; [b]Division of Metabolic and
Nutritional Medicine, Dr. von Hauner Children's Hospital, University of Munich Medical Centre – Klinikum
der Universität München, Munich, Germany; [c]Department of Pediatrics, Tel Aviv Medical Center, Tel Aviv
University, Tel Aviv, Israel; [d]Division of Neonatology, Pontifical Catholic University Medical School and Institute
of Nutrition Universidad de Chile, Santiago de Chile, Chile

Reviewed by Nicholas B. Embleton, Neonatal Service, Newcastle Hospitals, Institute of Health and Society,
Newcastle University, Newcastle upon Tyne, UK; Brenda Poindexter, Indiana University School of Medicine,
Indianapolis, Ind., USA

Abstract

Being up to date with current medical research in order to deliver the best possible care to patients
has never been easy, and it is not easy today. Still, clinical decision-making at all levels of medical care
needs to be made based on evidence. This chapter aims to provide tools for understanding how to
assess the medical literature. It starts with an overview of study designs. Each of the study designs
can provide useful information if applied in the appropriate situation, with the proper methods, and
if properly reported. The strengths and limitations of each study design, mainly in relation to the potential to establish causality, are presented. Then, the chapter provides a summary of the key elements
of practicing evidence-based medicine, the necessity of today's medicine. These key elements are as
follows: formulation of an answerable question (the problem); finding the best evidence; critical appraisal of the evidence, and applying the evidence to the treatment of patients. Special focus is placed
on critical appraisal of the evidence, as not all research is of good quality. Studies are frequently biased
and their results are incorrect. In turn, this can lead one to draw false conclusions. While an attempt
was made to discuss all of the issues in the context of studies conducted in neonatal nutrition, the
principles are applicable to practicing medicine in general.   © 2014 S. Karger AG, Basel

Being up to date with current medical research in order to deliver the best possible
care to patients has never been easy, and it is not easy today. It has been estimated that
there are 75 trials and 11 systematic reviews of trials published per day, and a plateau
in growth has not yet been reached [1]. One way of dealing with information overload
is to practice evidence-based medicine (EBM) [2].

This chapter starts with an overview of study designs and discusses their strengths
and limitations, mainly in relation to the potential to establish causality. Then, it pro-

vides an overview of four steps needed for practicing EBM, the necessity of today's medicine. These steps are as follows: (i) Formulation of an answerable question (the problem); (ii) Finding the best evidence; (iii) Critical appraisal of the evidence, and (iv) Applying the evidence to the treatment of patients. Finally, evidence-based guidelines and a grading system are presented. An attempt was made to discuss all of the issues in the context of studies conducted in neonatal nutrition. However, the principles are applicable to practicing medicine in general.

Study Designs in Clinical Research

Table 1 provides characteristics of the major types of study designs, and figure 1 shows an algorithm for classification of the major types of study design. In brief, based on whether the investigator assigns the exposure (e.g. treatment) or not, clinical research is divided into experimental and observational studies [3]. Experimental trials may be randomized (the intervention or exposure was assigned by randomization) or non-randomized. Observational studies are subdivided into two types: descriptive (these are studies without a comparison/control group; e.g. case report or case-series report) or analytical (there is a comparison/control group). Within analytical studies, the temporal (time) relationship between exposure and outcome determines the study design. If both exposures and outcomes are assessed at one time point, this is a cross-sectional study *('a snaphot in time')* [3]. If a study follows up two or more groups from exposure to outcome, it is defined as a cohort study *('looking forward in time')* [3]. Finally, case-control studies start with an outcome (e.g. a disease) and look backward in time for exposures/risk factors *('research in reverse')* [3]. All observational studies are susceptible to confounding (see below).

Table 2 provides the levels of evidence as proposed by the Oxford Centre for EBM [4]. Below, some study designs are discussed in more detail. The designs are listed in decreasing order of their capacity to document causality.

Systematic Review and Meta-Analysis
In the hierarchy of levels of evidence (table 2), the results of a systematic review, with or without a meta-analysis, are considered to be the evidence of the highest grade. Thus, if available, systematic reviews and meta-analyses should be used in support of clinical decision-making.

While the two terms, i.e. 'systematic review' and 'meta-analysis', are commonly used interchangeably, there is a distinction between them. A systematic review is *'a review of a clearly formulated question that uses systematic and explicit methods to identify, select and critically appraise relevant research, and to collect and analyze data from studies that are included in the review. Statistical methods may or may not be used to analyze and summarize the results of the included trials'* [5]. A meta-analysis is a name that is given to any review article when statistical techniques are used in a sys-

Szajewska · Koletzko · Mimouni · Uauy

Table 1. Study designs in decreasing order of their ability to document causality. Advantages and disadvantages [based on references 3, 17, 35]

Study design	Definition	Advantages	Disadvantages
Randomized controlled trial	An experiment in which two or more interventions are compared by being randomly allocated to participants	Internal validity Known and unknown confounding factors are equally balanced Causation can be established Effect size can be determined	Disease outcomes may not be apparent for a long time Need for presumed markers of later disease risk May be expensive (time and money) May be ethically inappropriate
Non-randomized trial	Any quantitative study estimating the effectiveness of an intervention (harm or benefit) that does not use randomization to allocate units to comparison groups	Use of a concurrent control group Uniform ascertainment of outcomes in both groups	Selection bias
Cohort study	An observational study in which a defined group of people (the cohort) is followed up over time	Accuracy of data collection with regard to exposures, confounders, and outcomes Large sample size is possible	Long-term follow-up required to study disease outcomes Need to use proxies for assessing risk of some diseases Confounding possible ? Causality High cost in time & money (long follow-up)
Case-control studies	A study that compares people with a specific disease or outcome of interest (cases) to people from the same population without that disease or outcome (controls), and which seeks to find associations between the outcome and prior exposure to particular risk factors	Useful for rare outcomes or those that take a long time to develop Short duration Small, inexpensive Can study several exposures	High confounding risk Selection of controls (controls should be similar to cases in all important respects except for not having the outcome in question) Survivor bias Recall bias (better recollection of exposures among the cases than among the controls) Cannot establish temporal sequence between exposure and outcome Limited to 1 outcome Cannot assess incidence/prevalence
Cross-sectional studies (other terms: frequency survey; prevalence study)	A study measuring the distribution of some characteristic(s) in a population at a particular point in time	Cheap and simple Ethically safe Many study multiple outcomes and exposures Short duration Can provide an estimate of prevalence of an outcome Less feasible for rare predictors or outcomes	Temporal sequence between exposure and outcome cannot be established ? Causality

Table 1. Continued

Study design	Definition	Advantages	Disadvantages
Ecological study	An observational study in which the associations between the occurrence of disease and exposure to known or suspected causes is assessed The unit of observation is the population or community (not an individual)	Cheap and quick to conduct May use data collected for other purposes	Confounding possible Does not allow one to establish causality Poor quality of data collected over time and from different places
Case report/case-series report	A study reporting observations on a single individual or observations on a series of individuals, usually all receiving the same intervention, with no control group	Inexpensive Convenient	? Causality (because of lack of comparison group) Does not allow assessment of associations

tematic review to combine the results of included trials to produce a single estimate of the effect of a particular intervention (i.e. a number or a graph) [5]. At least two primary studies are needed to perform a meta-analysis [5].

In 2004, Mike Clarke stated that *'nobody should do a trial without reviewing what is known'* [6]. A few years later, he reconfirmed his position by stating that *'clinical trials should begin and end with systematic reviews of relevant evidence'* [7]. In addition to these clear messages, the main formal objectives of performing a meta-analysis include the following: to increase power, i.e. the chance to reliably detect a clinically important difference if one actually exists; to increase precision in estimating effects, i.e. narrow the confidence interval around the effects; to answer questions not raised by individual studies; to resolve controversies arising from studies with conflicting results, and to generate new hypotheses for future studies [5].

Key components needed to conduct a systematic review include the following: formulation of the review question; searching for studies based on predefined inclusion and exclusion criteria; selecting studies, collecting data, and creating evidence-based tables, and assessing the risk of bias in the included trials. Usually the following criteria generally associated with good-quality studies are evaluated: adequacy of sequence generation, allocation concealment, and blinding of investigators, participants, outcome assessors, and data analysts; intention-to-treat analysis, and comprehensive follow-up ($\geq 80\%$). The final step is synthesizing data from the included studies and meta-analysis.

Is it always appropriate to pool the results? This is one of the important decisions to be made by the authors of any systematic reviews. The take-home message is that it is always appropriate to perform a systematic review, and every meta-analysis should be preceded by a systematic review. However, not every systematic review

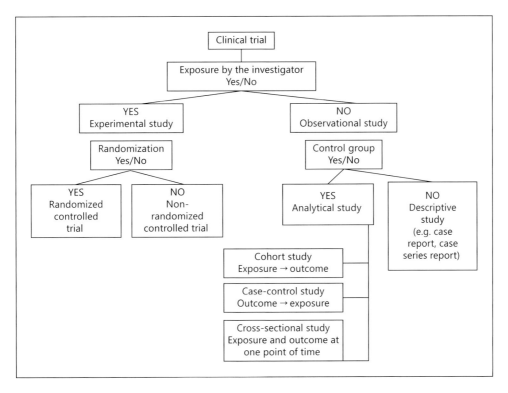

Fig. 1. Algorithm for classification of study designs [adapted from 3].

should be finalized with a meta-analysis; in fact, it is sometimes erroneous and even misleading to perform a meta-analysis [5]. While it is unrealistic to expect absolute similarity of all the studies, comparability is needed. In principle, data should only be pooled if they are homogeneous, i.e. the participants, intervention, comparison, and outcomes must be similar (homogeneous) or at least comparable [5].

In neonatal nutrition research, a large number of clinical questions have been addressed by a systematic review. One such example is a systematic review with a meta-analysis that evaluated the effect of maternal *(population)* omega–3 long-chain poly-unsaturated fatty acids (LC-PUFA) supplementation during pregnancy *(intervention)* on neurologic and visual development in the offspring *(outcomes)*. No evidence that conclusively supports or refutes the notion that omega–3 LC-PUFA supplementation during pregnancy improves cognitive or visual development was found [8]. Another example is a Cochrane review that aimed to compare the efficacy and safety of prophylactic enteral probiotics administration *(intervention)* versus placebo or no treatment *(comparison)* in the prevention of severe necrotizing enterocolitis (NEC) and/or sepsis *(outcomes)* in preterm infants *(population)*. The authors concluded that enteral supplementation with probiotics prevents severe NEC and all-cause mortality in preterm infants, and they believe available evidence supports a change in practice [9], although the latter remains controversial. The major concern with regard to these

Table 2. Oxford Centre for Evidence-Based Medicine 2011 Levels of Evidence

Question	Level 1*	Level 2*	Level 3*	Level 4*	Level 5
How common is the problem?	Local and current random sample surveys (or censuses)	SR of surveys that allow matching to local circumstances**	Local non-random sample**	Case series**	N/A
Diagnosis	SR of cross-sectional studies with consistently applied reference standard and blinding	Individual cross-sectional studies with consistently applied reference standard and blinding	Non-consecutive studies, or studies without consistently applied reference standards**	Case-control studies, or poor or non-independent standard	N/A
Prognosis	Systematic review of inception cohort studies	Inception cohort studies	Cohort study or control arm of RCT	Case-series report, case-control studies, or poor quality prognostic cohort study**	N/A
Treatment benefits	SR of RCT or n-of-1 trials	RCT or observational trial with dramatic effect	Non-randomized controlled cohort/follow-up study**	Case-series report, case-control studies, or historically controlled studies**	Mechanism-based reasoning
Treatment COMMON harms	SR of RCTs, SR of nested case-control studies, n-of-1 trial with the patient you are raising the question about, or observational study with dramatic effect	Individual RCT or (exceptionally) observational study with dramatic effect	Non-randomized controlled cohort/follow-up study (post-marketing surveillance) provided there are sufficient numbers to rule out a common harm. For long-term harms, the duration of follow-up must be sufficient	Case-series report, case-control studies, or historically controlled studies**	Mechanism-based reasoning
Treatment RARE harms	SR of RCTs or n-of-1 trial	RCT or (exceptionally) observational study with dramatic effect			
Screening	SR of RCTs	RCT	Non-randomized controlled cohort/follow-up study**	Case-series report, case-control studies, or historically controlled studies**	Mechanism-based reasoning

* Level may be graded down on the basis of study quality, imprecision, indirectness (study PICO does not match questions PICO), because of inconsistency between studies, or because the absolute effect size is very small; level may be graded up if there is a large or very large effect size.
** As always, a systematic review is generally better than an individual study.

meta-analyses, as with many other meta-analyses in the area of probiotics [10–13], is whether it is appropriate to pool data on different microorganisms [discussed in chapter by J. Neu, Necrotizing Enterocolitis].

If a meta-analysis is performed, the results from individual studies together with the combined result are graphically displayed as a forest plot. Figure 2 shows an interpretation of a forest plot from a hypothetical meta-analysis comparing the effect of a new infant formula supplemented with a novel ingredient with a standard infant formula for the prevention of the outcome.

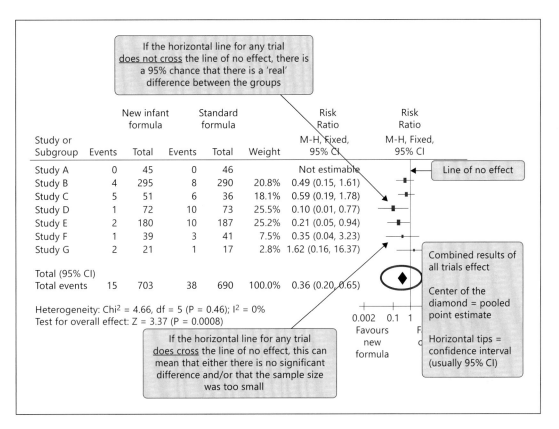

Fig. 2. Forest plot from a hypothetical meta-analysis comparing the effect of a new infant formula with a standard infant formula on the risk of an outcome. The relative risk of 0.36 suggests that, compared to use of the standard formula, the use of the new infant formula reduces the risk of the outcome in an infant (64% reduction). CI indicates confidence interval.

Recently, other types of meta-analyses are gaining popularity. First, reviews of *individual patient data* (IPD). Here, the original research data from each participant in each study are sought directly from the researchers responsible for that study. One such example is a review aimed at determining if supplementation of formula milk with LC-PUFA affects neurodevelopment at 18 months of age in term or preterm infants by an IPD meta-analysis. This IPD meta-analysis, based on the data of 870 children from 4 large randomized clinical trials (RCTs), found that LC-PUFA supplementation of infant formula does not have a clinically meaningful effect on neurodevelopment as assessed by Bayley scores at 18 months. The reviewers stated that inclusion of all relevant data should not have led to differing conclusions except, possibly, for very-low-birth-weight infants [14].

Second, *indirect comparisons* and *multiple-treatments meta-analysis* (MTM), known also as 'network meta-analysis' or 'mixed treatment comparisons', are other types of analysis that are gaining popularity. Indirect comparisons are comparisons that are made between interventions that have not been compared directly with each other [5]. MTM is an extension to indirect comparisons that allows the combination of direct with indirect comparisons and also the simultaneous analysis of the comparative effects of many interventions [5]. These are comparisons that are made between interventions that have not been compared directly with each other. It allows the comparison and the ranking of several treatments by considering them as a trial network [15].

Randomized Controlled Trials

A randomized controlled trial (RCT) is defined as an experiment in which two or more interventions are compared by being randomly allocated to participants. Well-designed and well-implemented RCTs are considered the gold standard for evaluating the efficacy of healthcare interventions (therapy or prevention).

RCTs are the best way to identify causal relationships. The fact that they are less likely to be biased by known and unknown confounders is an added strength relative to all other study designs. However, the following limitations need to be considered in analyzing results from RCTs in the evaluation of causation and prevention of neonatal conditions addressed in this book.

First, critically relevant outcomes that relate to neonatal nutritional practices may take years or decades to become apparent. Therefore, it is difficult to design and implement RCTs that last for a sufficient time to cover more than just a small fraction of the process leading to the final outcome.

Second, diet/nutritional and related exposures are complex and interrelated, and in most cases, short-term effects do not persist in the medium to long term. Most studies assess responses to single macro- or micronutrient changes, which may not reflect real-life conditions in which multiple exposures (deficiencies or potential excesses) co-exist and interact to define specific outcomes.

Third, the outcome of a trial is to show (or to fail in demonstrating) efficacy in achieving a desired outcome. Results of such trials can be simply and robustly interpreted in light of the specific intervention and the given study population. However, extrapolation to other populations or to interventions not exactly the same as those tested in the trial may be inappropriate.

The results of RCTs may change medical practice. In neonatal nutrition research, one example of a clinical question that has been addressed by an RCT is does the fortification of human milk with either human milk-based, human milk fortifier or bovine milk-based, human milk fortifier *(intervention)* have an effect on the risk of NEC *(outcome)* in extremely premature infants *(population)*? This RCT, involving 207 infants (birth weight 500–1,250 g), showed that the groups receiving exclusively human milk had a significantly reduced risk of NEC and NEC-needing surgical intervention. Lack of blinding was one of the limitations of the study. Still, the findings strongly support the use of human milk for reducing the risk of NEC in preterm infants [16].

Cohort Studies

In cohort studies, the diets, body compositions, and/or physical activity levels of a large group (the cohort) of participants are assessed, and the group is followed-up over a period of time. During the follow-up period, some members of the cohort will develop and be diagnosed with nutrition-related disorders or effects, while others will not. Comparisons can then be made between study participants who develop nutrition-related disease and those that do not in terms of their characteristics measured at the start of (and perhaps during) the study. Because measurements are made before any outcome condition has been identified, cohort studies are not subject to recall bias.

Cohort studies provide the opportunity to obtain repeated assessments of participants' diets at regular intervals, which may improve the assessment of dietary exposures. Also, in cohort studies, blood and tissue samples are often collected and stored for future analysis.

A cohort study is the best study design to identify the incidence and natural history of a disease [17]. It allows calculations of true incidence rates, relative risks, and attributable risks [3].

Cohort studies may need to be very large (up to tens of thousands of subjects) in order to yield enough statistical power to identify factors that may increase disease risk by as little as 20 or 30%. They are often expensive (though less so than many large trials). Therefore, these studies tend to be conducted in or for high-income countries. Also, in some cases (e.g. in malnutrition-related disease) the consequences take decades to develop. Thus, a long follow-up time is needed to identify enough cases to study the diet-disease relationship. In some circumstances, the cohort of people selected from the population at large may exhibit relatively little variability in dietary habits or physical activity, and this can mean that small effects may be missed.

Cohort studies can be historical. Historical cohort studies are conducted by using data collected in the past (e.g. existing dietary records) and relating these to subsequent records diagnosing nutrition-related disease. Because this study design uses past diet records prior to the diagnosis of an outcome, it is not subject to the same recall bias as case-control studies.

Cohort studies can be conducted on selected subgroups in a population, for example, people of a particular social class or with a particular occupation. Findings from these studies may not be generalizable to the population as a whole. It is possible to conduct a case-control study nested within a cohort study. In nested case-control studies, the cases and controls are drawn from the current existing population of the prospective cohort study. All of the cases and a sample of the unaffected subjects from the cohort become the control group. This design characterizes diet prior to outcome and so avoids problems of recall bias. Case-cohort studies are similar in that cases and controls are also drawn from the population of a prospective cohort. However, in case-cohort studies, the controls are a random sample of the entire cohort at enrollment rather than simply unaffected individuals identified later.

In the field of neonatal nutrition, the bulk of evidence on the effects of breastfeeding comes from prospective, observational, cohort studies with appropriate adjustment of potential confounders. One example of a question that has been addressed by a cohort study is does hospital re-admission within the first 2 months of life have an effect on the duration of predominant breastfeeding in late preterm or term infants? The authors found that hospital re-admission within the first 60 days of life does not have such an effect [18].

Case-Control Studies

A case-control study compares people with a specific disease or outcome of interest (cases) to people from the same population without that disease or outcome (controls). Well-designed case-control studies can produce useful initial evidence to generate hypotheses that can then be tested prospectively. However, in these studies, diet and nutritional exposures are measured after the outcome has occurred, thus they are susceptible to biased recording. The value of evidence from a case-control study is strengthened when bias is minimized and when cases and controls are selected from the same source population. Case-control studies are usually less expensive and can be conducted over shorter time periods than cohort studies. They are also more able than cohort studies to study rare outcomes, such as some nutrition-related outcomes. Some types of case-control studies are nested within existing cohort studies (as discussed above).

Cross-Sectional Studies

A cross-sectional study typically quantifies the relationship between exposure and outcome and, therefore, has an analytical character [3]. However, it may also be a study that is entirely descriptive (a simple survey assessing prevalence). Other terms used for a cross-sectional study are 'frequency survey' or 'prevalence study'.

A cross-sectional study measures the distribution of some characteristic(s) (e.g. diet) in a particular population at one point in time. Because cross-sectional studies investigate the characteristics of populations or individuals at a set point in time, this study type cannot differentiate between cause and effect (directionality). It is not possible on the basis of the associations alone to determine whether the characteristics of the diet or lifestyle are a result of the disease process or whether the characteristics of the diet or lifestyle cause the disease. Furthermore, the levels of exposure measured at the time of the study may not reflect those many years earlier when the disease process was initiated, or they may be biased by knowledge of the disease. As with other observational studies, cross-sectional studies are susceptible to confounding.

Ecological Studies

These studies search for associations between the occurrence of disease and exposure to identified or assumed causes. In ecological studies, the unit of observation is the population or community. The presence or absence of a specific risk factor is not related to individuals with or without disease, but rather to populations.

Szajewska · Koletzko · Mimouni · Uauy

In neonatology research, ecological studies may compare the occurrence of abnormal neonatal health conditions across populations or within populations over time. As with other types of observational studies, the results from ecological studies are often limited by confounding factors.

Population-level food disappearance data are used to assess diet in many ecological studies. This may introduce error because actual dietary intakes of relevant individuals are not specifically measured. Another problem is that the exposure or outcome may be relevant only to a subpopulation of individuals in the population. For example, an ecological study may show a correlation between alcohol consumption and risk of altered neonatal health conditions. However, all women are included in population alcohol consumption statistics, although the relevant groups are those that are potentially able to get pregnant, i.e. women of reproductive age.

In some cases, ecological studies collect data only on relevant population subgroups divided, for example, by sex or age. Some types of ecological studies cannot easily be independently reproduced. Replication is an important part of the scientific process and, therefore, this is a potential limitation of this study type.

Ecological studies have value and should be included in an integrated approach to evaluating the evidence. Variations in the range of intakes of foods and dietary constituents between different nations or populations are often wider than, or different from, variations within a particular nation or population. Levels of intake that modify disease risk may be above or below the ranges found in specific populations, or an effect may not be strong enough to be detected in a population with a relatively narrow range of intake (and hence a similar level of risk attributable to that exposure).

Ecological studies also have other strengths. The disease rates used in international ecological studies are often derived from relatively large populations and are, therefore, subject to only small random errors. However, the quality of assessment and recording of disease varies between countries and regions, and precise estimates that are wrong would be terribly misleading. Some ecological and cross-sectional studies are repeated at time intervals. These are called 'time series with multiple measurements' or 'secular trend' studies. Changes in patterns of disease within relatively short periods of time demonstrate that environmental factors, which include diet and physical activity, play a role in the causation of disease. Genetic and other susceptibilities also influence which particular individuals become affected within a population. Ecological studies can provide a valuable contribution to the overall evidence.

Mendelian Randomization

A technique called 'mendelian randomization' has been developed to address some of the issues relating to confounding found in observational studies. Mendelian randomization provides a method for studying nutritional influences on disease by examining the influence of genetic variation in nutrient metabolism [19].

Gene assortment from parents to their children is random. With growing knowledge of the human genome, many genes have been identified that are involved in nutrient metabolism. If a particular genetic variation is associated with perinatal nutrition-related disease and is also involved in the way the body handles an individual micronutrient, this provides strong evidence of a link between that micronutrient and the nutrition-related perinatal condition. In this case, the genetic randomization acts in the same way as random assortment in RCTs to eliminate potential confounding. However, it cannot be excluded that there may be unknown actions of the gene in question, or that the gene may be linked to another one nearby that is truly causal. One such example is the effect of polymorphisms in the fatty acid desaturase *(FADS)* genes that determine the efficiency how polyunsaturated fatty acids (PUFA) are metabolized. Recent gene-nutrition interaction studies indicate that these polymorphisms have a marked modulating effect on the relation of dietary PUFA intake on complex phenotypes such as cognitive outcomes and asthma risk in children [20]. For example, the benefit of postnatal breastfeeding, which provides LC-PUFA, on intelligence at the age of 8 years was significantly greater in children carrying *FADS* polymorphisms resulting in low LC-PUFA synthesis [21]. Similarly, breastfeeding did not have any significant effect on doctor's diagnosed asthma up to age of 10 years in children with the common *FADS* genotype resulting in more active LC-PUFA synthesis, whereas children heterozygous or homozygous for less common *FADS* genotype who have lower LC-PUFA-formation, longer breastfeeding providing preformed LC-PUFA led to about 60% less diagnosed asthma [22]. These results support the conclusion that postnatal PUFA status is causally related to long-term cognitive development and risk of asthma. These recent gene-nutrition interaction studies may well translate into future clinical practice.

Confounding

Confounding factors can limit the validity of findings from non-RCTs, including observational studies. A confounder is a factor that is related to the outcome being studied (e.g. growth rate) and is also associated with the exposure being studied (e.g. feeding tolerance or fat intake). Some confounders are well known. For instance, low birth weight (LBW) infants may have an increased risk of anemia due to low iron intake relative to greater iron needs. However, LBW infants are also likely to be receiving extra PUFA to achieve greater energy intake and thus are more likely to have red cell hemolysis due to the higher PUFA intake relative to antioxidant supply. Thus, unless data on these factors are available and/or the design of the study has adequately controlled for these factors, it is not possible to be sure that the increase in risk of anemia is due solely to low iron intake and not to the excess PUFA relative to tocopherol intake. In this example, the known confounder, the PUFA-to-tocopherol ratio, can be dealt with by analyzing the results adjusting for iron relative to PUFA intake and/or by analyzing the anemia relative to tocopherol/PUFA intake. Large, well-conducted, case-control or cohort studies generally control confounding in these ways. Problems arise when the confounding factors are unknown or cannot be accurately measured. It is not possible to know whether unknown confounders are having an effect on the risk estimates from epidemiological studies. Many studies do not properly correct for all known confounders, and this needs to be considered in assessing results of studies or evaluating conflicting evidence from apparently similar studies. RCTs of sufficient size can be interpreted with confidence that confounding is not a problem. This is because in large, well-designed and conducted trials, known and unknown confounders should be distributed evenly between the study groups. Confounding may cause bias in smaller randomized trials because of imbalances between treatment and control groups that occur by chance.

Standards for Reporting Clinical Research

There is evidence that incomplete and/or poor and/or inaccurate reporting of clinical research is a problem, thus reducing its role in clinical decision-making. Being aware of these reporting problems, journal editors, together with other stakeholders such as methodologists, researchers, clinicians, and members of professional organizations, have developed a number of standards for reporting clinical research to ensure that all details of design, conduct, and analysis are included in the manuscript. The editors now require that authors follow these standards when submitting a manuscript for publication. Among others, these standards include the following:

- CONSORT (Consolidated Standards of Reporting Trials) – a checklist and a flowchart for a randomized controlled trial (RCT); the CONSORT statement has several extension statements (e.g. for structured abstracts, cluster RCTs, pragmatic trials, and non-inferiority and equivalence RCTs) [23–27]. See http://www.consort-statement.org
- PRISMA (Preferred Reporting Items for Systematic reviews and Meta-Analyses) – a checklist and a flowchart for a systematic review or meta-analysis of RCTs [28]. See http://www.prisma-statement.org
- STARD (Standards for the Reporting of Diagnostic Accuracy Studies) – a checklist and flowchart for assessing diagnostic accuracy [29]. See http://www.stard-statement.org
- MOOSE (Meta-analysis of Observational Studies in Epidemiology) – a checklist for a meta-analysis of observational trials [30].

Practicing EBM

The following four steps are needed for practicing EBM: (1) Formulation of an answerable question (the problem); (2) Finding the best evidence; (3) Critical appraisal of the evidence, and (4) Applying the evidence to the treatment of patients.

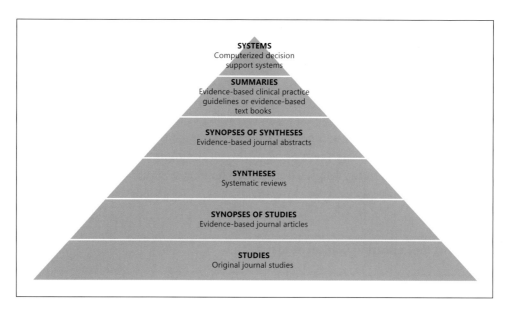

Fig. 3. The 6S hierarchy of evidence-based resources [31]. The search for evidence should begin at the highest possible layer.

Step 1: Formulation of an Answerable Question

The search for the best research answers to clinical uncertainties begins with formulation of an answerable question. In general, the key components of a research question should address the types of participants/patient problem/population (P), interventions (I), comparisons (C), and outcomes (O) of interest. The use of the acronym 'PICO' is helpful for developing a well-formulated question. Different research questions require different study designs – see table 2.

Step 2: Finding the Best Evidence

The clinician/investigator faced with a clinical or research issue is often faced with the challenging task of retrieving the correct available evidence. For this, we suggest using the hierarchy of pre-appraised evidence specified by DiCenso et al. [31] and called the 6S approach. This model is shown in figure 3 and consists of a pyramid with six levels of evidence that are used for decision-making.

At the base of the pyramid lie individual *original studies* (the first of the 6S). For this purpose, the reader will define appropriate key words and search individual studies using search engines such as PubMed (Medline) or Embase. The task might be enormous, as there may be hundreds of studies (or even more) on a single topic. For instance, a Medline search of all clinical trials on NEC performed on July 9, 2013 allowed the retrieval of 4,370 articles published since 1966, even after the exclusion of animal studies. The search requires the clinician to be fluent with the search engine being used, to be familiar with its tools (such as filters that enable restricting the number of articles to read), and to be able to interpret each study on his/her own without any expert opinion.

Thus the usefulness of *synopses of studies* (the second S and second stratum of the pyramid) that allow the use of resources that summarize the results of single studies. These resources save time, and they do not require the reader to have significant expertise related to the topic. Examples include Evidence-Based Medicine (http://ebm.bmj.com/), McMaster PLUS Database (http://hiru.mcmaster.ca/hiru/HIRU_McMaster_PLUS_Projects. aspx), Journal Watch (produced by the New England Journal of Medicine, http://www. jwatch.org/), AAP SmartBriefs (https://www2.smartbrief.com), or more specifically, SmartBriefs for Nutritionists (to be found at the internet address: https://www.smartbrief. com/signupSystem/subscribe.action?pageSequence = 1&briefName = nutritionists). The reviewers of these studies and the authors of the synopses tend to choose higher quality articles that are summarized and commented upon. It also means that a synopsis is not necessarily available for every study. AAP SmartBriefs, or SmartBriefs for Nutritionists, are routinely emailed on a daily basis without fee to readers that sign up for this service. To the best of our knowledge, at the present time, there is no such thing as 'Smartbrief for Neonatal Nutritionists' addressing specifically the issues of neonatal nutrition.

The third S, or third stratum of the pyramid, is *syntheses*, which consists of systematic reviews (usually, but not always, with meta-analyses) that allow one to integrate the information provided by individual studies in these reviews. The information from multiple individual studies is integrated according to specific inclusion and exclusion criteria, increasing greatly the power and precision. Most systematic reviews state the limitations of the studies, whether or not data are conclusive, and whether additional studies may be needed. They are, however, limited by the fact that they may be very complex and difficult to read and biased if mostly studies with positive results get published. Systematic reviews and meta-analyses can be specifically searched for and retrieved using databases such as PubMed (www.ncbi.nlm.nih.gov/pubmed), The Cochrane Library (www.thecochranelibrary.com/), or DynaMed (https://dynamed. ebscohost.com/). For instance, a Medline search performed on July 9, 2013 of all meta-analyses on NEC allowed the retrieval of 96 such articles since 1966. Obviously, not all aspects of NEC have been evaluated by these analyses.

The fourth stratum of the pyramid (4th S) is *synopses of syntheses*. These synopses are particularly useful when we want quick, pre-appraised information, but we do not have the time to read the whole meta-analysis. Resources that provide synopses of syntheses include the Cochrane reviews, Evidence-Based Medicine, DARE, DynaMed, and Journal Watch. These synopses summarize a systematic review in a critical manner as well and are particularly useful when they are available and current.

The fifth stratum of the pyramid (5th S) is *summaries*, which are needed when clinical decision-making is needed. These summaries are usually evidence-based clinical guidelines, which are usually found using the National Guidelines Clearinghouse (www.guideline.gov/), American College of Physicians Physicians' Information and Education Resource (PIER) (http://pier.acponline.org/index.html), UpToDate, or even Medline. Summaries need to be updated when evidence changes, and it is not uncommon to see that guidelines may differ according to the composition of their writers and their professional associations. A Medline search performed on July 9, 2013 of all clinical guidelines on NEC allowed the retrieval of only 11 such articles since 1966.

On top of the pyramid is the sixth stratum (6th S), which stands for *systems*. Systems are computerized health records with computerized decision support systems. They should allow for keeping up with the guidelines for each individual patient. Systems are not of widespread use, but we can predict that in the future they will become more and more available.

Step 3: Critical Appraisal of the Evidence

Not all research is of good quality. Studies are frequently biased and their results are incorrect. In turn, this can lead one to draw false conclusions. Thus, critical appraisal is necessary to identify unbiased valid studies, with true results, to guide clinical decision-making at all levels of medical care. Critical appraisal has been defined by the Cochrane Collaboration '*as the process of assessing and interpreting evidence by systematically considering its validity, results, and relevance*' [32].

Studies have two kinds of validity: internal and external. The internal validity is the extent to which the design and conduct of a study are likely to have prevented bias or systematic error. While there is no ideal study, i.e. a study free from any bias, strictly designed (and executed) trials are more likely to produce results that are nearer to the truth. The external validity of a study is the extent to which results may be generalized to other circumstances [33]. One such example is studies carried out in term infants with results that may not be extrapolated to very-low-birth-weight infants.

A number of organizations have developed checklists specific to particular study designs. Some of the most commonly used are those developed by the Critical Appraisal Skills Programme (CASP), and these checklists are freely available on the internet (http://www.casp-uk.net) [34]. These checklists involve answering a number of questions related to a specific research paper. However, the following three principal questions apply to all study designs: Are the results of the study valid? What are the results? Will the results help me locally? [35]. Below, we provide an overview of the basics of critical appraisal of scientific research.

Rapid Critical Appraisal of a Randomized Controlled Trial

The questions developed by CASP for rapid critical appraisal of an RCT are as follows [36]:
- *Are the results of the trial valid?*

(1) Did the trial address a clearly focused question [in terms of PICO: of the population (P), the intervention (I), the comparison (C), and the outcome(s) (O)]?

(2) Was the assignment of patients to treatments randomized (and was it done appropriately so)?

(3) Were all of the participants who entered the trial properly accounted for at its conclusion (i.e. was follow-up complete and were patients analyzed in the groups to which they were randomized)? Good studies will have at least 80% follow-up and will use intention-to-treat analysis. This means that all participants are included in the arm to which they were allocated, whether or not they received (or completed) the intervention given to that arm.

(4) Were participants, staff, and study personnel 'blind' to treatment?

(5) Were the groups similar at the start of the trial (i.e. did the randomization work properly and achieved comparable groups)? Each paper should have a table entitled 'Baseline characteristics', which demonstrates that both study groups were broadly comparable in regard to baseline factors such as age, sex, level of illness, etc.

(6) Aside from the experimental intervention, were the groups treated equally?
- *What are the results?*

(7) How large was the treatment effect?

(8) How precise was the estimate of the treatment effect? In clinical research, the use of p values is discouraged. Preference is given to the use of a confidence interval, which provides a range of values for a variable (e.g. relative risk) within which the 'true' value for the entire population is expected to be with a given degree of certainty (typically 95%) [3].
- *Will the results help me locally?*

(9) Can the results be applied to the local population?

(10) Were all clinically important outcomes considered so the results can be applied?

(11) Are the benefits worth the harms and costs?

Rapid Critical Appraisal of a Cohort Study

Rapid critical appraisal of a cohort study involves answering the following questions [37]:
- *Are the results of the study valid?*

(1) Did the study address a clearly focused issue (in terms of the population studied, the risk factors studied, and the outcomes considered)? Is it clear whether the study tried to detect a beneficial or harmful effect?

(2) Did the authors use an appropriate method to answer their question?

(3) Was the cohort recruited in an acceptable way?

(4) Was the exposure accurately measured to minimize bias?

(5) Was the outcome accurately measured to minimize bias?

(6) Have the authors identified all important confounding factors? Have they taken into account the confounding factors in the design and/or analysis?

(7) Was the follow-up of subjects complete enough? Was the follow-up of subjects long enough?

- *What are the results?*
  (8) What are the results of this study?
  (9) How precise are the results? How precise is the estimate of the risk?
  (10) Do you believe the results?
- *Will the results help me locally?*
  (11) Can the results be applied to the local population?
  (12) Do the results of this study fit with other available evidence?

Rapid Critical Appraisal of a Case-Control Study

Critical appraisal of a case-control study includes answering the following questions [38]:

- *Are the results of the study valid?*
  (1) Did the study address a clearly focused issue (in terms of the population studied, the risk factors studied, whether the study tried to detect a beneficial or harmful effect)?
  (2) Did the authors use an appropriate method to answer their question?
  (3) Were the cases recruited in an acceptable way?
  (4) Were the controls selected in an acceptable way?
  (5) Was the exposure accurately measured to minimize bias?
  (6) What confounding factors have the authors accounted for? Have the authors taken into account the potential confounding factors in the design and/or in their analysis?
- *What are the results?*
  (7) What are the results of this study?
  (8) How precise are the results? How precise is the estimate of risk?
  (9) Do you believe the results?
- *Will the results help me locally?*
  (10) Can the results be applied to the local population?
  (11) Do the results of this study fit with other available evidence?

Rapid Critical Appraisal of a Cross-Sectional Study

Critical appraisal of a cross-sectional study includes answering the following questions:

- *Are the results of the study valid?*
  (1) Did the study address a clearly focused issue?
  (2) Did the authors use an appropriate method to answer their question?
  (3) Were the subjects recruited in an acceptable way?
  (4) Were the measures accurately measured to reduce bias?
  (5) Were the data collected in a way that addressed the research issue?
  (6) Did the study have enough participants to minimize the play of chance?
- *What are the results?*
  (7) How are the results presented and what is the main result?
  (8) Was the data analysis sufficiently rigorous?

(9) Is there a clear statement of findings?
- *Will the results help me locally?*
  (10) Can the results be applied to the local population?

Rapid Critical Appraisal of a Systematic Review

As with other research, systematic reviews can be done very well, very poorly, or somewhere in between. Critical appraisal of a systematic review includes answering the following questions [39]:

- *Are the results of the review valid?*
  (1) Did the review ask a clearly focused question [in terms of PICO: the population (P), the intervention (I), the comparison(C), and the outcome(s) (O)]?
  (2) Did the review include the right type of studies (to address the review's question and have an appropriate study design)?
  (3) Did the reviewers try to identify all relevant studies? The more data sources that are searched, the more likely it is that none of the important trials will be missed.
  (4) Did the reviewers assess the quality of the included studies?
  (5) If the results of the studies have been combined, was it reasonable to do so? The Cochrane Handbook recommends that data only be pooled if the data summarized are homogeneous (i.e. the participants, intervention, comparison, and outcomes must be similar (homogeneous) or at least comparable) [5].
- *What are the results?*
  (6) How are the results presented and what is the main result? For interpretation of a forest plot (a graphical display used in a meta-analysis of results from individual studies together with the combined result), see figure 2.
  (7) How precise are these results (i.e. what are the confidence intervals)?
- *Will the results help me locally?*
  (8) Can the results be applied to the local population?
  (9) Were all important outcomes considered?
  (10) Should policy or practice change as a result of the evidence contained in this review?

Step 4: Applying the Evidence to the Treatment of Patients

The ultimate aim of practicing EBM is to integrate current best evidence from research with clinical expertise and the patient's features and values. Unfortunately, for a number of conditions and settings, a gap exists between the best available evidence and the management patients receive. Glasziou and Haynes [40] described a number of stages from evidence to action that need to be considered to apply evidence-based treatment at the right time, in the right place, and in the right way. The clinician needs to be aware, then accept, then adopt, and then act. The patient needs to agree to and adhere to the treatment. Last but not least, the intervention needs to be available.

Table 3. The GRADE system [41]

Quality of evidence	High quality	Further research is unlikely to change our confidence in the estimate of effect
	Moderate quality	Further research is likely to have an important impact on our confidence in the estimate of effect and may change the estimate
	Low quality	Further research is very likely to have an important impact on our confidence in the estimate of effect and is likely to change the estimate
	Very low quality	Any estimate of effect is very uncertain
Grade of recommen-dation	Strong	When the desirable effects of an intervention clearly outweigh the undesirable effects, or clearly do not
	Weak	When the trade-offs are less certain (either because of low quality of evidence or because evidence suggests that desirable and undesirable effects are closely balanced)

While efforts are being made to change it, the quote from Machiavelli *'It must be considered that there is nothing more difficult to carry out, nor more doubtful of success, nor more dangerous to handle, than to initiate a new order of things'* remains very true with regard to applying the evidence.

Evidence-Based Guidelines and Grading Criteria

One way of supporting the introduction of new knowledge into clinical practice and reducing the delivery of inappropriate care is through the use of evidence-based guidelines. These guidelines are based on a systematic review of published research. Often, high-quality evidence is not available, or evidence is not available at all. If so, expert opinion and/or description of usual practice may be included in the guidelines, but it should be clearly labeled as such. Many guidelines grade their recommendations. The GRADE system, developed by the Grading of Recommendations, Assessment, Development and Evaluations (GRADE) Working Group, is increasingly being used. In brief, the GRADE system offers four categories of the quality of the evidence (high, moderate, low, and very low) and two categories of the strength of recommendation (strong or weak; for the latter, terms such as 'conditional' or discretionary' are also used) [41] (table 3).

Summary

- Clinical decision-making at all levels of medical care is made based on evidence from medical research.
- Each of the study designs can provide useful information if applied in the appropriate situation, with the proper methods, and if properly reported.

- One way of dealing with information overload is to practice EBM.
- The key elements of practicing EBM are formulation of an answerable question (PICO), finding the evidence (e.g. using the 6S approach), critical appraisal of the evidence (using checklists), and applying the evidence to the treatment of patients.
- The extent to which one can draw conclusions from published clinical research depends on whether the data and results of the study are free of biases. If there are biases, the task is to consider how they might affect the results.

References

1 Bastian H, Glasziou P, Chalmers I: Seventy-five trials and eleven systematic reviews a day: how will we ever keep up? PLoS Med 2010;7:e1000326.

2 Straus SE, Sackett DL: Using research findings in clinical practice. BMJ 1998;317:339–342.

3 Grimes DA, Schulz KF: An overview of clinical research: the lay of the land. Lancet 2002;359:57–61.

4 OCEBM Levels of Evidence Working Group. Howick J, Chalmers I, Glasziou P, et al: The Oxford 2011 Levels of Evidence. Oxford Centre for Evidence-Based Medicine. http://www.cebm.net/index.aspx?o=565. Accessed on July 13, 2013.

5 Higgins JPT, Green S (eds): Cochrane Handbook for Systematic Reviews of Interventions Version 5.0.1 (updated September 2008). The Cochrane Collaboration, 2008. Available from www.cochrane-handbook.org.

6 Clarke M: Doing new research? Don't forget the old. PLoS Med 2004;1:e35.

7 Clarke M, Hopewell S, Chalmers I: Clinical trials should begin and end with systematic reviews of relevant evidence: 12 years and waiting. Lancet 2010; 376:20–21.

8 Gould JF, Smithers LG, Makrides M: The effect of maternal omega–3 (n–3) LCPUFA supplementation during pregnancy on early childhood cognitive and visual development: a systematic review and meta-analysis of randomized controlled trials. Am J Clin Nutr 2013;97:531–544.

9 Alfaleh K, Anabrees J, Bassler D, Al-Kharfi T: Probiotics for prevention of necrotizing enterocolitis in preterm infants. Cochrane Database Syst Rev 2011; 3:CD005496.

10 Deshpande G, Rao S, Patole S: Probiotics for prevention of necrotising enterocolitis in preterm neonates with very low birthweight: a systematic review of randomised controlled trials. Lancet 2007;369:1614–1620.

11 Alfaleh K, Bassler D: Probiotics for prevention of necrotizing enterocolitis in preterm infants. Cochrane Database Syst Rev 2008;1:CD005496.

12 Barclay AR, Stenson B, Simpson JH, et al: Probiotics for necrotizing enterocolitis: a systematic review. J Pediatr Gastroenterol Nutr 2007;45:569–576.

13 Deshpande G, Rao S, Patole S, et al: Updated meta-analysis of probiotics for preventing necrotizing enterocolitis in preterm neonates. Pediatrics 2010;125: 921–930.

14 Beyerlein A, Hadders-Algra M, Kennedy K, Fewtrell M, Singhal A, Rosenfeld E, Lucas A, Bouwstra H, Koletzko B, von Kries R: Infant formula supplementation with long-chain polyunsaturated fatty acids has no effect on Bayley developmental scores at 18 months of age – IPD meta-analysis of four large clinical trials. J Pediatr Gastroenterol Nutr 2010;50:79–84.

15 Salanti G, Higgins JP, Ades AE, Ioannidis JP: Evaluation of networks of randomized trials. Stat Methods Med Res 2008;17:279–301.

16 Sullivan S, Schanler RJ, Kim JH, Patel AL, Trawöger R, Kiechl-Kohlendorfer U, Chan GM, Blanco CL, Abrams S, Cotten CM, Laroia N, Ehrenkranz RA, Dudell G, Cristofalo EA, Meier P, Lee ML, Rechtman DJ, Lucas A: An exclusively human milk-based diet is associated with a lower rate of necrotizing enterocolitis than a diet of human milk and bovine milk-based products. J Pediatr 2010;156:562–567.e1.

17 Grimes DA, Schulz KF: Cohort studies: marching towards outcomes. Lancet 2002;359:341–345.

18 McNeil DA, Siever J, Tough S, Yee W, Rose MS, Lacaze-Masmonteil T: Hospital re-admission of late preterm or term infants is not a factor influencing duration of predominant breastfeeding. Arch Dis Child Fetal Neonatal Ed 2013;98:F145–F150.

19 Lawlor DA, Harbord RM, Sterne JA, Timpson N, Davey Smith G: Mendelian randomization: using genes as instruments for making causal inferences in epidemiology. Stat Med 2008;27:1133–1163.

20 Lattka E, Klopp N, Demmelmair H, Klingler M, Heinrich J, Koletzko B: Genetic variations in polyunsaturated fatty acid metabolism – implications for child health? Ann Nutr Metab 2012;60(suppl 3):8–17.

21 Steer CD, Davey Smith G, Emmett PM, Hibbeln JR, Golding J: *FADS2* polymorphisms modify the effect of breastfeeding on child IQ. PLoS One 2010;5: e11570.

22 Standl M, Sausenthaler S, Lattka E, Koletzko S, Bauer CP, Wichmann HE, et al: *FADS* gene cluster modulates the effect of breastfeeding on asthma. Results from the GINIplus and LISAplus studies. Allergy 2012;67:83–90.

23 Moher D, Hopewell S, Schulz KF, Montori V, Gøtzsche PC, Devereaux PJ, Elbourne D, Egger M, Altman DG: CONSORT 2010 explanation and elaboration: updated guidelines for reporting parallel group randomised trials. BMJ 2010;340:c869.

24 Campbell MK, Piaggio G, Elbourne DR, Altman DG; CONSORT Group: Consort 2010 statement: extension to cluster randomised trials. BMJ 2012;345: e5661.

25 Hopewell S, Clarke M, Moher D, Wager E, Middleton P, Altman DG, Schulz KF; CONSORT Group: CONSORT for reporting randomized controlled trials in journal and conference abstracts: explanation and elaboration. PLoS Med 2008;5:e20.

26 Zwarenstein M, Treweek S, Gagnier JJ, Altman DG, Tunis S, Haynes B, Oxman AD, Moher D; CONSORT Group; Pragmatic Trials in Healthcare (Practihc) Group: Improving the reporting of pragmatic trials: an extension of the CONSORT statement. BMJ 2008; 337:a2390.

27 Piaggio G, Elbourne DR, Pocock SJ, Evans SJ, Altman DG; CONSORT Group: Reporting of non-inferiority and equivalence randomized trials: extension of the CONSORT 2010 statement. JAMA 2012;308: 2594–2604.

28 Liberati A, Altman DG, Tetzlaff J, Mulrow C, Gøtzsche PC, Ioannidis JP, Clarke M, Devereaux PJ, Kleijnen J, Moher D: The PRISMA statement for reporting systematic reviews and meta-analyses of studies that evaluate healthcare interventions: explanation and elaboration. BMJ 2009;339:b2700.

29 Bossuyt PM, Reitsma JB, Bruns DE, Gatsonis CA, Glasziou PP, Irwig LM, Lijmer JG, Moher D, Rennie D, de Vet HC; Standards for Reporting of Diagnostic Accuracy: Towards complete and accurate reporting of studies of diagnostic accuracy: the STARD initiative. BMJ 2003;326:41–44.

30 Stroup DF, Berlin JA, Morton SC, Olkin I, Williamson GD, Rennie D, Moher D, Becker BJ, Sipe TA, Thacker SB: Meta-analysis of observational studies in epidemiology: a proposal for reporting. Meta-analysis of Observational Studies in Epidemiology (MOOSE) group. JAMA 2000;283:2008–2012.

31 DiCenso A, Bayley L, Haynes RB: ACP Journal Club. Editorial: Accessing preappraised evidence: fine-tuning the 5S model into a 6S model. Ann Intern Med 2009;151:JC3–2, JC3–3.

32 http://www.cochrane.org/glossary/5#letterc. Accessed on February 25, 2013.

33 http://www.cochrane.org/glossary. Accessed on March 8, 2013.

34 http://www.casp-uk.net. Accessed on March 2, 2013.

35 Guyatt G, Rennie D (eds): User's guides to the medical literature. A manual for evidence-based clinical practice. AMA 2002.

36 http://www.casp-uk.net/wp-content/uploads/2011/11/CASP_RCT_Appraisal_Checklist_14oct10.pdf. Accessed on March 2, 2013.

37 http://www.casp-uk.net/wp-content/uploads/2011/11/CASP_Cohort_Appraisal_Checklist_14oct 10.pdf. Accessed on March 8, 2013.

38 http://www.casp-uk.net/wp-content/uploads/2011/11/CASP_Case-Control_Appraisal_Checklist_14oct10.pdf.

39 http://www.casp-uk.net/wp-content/uploads/2011/11/CASP_Systematic_Review_Appraisal_Checklist_14oct10.pdf. Accessed on March 10, 2013.

40 Glasziou P, Haynes B: The paths from research to improved health outcomes. Evid Based Nurs 2005;8: 36–38.

41 Guyatt GH, Oxman AD, Vist GE, Kunz R, Falck-Ytter Y, Alonso-Coello P, Schünemann HJ; GRADE Working Group. GRADE: an emerging consensus on rating quality of evidence and strength of recommendations. BMJ 2008;336:924–926.

Hania Szajewska, MD
Department of Paediatrics
The Medical University of Warsaw
Dzialdowska 1, PL–01-184 Warsaw (Poland)
E-Mail hania@ipgate.pl

Koletzko B, Poindexter B, Uauy R (eds): Nutritional Care of Preterm Infants: Scientific Basis and Practical Guidelines.
World Rev Nutr Diet. Basel, Karger, 2014, vol 110, pp 49–63 (DOI: 10.1159/000358458)

Amino Acids and Proteins

Johannes B. van Goudoever[a, b] • Hester Vlaardingerbroek[a] •
Chris H. van den Akker[d] • Femke de Groof[e] •
Sophie R.D. van der Schoor[c]

[a]Department of Pediatrics, Emma Children's Hospital – AMC, [b]Department of Pediatrics, VU University Medical
Center, [c]Department of Pediatrics, Onze Lieve Vrouwe Gasthuis, Amsterdam, [d]Department of Pediatrics,
Sophia Children's Hospital – Erasmus MC, Rotterdam, and [e]Department of Pediatrics, Medisch Centrum
Alkmaar, Alkmaar, The Netherlands

Reviewed by Alexandre Lapillonne, Paris Descartes University, APHP Necker Hospital, Paris, France;
Ekhard Ziegler, Department of Pediatrics, University of Iowa, Coralville, Iowa, USA

Abstract

Amino acids and protein are key factors for growth. The neonatal period requires the highest intake
in life to meet the demands. Those demands include amino acids for growth, but proteins and
amino acids also function as signalling molecules and function as neurotransmitters. Often the nutritional requirements are not met, resulting in a postnatal growth restriction. However, current
knowledge on adequate levels of both amino acid as well as protein intake can avoid under nutrition in the direct postnatal phase, avoid the need for subsequent catch-up growth and improve
later outcome.   © 2014 S. Karger AG, Basel

For neonatologists, the ultimate goal of feeding preterm infants is to ameliorate the
outcome of these infants to a level that is comparable to healthy term born infants.
That is a postnatal growth rate that comes close to fetal growth rate with comparable
tissue composition and a functional outcome similar to that of healthy term-born infants, as stated by the European Society for Paediatric Gastroenterology, Hepatology,
and Nutrition (ESPGHAN) Committee on Nutrition and the American Academy of
Pediatrics Committee on Nutrition [1–4]. In daily practice, outcome is based on several criteria, such as postnatal growth in comparison to intrauterine growth charts [5]
or to growth charts obtained from preterm infants [6–8], incidence of specific neonatal diseases, duration of hospital stay and neurodevelopmental outcome. Feeding efficacy is however frequently based on solely weight gain rates. Length is not measured
on a regular basis and has a large interindividual accuracy range, while head circumference growth rate is not easily assessed due to the use of several devices to supply

ventilatory support. Other functional outcomes such as cardiovascular or endocrine parameters are hard to assess during the neonatal period, and are usually not registered during follow-up. Neurocognitive outcomes are reliable from to the age of 2 years onwards, leaving most neonatologists with only weight gain to assess feeding efficacy during the neonatal period. The present chapter will describe the role of proteins and amino acids, the ways to assess requirements and practical recommendations what preterm infants need in the parenteral phase and during the enteral phase. Individual infants may require different amounts as their health condition may demand specific substrates. The recommendations provided in this chapter are for the general population preterm infants.

Proteins

Proteins are the driving source for weight gain [9] and anabolism can be achieved at low levels of energy intake [10], whenever amino acids or proteins are provided in adequate amounts. Amino acids are used for parenteral solutions, whereas most infant formulas contain intact proteins, although hydrolyzed formulas are available.

Protein is the major functional and structural component of all the cells of the body. The defining characteristic of protein or amino acid is its requisite amino nitrogen group. This nitrogen group distinguishes an amino acid from for example a sugar. Proteins are macromolecules consisting of long chain of amino acid subunits. In the protein molecule, the amino acids are joined together by peptide bonds. In biological systems, the chains formed might be anything from a few amino acids (di-, tri- or oligopeptide) to thousands of units (polypeptide). The sequence of amino acids in the chain is known as the primary structure. A critical feature of proteins is the complexity of their physical structures. Polypeptide chains do not exist as long chains but they fold in a three-dimensional structure. The chains of amino acids tend to coil into helices (secondary structure). Sections of the helices may fold on each other due to hydrophobic interactions between non-polar side chains and, in some proteins, to disulfide bonds so that the overall molecule might be globular or rod-like (tertiary structure). Their exact shape depends on their function and for some proteins, their interaction with other molecules (quaternary structure) [11].

Amino Acids

The amino acids that are incorporated into mammalian protein are α-amino acids. This means that amino acids have a carboxyl group, an amino nitrogen group, and a side chain attached to a central α-carbon (fig. 1). Proline is the only exception, being unique among the 20 protein-forming amino acids in that the amine nitrogen is bound to not one but two alkyl groups, thereby making it an α-imino acid. Function-

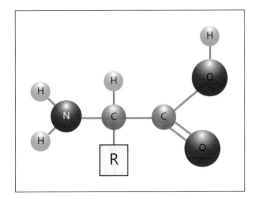

Fig. 1. An amino acid: an amino (NH_2) group, a carboxyl group (COOH) and a side chain attached to a central α-carbon (R).

al differences among the amino acids lie in the structure of their side chains. Functional differences among the amino acids lie in the structure of their side chains. Classification of amino acids was initially based on the classic studies of Rose and co-workers [12, 13]. These studies were based on the qualitative significance of each amino acid in human nutrition. Rose defined amino acids as essential or non-essential based on their capacity to maintain nitrogen balance in young men. Holt and Snyderman [14], Snyderman et al. [15–17], and Fomon [18] extended Rose's studies to the pediatric population. In their studies (of which only a few are referenced here), they demonstrated that only the 'essential' amino acids were needed to maintain growth in young infants and therefore conformed according to the original definition of 'essentiality of amino acids'. Through the following decades it became evident that Rose's classification was limited and that a distinction between essential and non-essential amino acids was complex and could not be defined based solely on the nutritional criteria of maintenance of nitrogen balance or growth [19]. For example, histidine, an non-essential amino acid in the rat that was considered non-essential in humans in the original Rose classification, has been proven to be essential in health and disease, and was included as an essential amino acid by the Food Agricultural Organization/World Health Organization/United Nations University (FAO/WHO/UNU) expert report in 1985 and subsequent reports [20].

Over the past decades the concept of essentiality based on maintenance of growth or of nitrogen equilibrium has been revisited and with contributions by many [21–25] the concept of amino acid essentially has changed. Mitchell [26] considered a more dynamic concept of 'essentiality' based on the ratio of supply to demand, rather than on the maintenance of nitrogen balance or growth. The term 'conditionally indispensable' has been used to refer to those non-essential or dispensable amino acids that become essential or indispensable under pathophysiologic conditions. Because the carbon skeleton of the amino acid is the moiety that determines its nutritional indispensability, some classification of amino acids has been based on the ability to synthesize and/or aminate the carbon skeleton [23]. In metabolic terms, the amino acids that are generally considered to be nutritionally essential contain specific chemical structures, the synthesis of which cannot be catalyzed by mammalian enzymes, such as the branch aliphatic side chain of leucine, isoleucine, or valine; the primary amine of lysine; the secondary alcohol of threonine; the secondary thiol of methionine; the indole ring of tryptophan; the aromatic ring of phenylalanine, or the imidazole ring of histidine. It is important, however, to remember that an amino acid classification should not be based solely on nutritional (growth and maintenance), metabolic (de novo synthesis, tissue utilization, and catabolism), or chemical aspects of the amino acids, but also, and perhaps most importantly, on the maintenance of amino acid function. Some amino acids that would be considered truly dispensable in nutritional, metabolic, and chemical terms are utilized as precursors of other amino acids that maintain important physiologic functions, such as glutamate and serine, which serve, respectively, as precursors of glutamine and cystathionine. Other dispensable amino acids like alanine and aspartate contribute to physiologic and pathophysiologic events [27, 28].

With new knowledge emerging on non-nutritional function as well as the physiological and pharmacological properties of amino acids, the concept of amino acid requirement has changed from the traditional nutritional criteria based on growth or weight maintenance, to a broader functional outcome. Therefore, 'adequacy' of nutritional support is ill defined and conditional to the end goals to be achieved. Based on this new knowledge about non-nutritional functions of amino acids [21, 23], a key question regarding nutritional adequacy is 'What is the objective to be achieved?' Is the objective to promote growth and weight maintenance? To maintain non-nutritional functions? To prevent pathophysiologic events? To act as pharmacological agent(s)? To induce gene expression? Or for nutritional rescue? These important questions are just beginning to be explored and will be better answered in the future.

Protein Metabolism and Distribution

Most proteins in the body are constantly being synthesized from amino acids and degraded back to them. The turnover rate of proteins in neonates is three times higher than in adults, resulting in a higher energy demand for infants per kilogram body weight than for adults.

The 'pool' of amino acids is in dynamic equilibrium with tissue protein as depicted in figure 2. Amino acids are continually taken from the pool for protein synthesis and replaced by the hydrolysis of dietary and tissue protein. The distribution of protein among the different organs varies with developmental age. Infants have, proportionally, a larger amount of visceral (liver, kidney, brain, heart, and lung) protein than in the skeletal muscle, while in adults protein constitutes about 15% of their weight. Not all proteins in the body have a similar turnover rate. Figure 3 shows the protein synthesis rate of different tissues in neonatal pigs and rodents, expressed as % of the protein pool of a specific organ that is synthesized per day. Despite the high fractional turnover rate of gut proteins, most protein synthesis and degradation occurs in the

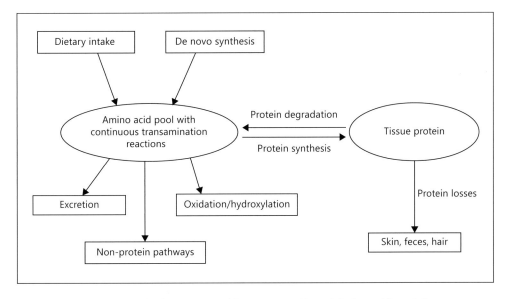

Fig. 2. Exchange between body protein and free amino acid pools [adapted from 11].

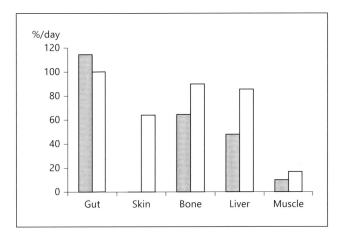

Fig. 3. Fractional protein synthesis rates of different organs expressed as % per day in pigs (hatched bars) and rats (open bars) [85–88].

muscle because of the large pool size. Nevertheless, the relative high turnover rate of the gut indicates that the intestines are metabolically a very active organ. This is illustrated by the fact that first-pass uptake or splanchnic utilization is high.

Digestion and Absorption of Proteins

Proteins are digested and absorbed along the upper part of the intestinal tract, with for human milk proteins an almost complete removal from the lumen. Proteins are broken down in the stomach to smaller polypeptide chains via hydrochloric acid and

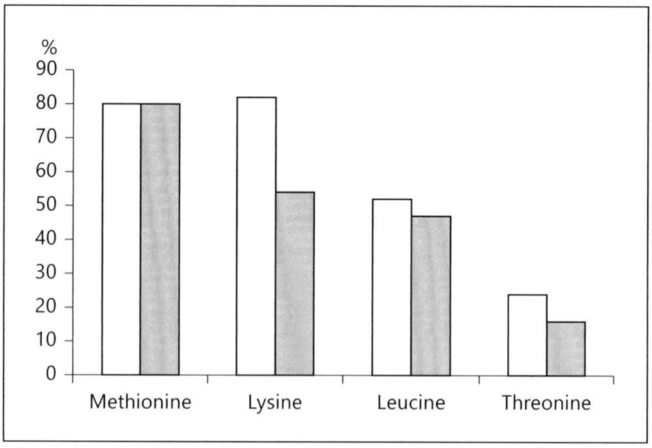

Fig. 4. Systemic availability (expressed as percentage of intake) of enterally ingested amino acids in newborn pigs (following utilization in portal drained viscera, open bars) and preterm infants (following first-pass utilization, filled bars) [32, 67, 89, 90].

proteases in the duodenum and jejunum. Peptides and free amino acids can be absorbed by the enterocyte. However the systemic availability of amino acids is not 100% because a significant portion of the amino acids is utilized within the intestine. These amino acids are used as substrate for (glycol-)protein synthesis and as energy source during high protein intakes [29–33]. The rate of first-pass utilization is different for each individual amino acid as is shown in figure 4. Some of the individual amino acids are utilized to a great extent, such as threonine. Threonine is an important amino acid in the peptide backbone of secretory mucin 2 (MUC2). MUC2 is secreted by goblet cells of the intestine and gives intestinal mucus a high density and viscoelasticity.

Approaches to Determine Amino Acid Requirements for Preterm Infants

Fetal Approach

Different approaches can be used in determining the adequate amino acid requirements for preterm infants. First, the intake of the fetus of a similar gestational age can be regarded as suitable. Information about fetal protein requirements and metabolism is limited and most information comes from animal studies, in particular fetal sheep. Under physiological conditions in pregnant ewes, the fetal amino acid uptake exceeds the amount required for protein synthesis. The excess amount of amino acids is oxidized and contributes considerably to fetal energy generation [34, 35]. These quantitative balance studies required blood sampling from both the venous and arterial umbilical vessels and measuring flow rates. In humans, this can only be performed safely around birth. Around elective cesarean section human studies on fetal leucine, valine, phenylalanine, and tyrosine kinetics were performed [36–38]. Results demonstrate that the amino acid uptake exceeded the amount that would be necessary for net protein accretion, which indicates that also the human fetus oxidizes amino acids to gen-

van Goudoever · Vlaardingerbroek · van den Akker · de Groof · van der Schoor erate energy [36]. However, this method has been applied in a limited number of fetuses while many methodological assumptions are made, which reduces the reliability of the obtained results.

Factorial Approach
A second method to determine the requirements is the factorial approach. The factorial approach combines the estimated growth rate of a fetus of a certain gestational age with the composition of newly formed tissue. Some drawbacks of the use of fetal metabolism as a reference standard for preterm infants can be pointed out. The extrauterine environment has different physical and physiological properties than the intrauterine environment. In addition, nutrients not used for tissue deposition, but used for energy generation or other functions, are not taken into account. Also, at birth, most preterm infants are ill, requiring ventilatory support, antibiotic therapy and sometimes cardiac support. In these conditions, energy and protein needs and metabolism might differ from those in the physiological intrauterine situation. Despite these limitations, the factorial approach is commonly used to determine requirements.

Human Milk Approach
A third approach is to base the requirements on the composition of human milk. However, the composition of human milk varies at different gestational ages, stages of lactation and between lactating mothers [39]. Very low birth weight (VLBW) infants fed their own mother's milk may become growth restricted if milk is not supplemented with so-called fortifiers, indicating that human milk composition is not adequately adapted to the nutritional need of the preterm infant below 32 weeks of gestation [40].

Clinical Study Approach
As all described methods (placental/fetal measurements, the factorial approach and (preterm) human milk analysis) have their drawbacks for the determination of the nutritional requirements of preterm infants, a trial and error approach has been used as well. Different amino acid and protein intakes in clinical studies have been assessed to indicate the adequacy of the intake. Those assessments include anthropometry (weight and length gain), nitrogen balance, metabolic indices (e.g. amino acid concentration, albumin, pre-albumin, total protein concentrations, plasma urea concentration), whole-body nitrogen kinetics, specific amino acid kinetics and the indicator amino acid method [41]. For determination of the requirement of individual amino acids in neonates, the indicator amino acid method is an accurate method [42]. Recently, some individual essential amino acid requirements for neonates born at term became available [43, 44]. For estimations of the total amino acid or protein requirement, the most widely used method is the nitrogen balance method. As summarized in the ESPGHAN guidelines, a minimum amino acid intake of

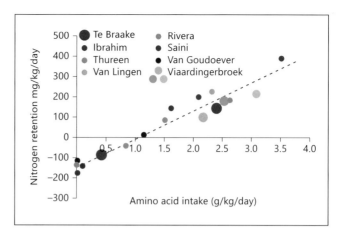

Fig. 5. Relationship of parenteral amino acid intakes and nitrogen retention during the first few days of life of preterm infants. Size of bullet resembles the number of infants included in the clinical trial.

1.5 g/(kg·day) is necessary to prevent a negative nitrogen balance in parenterally fed preterm neonates [41]. Higher intakes are needed to achieve physiological protein accretion and thus growth.

Timing and Amount of Parenteral Amino Acid Administration

In early studies on parenteral amino acid administration to preterm infants, amino acid administration was initiated several days after birth [45, 46]. During the last decades, multiple studies have demonstrated that earlier parenteral amino acid administration at amounts of 1.0–3.5 g/(kg·day) can reverse a negative nitrogen or stable isotope balance, which is indicative of protein accretion and thus growth, even at low caloric intake (fig. 5) [10, 46–56]. This policy also increased plasma amino acid concentrations to reference values [47, 50] and has been associated with improved neurodevelopmental outcomes compared to infants who received no amino acids during the first postnatal days [57]. Our own 2-year follow-up of the comparison of 2.4 g/(kg·day) versus no amino acids during the first few days of life in 111 very low birth infants revealed no differences in anthropometry and showed that boys, but not girls, survived without major disabilities at a higher rate (fig. 6). None of the studies with early amino acid administration up to 2.3 g/(kg·day) reported metabolic acidosis or hyperaminoacidemia. In addition, plasma concentrations of all essential amino acids and of most non-essential amino acids increased and were more in concordance with reference ranges from healthy fetuses or breast-fed term infants [10, 55].

Early higher-dose amino acid administration has beneficial effects on the synthesis of specific proteins as well. For example, upregulation of albumin synthesis with infusion of 2.4 g amino acids/(kg·day) from birth onwards has been demonstrated [58]. However, they were still lower than those measured in utero in fetuses between 28 and 35 weeks of gestation [59]. Besides raising albumin synthesis rates, early higher-dose

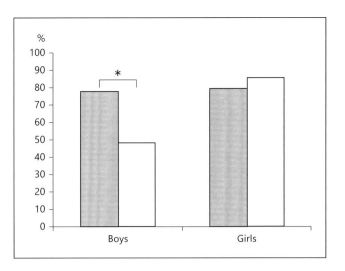

Fig. 6. Effect of early amino acid administration on the percentage of former preterm infants who are alive without major disabilities at a corrected age of 2 years. Hatched bars represent the intervention group, receiving 2.4 g amino acids/(kg·day) for the first 2 days of life, whereas the controls received dextrose only. * Significance with crude and adjusted ORs (adjusted for antenatal steroids, birth weight, gestational age, and 5-min Apgar scores) of 3.8 and 6.2, respectively.

amino acid administration also raised the concentration and absolute synthesis rates of glutathione, the major intracellular antioxidant [60]. Potential negative side effects observed with early high-dose amino acid infusion – such as increased mean peak serum indirect bilirubin, lower base excess, lower concentrations of bicarbonate, and increased plasma urea nitrogen – were without clinical implications [10, 54]. Overall, the studies with early high-dose amino acid administration show good efficacy during short-term follow-up without major side effects. However, it is important to stress that no studies are published that show beneficial effects during long term follow-up.

Practical Implications with Regard to Parenteral Amino Acid Administration

Starting doses of 1.5–3 g/(kg·day) are recommended, with increments to a maximum dose of 4 g/(kg·day) in the next few days [41, 61, 62]. Most neonatal intensive care units (NICUs) start amino acid infusion in preterm infants between 0 and 36 h postnatally. Starting doses vary widely: from as low as 0.5–1.0 g/(kg·day) up to 3.5 g/(kg·day). Some NICUs apply a stepwise procedure to reach the target dose of amino acids [63–66]. However, the preference for a stepwise procedure is solely empirical, non-evidence-based but based on fluid limitations, worries about intolerance, and fear of hyperglycemia in case of mixed glucose/amino acid solutions.

Enteral Protein Requirements of Preterm Neonates

Before reaching the systematic circulation and becoming available for growth, proteins in the gut have to be digested, absorbed and pass the gut and liver. Although rates of digestion and absorption of milk proteins are considered to be high, the utilization rate in first pass is high as well. Stable isotope tracer studies have indicated that first-pass amino acid utilization rates vary between 15 and 85%, depending on the amino acid [32, 67–70]. In addition, the utilization rate is not a percentage of the intake, at lower enteral intakes the utilization rate is relatively higher. The implications of these studies are huge. While increasing the enteral intake, parenteral supplementation is usually lowered in daily practice. However, a substantial part of the enteral protein intake does not reach the systemic circulation and is not immediately available for the growth of other tissues. Therefore, infants with a reduced tolerance to enteral feeding (most frequently extremely low birth weight (ELBW) infants), who remain for a long term on partial enteral nutrition, are at high risk for developing protein malnutrition. A practical solution is to supply infants a relatively high dose of parenteral amino acids, while increasing the enteral intake. Our current feeding protocol does not allow tapering down parenteral amino acids before reaching at least 75 ml/(kg·day) of enteral nutrition.

Present protein requirements are 3.5–4.5 g/(kg·day) when on full enteral feeding for the ELBW infant, gradually declining to 2–2.5 g/(kg·day) at term age [1, 71]. No differentiation is made between infant requirements when fed own mother's milk, pasteurized milk or infant formula, since no systematic evaluation has occurred yet.

Proteins in Infant Formulas and Human Milk

The amino acid content of cow milk proteins is different than that of human milk. Both milks are composed of two classes of proteins, casein or acid-precipitable proteins and whey or acid-soluble proteins. The whey:casein ratio in colostrum is 80:20 and changes to 55:45 in mature milk [72]. Casein-dominant cow milk-based infant formulas are made with non-fat dry milk and contain about 82% bovine casein and 18% bovine whey proteins. During the manufacturing process of infant formulas, whey is added to cow milk to obtain a whey:casein ratio of 60:40 which is more similar to human milk. However, human milk proteins differ from bovine proteins in concentrations of the proteins present and in amino acid composition of these proteins. So adding bovine whey proteins does not make the formula identical to the amino acid composition of human milk. In casein-dominant formula, especially methionine and tyrosine are elevated. In whey-dominant formula, methionine, threonine and lysine are elevated. The sum of the branched-chain amino acids is much higher in formulas than human milk: infants fed formula have higher concentrations of branched-chain amino acids than human milk-fed infants, suggesting that levels of these amino acids are more closely related to protein quantity than protein quality [73, 74].

In studies of protein quality, the assessment of the protein and amino acid compositions of various formula preparations is usually conducted by comparing them to human milk. This assessment must consider that cow milk formula contains more protein per volume than human milk and that there are differences in the composition of both whey and casein from the two species [75]. Whey-dominant infant for-

van Goudoever · Vlaardingerbroek · van den Akker · de Groof · van der Schoor mula produces concentrations of plasma free amino acids that are more like those in infants fed pooled human milk than does casein-predominant formula [76]. According to some, the standard for protein quality should be such that reflects the plasma amino acid pattern of optimally growing low birth weight infants fed only human milk proteins [75, 77]. One could argue whether other standards like amino acid composition of human milk or plasma amino acid levels of healthy breast-fed term neonates should be the standard, or that functional outcome measurements like neurodevelopmental outcome and development of metabolic syndrome should be taken into account, or even made the superior standard.

The nutritional implications of the differences in amino acid content of different proteins or mixtures of proteins can be evaluated by comparing the amino acid composition of the protein source with a suitable reference amino acid pattern by use of an amino acid scoring pattern. These scoring systems use the amino acid requirement in humans to develop reference amino acid patterns for purposes of evaluating the quality of food proteins or their capacity to efficiently meet both the nitrogen and indispensable amino acid requirement of the individual [11]. The scoring systems use the limiting essential amino acid in the test protein, divide it by the amount of amino acid in a reference protein and correct it for true digestibility. The indispensable amino acid composition of the specific protein source is compared to that of that of a reference amino acid composition profile. Earlier the amino acid composition of protein from eggs was used, which is regarded as being well balanced in amino acid content in relation to human needs [78]. Later the amino acid content of human milk was used as reference pattern [79, 80] since adequate growth and development are known to occur in infants provided human milk and plasma amino acid profiles of infants have been shown to reflect the amino acid composition of human milk. The Life Sciences Research Office report concluded that the amino acid scoring pattern of human milk is an accurate and an appropriate standard for assessing the protein quality of infant formulas [81]. The difficulty in composing infant nutrition is that even if the amino acid composition of infant formula could be made very similar to that of human milk, digestibility and absorption of amino acids and peptides could be quite different from that of breast milk, thus resulting in different plasma amino acid profiles. However, most recommendations just refer to absolute protein intakes, while quality of the proteins used is not taken into consideration.

Human milk contains (glycol-)proteins that are not only important from a nutritional point of view, but have been shown to be bioactive. These bioactivities include enzyme activities, enhancement of nutrient absorption, growth stimulation, modulation of the immune system and defense against pathogens. Among the bioactive (glycol-)proteins are lactoferrin, lysozyme, secretory immunoglobulin A, haptocorrin, lactoperoxidase, α-lactalbumin, bile salt stimulated lipase, β- and κ-casein, and tumor growth factor β. Clinical beneficial effects of providing human milk-based nutrition include reduction in sepsis and necrotizing enterocolitis [82–84]. When provided by the own mother, most infants receive fresh or unpasteurized previously frozen milk. Human donor milk is usually pasteurized, altering the bioactivity of most of these proteins, but that does not prevent being the second best choice following own mother's milk. To meet protein requirements, protein fortification of human milk is advised. Preterm formula is a good alternative.

Practical Considerations with Regard to Enteral Protein Supplementation

The transition from parenteral to enteral nutrition in preterm infants is a period where protein malnutrition can develop easily. Therefore, the initiation of tapering off parenteral amino acid intake should not start before at least 75 ml/(kg·day) of enteral nutrition is reached. When no growth faltering has occurred in the period before, aiming for 3.5–4.0 g protein/(kg·day) is advised for ELBW and VLBW infants. When catch-up growth is needed, intakes up to 4.5 g protein/(kg·day) are advised.

Conclusion

Amino acids and proteins are the major driving force for growth and therefore long-term outcome. Short-term studies show benefits of immediate commencement of amino acid supplementation to preterm infants following birth.

Initial safe intake is at least 2.0–2.5 g/(kg·day), with a gradual increase to level of 3.5 g/(kg·day). Infants at full enteral nutrition need 3.5–4.5 g protein/(kg·day), either with supplemented human (donor) milk or, second best, formula. With these recommendations, the risk of developing growth retardation at the NICU becomes rare, and the discussion on the need of additional supplementation to establish catch-up growth becomes futile.

Disclosure Statement

The authors have no conflicts of interest to disclose.

References

1 Agostoni C, Buonocore G, Carnielli VP, et al: Enteral nutrient supply for preterm infants: commentary from the European Society of Paediatric Gastroenterology, Hepatology and Nutrition Committee on Nutrition. J Pediatr Gastroenterol Nutr 2010;50: 85–91.
2 American Academy of Pediatrics Committee on Nutrition: Nutritional needs of low-birth-weight infants. Pediatrics 1985;75:976–986.
3 Hay WW Jr, Lucas A, Heird WC, et al: Workshop summary: nutrition of the extremely low birth weight infant. Pediatrics 1999;104:1360–1368.
4 Koletzko B, Goulet O, Hunt J, Krohn K, Shamir R: 1. Guidelines on Paediatric Parenteral Nutrition of the European Society of Paediatric Gastroenterology, Hepatology and Nutrition (ESPGHAN) and the European Society for Clinical Nutrition and Metabolism (ESPEN), Supported by the European Society of Paediatric Research (ESPR). J Pediatr Gastroenterol Nutr 2005;41(suppl 2):S1–S87.

5 Fenton TR: A new growth chart for preterm babies: Babson and Benda's chart updated with recent data and a new format. BMC Pediatr 2003;3:13.

6 Christensen RD, Henry E, Kiehn TI, Street JL: Pattern of daily weights among low birth weight neonates in the neonatal intensive care unit: data from a multihospital health-care system. J Perinatol 2006; 26:37–43.

7 Ehrenkranz RA, Younes N, Lemons JA, et al: Longitudinal growth of hospitalized very low birth weight infants. Pediatrics 1999;104:280–289.

8 Pauls J, Bauer K, Versmold H: Postnatal body weight curves for infants below 1,000 g birth weight receiving early enteral and parenteral nutrition. Eur J Pediatr 1998;157:416–421.

9 Kashyap S, Schulze KF, Ramakrishnan R, Dell RB, Heird WC: Evaluation of a mathematical model for predicting the relationship between protein and energy intakes of low-birth-weight infants and the rate and composition of weight gain. Pediatr Res 1994;35: 704–712.

10 Te Braake FW, van den Akker CH, Wattimena DJ, Huijmans JG, van Goudoever JB: Amino acid administration to premature infants directly after birth. J Pediatr 2005;147:457–461.

11 Institute of Medicine Food and Nutrition Board. Dietary Reference Intakes for Macronutrients. Washington, National Academy Press, 2005.

12 Rose WC: Amino acid requirements of man. Fed Proc 1949;8:546–552.

13 Rose WC: The amino acid requirements of adult man. Nutr Abstr Rev 1957;27:631–647.

14 Holt LE Jr, Snyderman SE: Protein and amino acid requirements of infants and children. Nutr Abstr Rev 1965;35:1–13.

15 Snyderman SE, Pratt EL, Cheung MW, et al: The phenylalanine requirement of the normal infant. J Nutr 1955;56:253–263.

16 Snyderman SE, Holt LE Jr, Smellie F, Boyer A, Westall RG: The essential amino acid requirements of infants: valine. AMA J Dis Child 1959;97:186–191.

17 Snyderman SE, Boyer A, Roitman E, Holt LE Jr, Prose PH: The histidine requirement of the infant. Pediatrics 1963;31:786–801.

18 Fomon SJ: Requirements and recommended dietary intakes of protein during infancy. Pediatr Res 1991; 30:391–395.

19 FAO/WHO: Energy and protein requirements: Report of a joint FAO/WHO ad hoc expert committee. Geneva, WHO, 1971.

20 WHO/FAO/UNU: Protein and Amino Acid Requirements in Human Nutrition. Publ Health Nutr 2005;8:7(A).

21 Reeds PJ: Dispensable and indispensable amino acids for humans. J Nutr 2000;130:1835S–1840S.

22 Chipponi JX, Bleier JC, Santi MT, Rudman D: Deficiencies of essential and conditionally essential nutrients. Am J Clin Nutr 1982;35(5 suppl):1112–1116.

23 Reeds PJ, Biolo G: Non-protein roles of amino acids: an emerging aspect of nutrient requirements. Curr Opin Clin Nutr Metab Care 2002;5:43–45.

24 Jackson AA: Amino acids: essential and non-essential? Lancet 1983;1:1034–1037.

25 Laidlaw SA, Kopple JD: Newer concepts of the indispensable amino acids. Am J Clin Nutr 1987;46:593–605.

26 Mitchell H: Comparative Nutrition of Man and Domestic Animals. New York, Academic Press, 1962, pp 166–172.

27 Skolnick P: Modulation of glutamate receptors: strategies for the development of novel antidepressants. Amino Acids 2002;23:153–159.

28 Tsai G, Coyle JT: N-acetylaspartate in neuropsychiatric disorders. Prog Neurobiol 1995;46:531–540.

29 Van Goudoever JB, Stoll B, Henry JF, Burrin DG, Reeds PJ: Adaptive regulation of intestinal lysine metabolism. Proc Natl Acad Sci USA 2000;97:11620–11625.

30 Van der Schoor SR, van Goudoever JB, Stoll B, et al: The pattern of intestinal substrate oxidation is altered by protein restriction in pigs. Gastroenterology 2001;121:1167–1175.

31 Van der Schoor SR, Reeds PJ, Stoll B, et al: The high metabolic cost of a functional gut. Gastroenterology 2002;123:1931–1940.

32 Van der Schoor SR, Reeds PJ, Stellaard F, et al: Lysine kinetics in preterm infants: the importance of enteral feeding. Gut 2004;53:38–43.

33 Schaart MW, Schierbeek H, van der Schoor SR, et al: Threonine utilization is high in the intestine of piglets. J Nutr 2005;135:765–770.

34 Lemons JA, Adcock EW 3rd, Jones MD Jr, Naughton MA, Meschia G, Battaglia FC: Umbilical uptake of amino acids in the unstressed fetal lamb. J Clin Invest 1976;58:1428–1434.

35 Van Veen LC, Teng C, Hay WW Jr, Meschia G, Battaglia FC: Leucine disposal and oxidation rates in the fetal lamb. Metabolism 1987;36:48–53.

36 Van den Akker CH, Schierbeek H, Minderman G, et al: Amino acid metabolism in the human fetus at term: leucine, valine, and methionine kinetics. Pediatr Res 2011;70:566–571.

37 Van den Akker CH, Schierbeek H, Dorst KY, et al: Human fetal amino acid metabolism at term gestation. Am J Clin Nutr 2009;89:153–160.

38 Chien PF, Smith K, Watt PW, Scrimgeour CM, Taylor DJ, Rennie MJ: Protein turnover in the human fetus studied at term using stable isotope tracer amino acids. Am J Physiol 1993;265:E31–E35.

Amino Acids and Proteins

39 Molto-Puigmarti C, Castellote AI, Carbonell-Estrany X, Lopez-Sabater MC: Differences in fat content and fatty acid proportions among colostrum, transitional, and mature milk from women delivering very preterm, preterm, and term infants. Clin Nutr 2011; 30:116–123.

40 Kuschel CA, Harding JE: Multicomponent fortified human milk for promoting growth in preterm infants. Cochrane Database Syst Rev 2004;1:CD000343.

41 Koletzko B, Goulet O, Hunt J, Krohn K, Shamir R: 3. Amino acids. Guidelines on Paediatric Parenteral Nutrition of the European Society of Paediatric Gastroenterology, Hepatology and Nutrition (ESPGHAN) and the European Society for Clinical Nutrition and Metabolism (ESPEN), Supported by the European Society of Paediatric Research (ESPR). J Pediatr Gastroenterol Nutr 2005;41(suppl 2):S12–S18.

42 De Groof F, Huang L, Twisk JW, et al: New insights into the methodological issues of the indicator amino acid oxidation method in preterm neonates. Pediatr Res 2013;73:679–684.

43 Huang L, Hogewind-Schoonenboom JE, van Dongen MJ, et al: Methionine requirement of the enterally fed term infant in the first month of life in the presence of cysteine. Am J Clin Nutr 2012;95:1048–1054.

44 Huang L, Hogewind-Schoonenboom JE, de Groof F, et al: Lysine requirement of the enterally fed term infant in the first month of life. Am J Clin Nutr 2011; 94:1496–1503.

45 Yu VY, James B, Hendry P, MacMahon RA: Total parenteral nutrition in very low birth weight infants: a controlled trial. Arch Dis Child 1979;54:653–661.

46 Van Lingen RA, van Goudoever JB, Luijendijk IH, Wattimena JL, Sauer PJ: Effects of early amino acid administration during total parenteral nutrition on protein metabolism in pre-term infants. Clin Sci (Lond) 1992;82:199–203.

47 Anderson TL, Muttart CR, Bieber MA, Nicholson JF, Heird WC: A controlled trial of glucose versus glucose and amino acids in premature infants. J Pediatr 1979;94:947–951.

48 Rivera A Jr, Bell EF, Bier DM: Effect of intravenous amino acids on protein metabolism of preterm infants during the first three days of life. Pediatr Res 1993;33:106–111.

49 Saini J, MacMahon P, Morgan JB, Kovar IZ: Early parenteral feeding of amino acids. Arch Dis Child 1989;64:1362–1366.

50 Van Goudoever JB, Colen T, Wattimena JL, Huijmans JG, Carnielli VP, Sauer PJ: Immediate commencement of amino acid supplementation in preterm infants: effect on serum amino acid concentrations and protein kinetics on the first day of life. J Pediatr 1995;127:458–465.

51 Thureen PJ, Anderson AH, Baron KA, Melara DL, Hay WW Jr, Fennessey PV: Protein balance in the first week of life in ventilated neonates receiving parenteral nutrition. Am J Clin Nutr 1998;68:1128–1135.

52 Blanco CL, Falck A, Green BK, Cornell JE, Gong AK: Metabolic responses to early and high protein supplementation in a randomized trial evaluating the prevention of hyperkalemia in extremely low birth weight infants. J Pediatr 2008;153:535–540.

53 Clark RH, Chace DH, Spitzer AR: Effects of two different doses of amino acid supplementation on growth and blood amino acid levels in premature neonates admitted to the neonatal intensive care unit: a randomized, controlled trial. Pediatrics 2007;120:1286–1296.

54 Ibrahim HM, Jeroudi MA, Baier RJ, Dhanireddy R, Krouskop RW: Aggressive early total parental nutrition in low-birth-weight infants. J Perinatol 2004;24: 482–486.

55 Thureen PJ, Melara D, Fennessey PV, Hay WW Jr: Effect of low versus high intravenous amino acid intake on very low birth weight infants in the early neonatal period. Pediatr Res 2003;53:24–32.

56 Vlaardingerbroek H, Vermeulen MJ, Rook D, et al: Safety and efficacy of early parenteral lipid and high-dose amino acid administration to very low birth weight infants. J Pediatr 2013;163:638–644.e1–e5.

57 Stephens BE, Walden RV, Gargus RA, et al: First-week protein and energy intakes are associated with 18-month developmental outcomes in extremely low birth weight infants. Pediatrics 2009;123:1337–1343.

58 Van den Akker CH, Te Braake FW, Schierbeek H, et al: Albumin synthesis in premature neonates is stimulated by parenterally administered amino acids during the first days of life. Am J Clin Nutr 2007;86: 1003–1008.

59 Van den Akker CH, Schierbeek H, Rietveld T, et al: Human fetal albumin synthesis rates during different periods of gestation. Am J Clin Nutr 2008;88: 997–1003.

60 Te Braake FW, Schierbeek H, de Groof K, et al: Glutathione synthesis rates after amino acid administration directly after birth in preterm infants. Am J Clin Nutr 2008;88:333–339.

61 Ehrenkranz RA: Early, aggressive nutritional management for very low birth weight infants: what is the evidence? Semin Perinatol 2007;31:48–55.

62 Simmer K: Aggressive nutrition for preterm infants – benefits and risks. Early Hum Dev 2007;83: 631–634.

63 Lapillonne A, Kermorvant-Duchemin E: A systematic review of practice surveys on parenteral nutrition for preterm infants. J Nutr 2013;143:2061S–2065S.

64 Collins CT, Chua MC, Rajadurai VS, et al: Higher protein and energy intake is associated with increased weight gain in pre-term infants. J Paediatr Child Health 2010;46:96–102.

65 Lapillonne A, Fellous L, Mokthari M, Kermorvant-Duchemin E: Parenteral nutrition objectives for very low birth weight infants: results of a national survey. J Pediatr Gastroenterol Nut 2009;48:618–626.

66 Lapillonne A, Carnielli VP, Embleton ND, Mihatsch W: Quality of newborn care: adherence to guidelines for parenteral nutrition in preterm infants in four European countries. BMJ Open 2013;3:e003478.

67 Van der Schoor SR, Wattimena DL, Huijmans J, Vermes A, van Goudoever JB: The gut takes nearly all: threonine kinetics in infants. Am J Clin Nutr 2007;86:1132–1138.

68 Van der Schoor SR, Schierbeek H, Bet PM, et al: Majority of dietary glutamine is utilized in first pass in preterm infants. Pediatr Res 2010;67:194–199.

69 Corpeleijn WE, Riedijk MA, Zhou Y, et al: Almost all enteral aspartate is taken up in first-pass metabolism in enterally fed preterm infants. Clin Nutr 2010;29: 341–346.

70 Riedijk MA, de Gast-Bakker DA, Wattimena JL, van Goudoever JB: Splanchnic oxidation is the major metabolic fate of dietary glutamate in enterally fed preterm infants. Pediatr Res 2007;62:468–473.

71 Lapillonne A, O'Connor DL, Wang D, Rigo J: Nutritional recommendations for the late-preterm infant and the preterm infant after hospital discharge. J Pediatr 2013;162(suppl):S90–S100.

72 Raiha NC: Milk protein quantity and quality in term infants: intakes and metabolic effects during the first six months. Acta Paediatr Scand Suppl 1989;351:24–28.

73 Raiha NC: Milk protein quantity and quality and protein requirements during development. Adv Pediatr 1989;36:347–368.

74 Socha P, Grote V, Gruszfeld D, et al: Milk protein intake, the metabolic-endocrine response, and growth in infancy: data from a randomized clinical trial. Am J Clin Nutr 2011;94:1776S–1784S.

75 Klein CJ: Nutrient requirements for preterm infant formulas. J Nutr 2002;132(suppl 1):1395S–1577S.

76 Rassin DK, Gaull GE, Heinonen K, Raih NC: Milk protein quantity and quality in low-birth-weight infants. II. Effects on selected aliphatic amino acids in plasma and urine. Pediatrics 1977;59:407–422.

77 Polberger SK, Axelsson IE, Raiha NC: Urinary and serum urea as indicators of protein metabolism in very low birth weight infants fed varying human milk protein intakes. Acta Paediatr Scand 1990;79:737–742.

78 FAO/WHO: Energy and Protein Requirements. Report of a Joint FAO/WHO Ad Hoc Expert Committee. Geneva, WHO, 1973.

79 Consultation JFWUE: Energy and Protein Requirements, 1985.

80 FAO/WHO: Protein Quality Evaluation in Human Diets. Report of a Joint FAO/WHO Expert Consultation, 1991.

81 Raiten DJ Talbot JM, Waters JH: Life Sciences Research Office Report: Executive Summary for the Report: Assessment of nutrient requirements for infant formulas. J Nutr 1998;128:2059S–2294S.

82 Corpeleijn WE, Kouwenhoven SM, Paap MC, et al: Intake of own mother's milk during the first days of life is associated with decreased morbidity and mortality in very low birth weight infants during the first 60 days of life. Neonatology 2012;102:276–281.

83 Sullivan S, Schanler RJ, Kim JH, et al: An exclusively human milk-based diet is associated with a lower rate of necrotizing enterocolitis than a diet of human milk and bovine milk-based products. J Pediatr 2010; 156:562–567.e1.

84 Cristofalo EA, Schanler RJ, Blanco CL, et al: Randomized trial of exclusive human milk versus preterm formula diets in extremely premature infants. J Pediatr 2013;163:1592–1595.e1.

85 Garlick PJ, Fern M, Preedy VR: The effect of insulin infusion and food intake on muscle protein synthesis in postabsorptive rats. Biochem J 1983;210:669–676.

86 Seve B, Reeds PJ, Fuller MF, Cadenhead A, Hay SM: Protein synthesis and retention in some tissues of the young pig as influenced by dietary protein intake after early-weaning. Possible connection to the energy metabolism. Reprod Nutr Dev 1986;26:849–861.

87 Burrin DG, Davis TA, Fiorotto ML, Reeds PJ: Stage of development and fasting affect protein synthetic activity in the gastrointestinal tissues of suckling rats. J Nutr 1991;121:1099–1108.

88 McNurlan MA, Garlick PJ: Rates of protein synthesis in rat liver and small intestine in protein deprivation and diabetes. Proc Nutr Soc 1979;38:133A.

89 Van Goudoever JB, van der Schoor SR, Stoll B, et al: Intestinal amino acid metabolism in neonates. Nestle Nutrition Workshop Series Paediatric Programme 2006;58:95–102; discussion 102–108.

90 Riedijk MA, Stoll B, Chacko S, et al: Methionine transmethylation and transsulfuration in the piglet gastrointestinal tract. Proc Natl Acad Sci USA 2007; 104:3408–3413.

J.B. van Goudoever
Emma Children's Hospital – AMC, c/o Room H7-276
PO Box 22660
NL–1100 DD Amsterdam (The Netherlands)
E-Mail h.vangoudoever@amc.uva.nl

Koletzko B, Poindexter B, Uauy R (eds): Nutritional Care of Preterm Infants: Scientific Basis and Practical Guidelines.
World Rev Nutr Diet. Basel, Karger, 2014, vol 110, pp 64–81 (DOI: 10.1159/000358459)

Energy Requirements, Protein-Energy Metabolism and Balance, and Carbohydrates in Preterm Infants

William W. Hay, Jr.[a] · Laura D. Brown[a] · Scott C. Denne[b]

[a]Department of Pediatrics, Section of Neonatology, Perinatal Research Center, University of Colorado School of Medicine, Aurora, Colo. and [b]Department of Pediatrics, University of Indiana School of Medicine, Indianapolis, Ind., USA

Reviewed by Josef Neu, Department of Pediatrics, University of Florida, Gainsville, Fla., USA; Nicholas B. Embleton, Neonatal Service, Newcastle Hospitals, Institute of Health and Society, Newcastle University, Newcastle upon Tyne, UK

Abstract

Energy is necessary for all vital functions of the body at molecular, cellular, organ, and systemic levels. Preterm infants have minimum energy requirements for basal metabolism and growth, but also have requirements for unique physiology and metabolism that influence energy expenditure. These include body size, postnatal age, physical activity, dietary intake, environmental temperatures, energy losses in the stool and urine, and clinical conditions and diseases, as well as changes in body composition. Both energy and protein are necessary to produce normal rates of growth. Carbohydrates (primarily glucose) are principle sources of energy for the brain and heart until lipid oxidation develops over several days to weeks after birth. A higher protein/energy ratio is necessary in most preterm infants to approximate normal intrauterine growth rates. Lean tissue is predominantly produced during early gestation, which continues through to term. During later gestation, fat accretion in adipose tissue adds increasingly large caloric requirements to the lean tissue growth. Once protein intake is sufficient to promote net lean body accretion, additional energy primarily produces more body fat, which increases almost linearly at energy intakes >80–90 kcal/kg/day in normal, healthy preterm infants. Rapid gains in adiposity have the potential to produce later life obesity, an increasingly recognized risk of excessive energy intake. In addition to fundamental requirements for glucose, protein, and fat, a variety of non-glucose carbohydrates found in human milk may have important roles in promoting growth and development, as well as production of a gut microbiome that could protect against necrotizing enterocolitis.   © 2014 S. Karger AG, Basel

Energy Intake and Production

Energy is necessary for all vital functions of the body at molecular, cellular, organ, and systemic levels. Nutritional energy is the electrochemical potential in dietary carbohydrates, lipids, and protein. The energy provided by dietary substrates is 4 kcal/g of

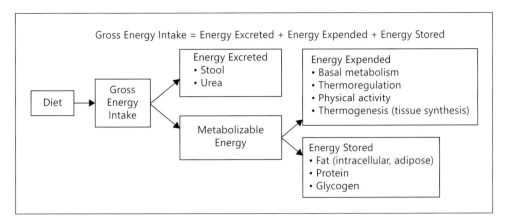

Fig. 1. Schematic of energy intake, excretion, metabolism, and storage.

protein, 4 kcal/g of carbohydrate, and 9 kcal/g of fat. The energy in these substrates is converted to ATP by oxidation in mitochondria or lost as heat production. Energy for maintaining vital functions, including storage and growth, is produced by hydrolysis of ATP (adenosine triphosphate) to ADP (adenosine diphosphate).

Dietary energy intake is balanced with energy requirements according to the energy balance equation:

Gross Energy Intake = Energy Excreted + Energy Expended + Energy Stored.

Gross Energy Intake is the total energy provided by the diet. Energy Excreted includes the energy lost in stool, mostly as fat but with small contributions from carbohydrate and protein, and in urine as urea. The term *digestible energy* refers to Gross Energy Intake minus the energy lost in stool. The term *metabolizable energy* refers to Gross Energy Intake minus Energy Excreted. Energy Expended includes energy for basal or resting metabolism, thermoregulation, physical activity, and diet-induced thermogenesis (DIT or energy expended in the synthesis of new tissue). Energy Stored includes primarily fat (intracellular as well as in adipose tissue) and protein (structural components of all tissues), with smaller amounts in glycogen (derived from glucose and other carbohydrates) (fig. 1) [1, 2].

Energy Requirements in the Fetus
Energy requirements for preterm infants have been derived from measured changes in energy metabolism in the human fetus, as well as from body composition analysis of the sheep fetus, which has a similar lean body mass composition as the human fetus at the same fractional gestational age but much less body fat. Table 1 compares carbon and energy balance data from fetal sheep with estimated values for human fetuses, as well as the nutrient supplies to produce such balances [3].

A second approach to determine energy requirements of the normally growing human fetus (and thus the preterm infant of the same gestational age) is based on the

Table 1. Nutrient substrate and carbon and calorie balance in late gestation fetal sheep and humans [adapted from 3]

Carbon-calorie balance	Carbon, g/kg/day	Calories, kcal/kg/day
Requirement		
Accretion in body: non-fat (sheep)	3.2	32
Accretion in body: non-fat (human)	3.2	32
Accretion in body: fat (human)	3.5	33
Excretion as CO_2	4.4	0
Excretion as urea	0.2	2
Excretion as glutamate	0.3	2
Heat (measured as O_2 consumption)	0.0	50
Total		
Without fat (sheep)	8.1	86
With fat (human)	11.6	119
Uptake		
Amino acids (sheep and human)	3.9	45
Glucose (sheep)	2.4	17
Glucose (human)	3.7	26
Lactate (sheep)	1.4	14
Lactate (human)	1.7	21
Fructose (sheep)	1.0	7
Acetate (sheep)	0.2	3
Fatty acids (human)	1.1–2.2	17–34
Total		
Sheep	8.9	86
Human	10.4–11.5	109–126

change in body composition and standard energy requirements for nutrient accretion and weight gain of a reference fetus. This approach has estimated caloric requirements for energy accretion of ~24 kcal/kg/day between 24 and 28 weeks' gestation, increasing slightly to ~28 kcal/kg/day for the remainder of gestation [4]. Lean tissue production begins during early gestation and continues through to term. During later gestation, fat accretion in adipose tissue adds an increasingly large caloric requirement to the lean tissue growth. Because of the greater caloric density of fat compared to lean tissue, the fractional rate of weight gain diminishes from ~18 g/kg/day at 24–28 weeks to ~15–16 g/kg/day at 32–36 weeks. The relatively large amount of fat that accumulates in normal human fetuses by term is unique among land mammals. Presumably, this unique fat content has some evolutionary advantage, but functionally, the role or value of such large amounts of fat in the normal human fetus and newborn infant is not known. There also is no rationale, other than its occurrence in normal fetuses, to support recapitulating this fetal developmental pattern in preterm infants. Most diets in preterm infants, however, actually produce large amounts of body fat by term gestation, even though much of this fat is intra-abdominal rather than in the usual fetal subcutaneous regions [5, 6]. Such fat in preterm infants also is produced from a much different mix of lipid products than probably occurs in the fetus and there is no information about

Table 2. Calorie needs (kcal/kg/day) for preterm infants to achieve normal growth rates

Study	Calorie needs, kcal/kg/day
American Academy of Pediatrics Committee on Nutrition [adapted from 65]	
Enterally fed infants	
Resting energy expenditure	50
Activity (0–30% above REE)	0–15
Thermoregulation	5–10
Thermic effect of feeding (synthesis)	10
Fecal loss of energy	10
Energy storage (growth)	25–35
Total	100–130
Intravenously fed infants	
Resting energy expenditure	50
Activity	0–5
Thermoregulation	0–5
Thermic effect of feeding (synthesis)	10
Energy storage (growth)	25
Total	85–95
ESPGHAN Committee on Nutrition [66]	
Energy intake recommended for preterm infants to achieve normal growth rates	115–130

whether such a different fat composition produced in preterm infants is healthy or not. Caution should be exercised, therefore, in producing body fat content in preterm infants that is in excess of the fat content that develops in the normal human fetus.

Energy Requirements in the Preterm Infant

Preterm infants have minimum energy requirements for basal metabolism and growth, but also have requirements for unique physiology and metabolism that influence energy expenditure. These include body size, postnatal age, physical activity, dietary intake, environmental temperatures, energy losses in the stool and urine, and clinical conditions and diseases, as well as changes in body composition. Table 2 provides estimates of energy requirements of milk or formula fed and intravenously fed preterm infants; the latter are assumed to be smaller, less physically active, kept warm in incubators, and not losing as much energy through fecal losses because their enteral intakes are generally quite low [1, 2, 7] (Evidence: moderate quality).

Age

Relationships between demographic factors, nutrient intake, and severity of illness assessments and measurements of total energy expenditure (TEE), oxygen consumption rates (VO_2), and carbon dioxide production rates (VCO_2) have been studied in preterm infants by indirect calorimetry [8]. Although VO_2, VCO_2, and TEE tend to increase over the first 3 weeks of life [9], there is a wide range of these values (Evi-

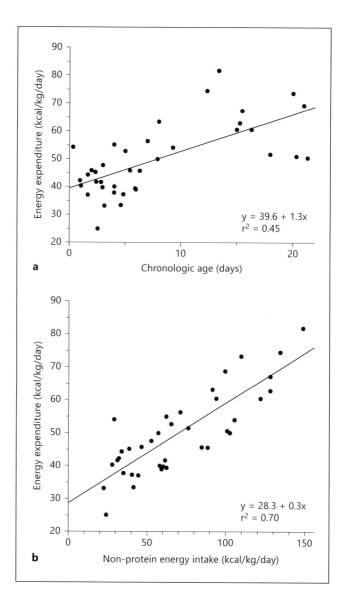

Fig. 2. Energy expenditure versus postnatal age (**a**) and non-protein energy intake (**b**) in 38 studies performed in 18 preterm infants [reproduced from 10].

dence: moderate quality). Energy expenditure is best predicted by non-protein calorie intake and postnatal age (fig. 2), while there is no correlation with birth weight, gestational age, protein intake, or severity of illness. Thus, the strong associations among postnatal age, energy intake, and energy expenditure most likely represent the routine clinical practice of daily increments in nutritional substrate intake in preterm infants.

Physical Activity

Some increase in energy expenditure is due to physical activity (energy expenditure of activity or EEA), particularly in infants with persistent respiratory distress. Earlier estimates ranged from 5 to 17% of TEE, but a more recent study uniquely determined

Hay Jr. · Brown · Denne

that physical activity accounts for only a very small contribution, ~3%, to TEE. By use of a force plate that measured work outputs, plus indirect calorimetry, TEE and EEA were measured and correlated with activity state in 24 infants with gestational ages of ~32 weeks and postnatal ages of ~25 days. TEE and EEA were 69 ± 2 and 2 ± 0.2 kcal/kg/day, respectively [10] (Evidence: moderate quality). Most extremely preterm infants have even less activity and thus lower rates of EAA. Whether there are differences between infants who are intubated and ventilated versus those managed with nasal continuous positive airway pressure (NCPAP) who appear to have greater breathing effort warrants further evaluation.

Dietary Intake

Dietary nutrients cause energy expenditure through mechanisms such as digestion, absorption, nutrient substrate transport across membranes, mechanical activities (heart rate/cardiac output, respiratory rate/minute ventilation), metabolism (including the energy needed to synthesize protein), and storage (fat, glycogen). Such energy expenditure has been referred to as the thermic effect of food, DIT, or specific dynamic action. In preterm infants, this value is determined as the difference between the baseline (fasting) rate of energy expenditure and the sum (or area under the curve) of energy expenditure measured following a meal, but over a specified period. Because of frequent (or even continuous) feedings, there seldom is a true fasting state in preterm infants; thus, estimates of DIT are likely underestimated. DIT generally increases resting energy expenditure by 10–15% in larger, more mature, late preterm infants. The magnitude of DIT is directly correlated with dietary energy intake and weight gain [11] (Evidence: moderate quality).

Environmental Temperature

Both hot and cold environments increase energy expenditure in the preterm infant. However, changes in environmental temperature are not always associated with such immediate changes in core body or even axillary temperature, indicating that some infants have the capacity to adapt to environmental temperature changes by varying energy expenditure. The environmental temperature that produces the least energy expenditure, determined as the lowest rate of oxygen consumption in relation to the immediate environmental temperature, is defined as the thermal neutral environmental temperature. Thermal neutral conditions and environmental temperature influences are subject to positioning (prone vs. lateral vs. supine), which influences physical activity and exposure of body surfaces to the environment [12]. Plastic wraps in the delivery room and warm blankets, overhead warmers, and shielding from colder areas of the NICU with barriers during nursing and medical or surgical care help reduce conduction and convection energy losses and the need for energy production by the infant from increased nutrient supply and metabolism.

Body Size

Body weight-specific measurements of energy expenditure vary considerably among preterm infants and larger, more normally grown infants [13]. Factors that influence this variability include body weight and proportions, the diet (generally less in preterm infants), growth rates (generally slower in preterm), and physical activity (generally greater in older, larger infants). Preterm infants generally have a greater brain size/body weight ratio, which increases body weight-specific energy expenditure; the opposite occurs in macrosomic infants who have excessive body fat content. Normally grown and macrosomic infants, however, generally have more muscle mass per bone length and body weight than do preterm infants. Body weight alone, therefore, is not necessarily the best indicator of energy expenditure or the best denominator for referencing metabolic rates among different populations of infants. Future technology that accurately measures body composition (e.g. muscle mass, bone content, brain size, fat mass) should eventually replace body weight as the reference for such metabolic measurements.

Clinical Conditions

Large increases in energy expenditure of 20–50% have been measured in term and preterm infants with sepsis. The increase in energy expenditure in sepsis is presumed secondary to systemic inflammatory responses. However, variable or even contradictory, measurements of energy expenditure in septic preterm infants have been made [14] (Evidence: low quality). For example, while increased energy expenditure with increased respiratory support has been reported [15], decreased energy expenditure has been observed with NCPAP. Increased energy expenditure also has been associated with chronic lung disease, possibly due to increased work of breathing, although this is not always clinically apparent. There is no evidence that infants with chronic lung disease benefit from increased energy intake [16] (Evidence: low quality). Use of caffeine for apnea of prematurity also has been associated with increases in energy expenditure by some investigators [17], though not by others [18] (Evidence: low quality). Such measurements in extremely preterm, extremely low birth infants are more limited [19].

Protein-Energy Metabolism and Balance

Protein-energy balance studies in preterm infants have provided data to guide recommendations for protein-energy intakes for specific short-term goals [20]. Effects of these intakes on long-term outcomes, such as growth (body weight), body composition, neurodevelopment, and clinical susceptibility to adult-onset diseases (e.g. the metabolic syndrome of obesity and insulin resistance) are still lacking. However, there is increasing evidence that early protein intake has benefits for reducing the number of infants with weights, lengths, and head circumferences <10th centile [21] (Evi-

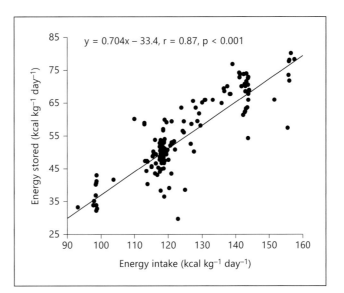

Fig. 3. Relationship between gross energy intake and energy stored of low birth weight infants enrolled in enteral feeding studies (based on data from Kashyap et al. as reported in references 24–26).

The plot shows: $y = 0.704x - 33.4$, $r = 0.87$, $p < 0.001$, with y-axis "Energy stored (kcal kg^{-1} day^{-1})" and x-axis "Energy intake (kcal kg^{-1} day^{-1})".

dence: moderate quality). Both energy and protein intakes are beneficial for growth of body weight, length, and head circumference, even when taking into account gestational age, baseline anthropometrics, and severity of illness [22].

Energy Cost of Growth
Energy storage, principally in fat, increases almost linearly at energy intakes >80–90 kcal/kg/day in normal, healthy preterm infants (fig. 3) [2]. Once protein intake is sufficient to promote net lean body accretion, additional energy primarily produces more fat gain (e.g. as measured by increased triceps skin fold thickness) as well as weight gain, but does not produce greater head circumference or length gain (the major components of lean body mass) (Evidence: moderate quality).

Energy Cost of Protein and Tissue Synthesis
The energy cost of protein and tissue synthesis cannot be determined directly. Estimates from studies of weight gain, macronutrient storage, and energy expenditure in preterm infants have shown that the energy expenditure of growing preterm infants is strongly related to their rate of weight gain; since this is a direct, linear relationship, the rate of energy expenditure versus weight gain provides an estimate of the energy required for tissue deposition or synthesis. The energy cost of weight gain, as estimated from this regression relationship, has been reported to be between 0.23 and 0.68 kcal/g, with the large variation dependent on water balance [23].

Rates of energy expenditure for protein and fat synthesis in preterm infants range from approximately 5–8 and 1.5–1.6 kcal/g, respectively, higher than the rates of energy cost of weight gain due to the inclusion of water in the measurements of body weight. From these values for protein and fat synthesis, the energy cost of growth can be estimated as the sum of energy stored and the energy cost of tissue synthesis and deposition. Rates for such energy cost of growth in growing preterm infants are quite large, with mean values as high as 74 kcal/kg/day. Approximately 75% of this energy cost of growth includes stored energy in body protein and fat and ~25% includes energy expended in the synthesis and deposition of protein and fat [1, 2] (Evidence: low quality).

Effect of Varying Energy and Protein Intake on Nitrogen Balance
A series of controlled enteral feeding studies in preterm infants examined the effects of independent and systematic variations in the absolute amount and relative proportion of protein and energy intake on the rate and composition of weight gain and metabolic response [24]. These studies demonstrated that metabolic indices, energy balance, and composition of weight gain were close to a normally growing human fetus in late gestation when feeding 115 kcal/kg/day and 3.6 g/kg/day of protein (Evidence: moderate quality). The studies indicate that a caloric intake of 115–120 kcal/kg/day will appropriately support a protein intake of 3.5–4 g/kg/day; more energy produced more body fat gain, but more protein than 4 g/kg/day did not independently increase lean body mass gain.

The data from the same series of studies also demonstrated that the relative composition of the weight gained as protein and fat stored was dependent on the protein/energy ratio of the diet. Relatively more protein was synthesized and deposited in growing lean tissue at higher protein intakes and more fat was synthesized and deposited in growth of adipose tissue at higher energy intakes. Energy is particularly important to promote protein balance at lower energy intakes, as amino acids are increasingly used for oxidative metabolism when non-protein energy is limited [25]. Regardless of energy intake, however, net protein balance requires increased protein intake.

To the extent that mimicking in utero fat gain is important, the composition of the newly formed tissue in preterm infants fed normal or low energy intakes has less fat accretion in AGA and SGA infants fed 100 kcal/kg/day than observed in normal fetuses growing in utero. Thus, preterm infants need a minimum of 110 kcal/kg/day to maintain the growth of fat in adipose tissue that is observed in the normally growing human fetus [26] (Evidence: moderate quality). Slightly higher amounts of energy will be needed to promote lean body growth at the in utero rate (table 2). However, most studies of changes in body composition in preterm infants during their NICU days demonstrate a relatively greater gain in body fat than would have occurred had these infants remained in utero at normal rates of nutrition and growth and change in body composition [4, 5]. These observations probably account for recent efforts to enhance the protein/energy ratio of the diets of preterm infants, particularly to add more protein supplements to maternal and especially mature donor breast milk [27].

While there is reasonable evidence that carbohydrate is more effective than fat in promoting nitrogen retention in animal models and older humans as well as preterm infants [24], there also is no apparent benefit of an energy intake, including carbohydrates, in excess of that necessary to assure utilization of the concomitant protein intake. Excessive energy and carbohydrate intakes simply result in excessive fat deposition relative to protein deposition. The potential for such rapid gains in adiposity to produce later life obesity is increasingly seen as an unwarranted risk [28].

Adding intravenous lipid infusions to total intravenous (parenteral) nutrition (TPN) reduces glucose oxidation and the production of CO_2, possibly beneficial for infants with respiratory distress. While most studies have shown increased nitrogen balance in response to glucose versus lipid, results vary among studies, with some showing that adding lipid to glucose and amino acid infusions improves nitrogen balance when caloric intakes are equivalent to glucose and amino acid infusions alone [29–31] (Evidence: moderate quality).

Effect of Other Nutrients and Growth Factors on Nitrogen Balance

Inadequate intake of any nutrient required for new tissue synthesis will also limit the extent to which protein can be deposited as new tissue. Significant correlations between growth or nitrogen retention (or protein balance) and the intake of electrolytes (sodium, potassium) and minerals (calcium, phosphorous) have been reported in preterm infants, [19] indicating that an inadequate intake of any nutrient required for production of new tissue is likely to interfere with the preterm infant's utilization of protein and/or amino acid intake for growth of lean body mass in new tissue, regardless of the concomitant energy intake (Evidence: moderate quality).

Insulin

There is no evidence that early insulin therapy in very low birth weight (VLBW) infants is beneficial for growth. A large randomized controlled trial demonstrated no improvement in growth in infants who received insulin, and there was a suggestion of increased mortality in the insulin group [32] (Evidence: high quality).

Carnitine

Carnitine has been used to promote fat oxidation, but there is no evidence that supplemental carnitine has clinically measurable impact on growth unless the infant remains on TPN for long periods (>2–3 weeks) [33] (Evidence: moderate quality).

Carbohydrate Intake

Under normal circumstances, carbohydrates are not produced in the fetus, but come exclusively via placental transport from the maternal circulation. However, non-glucose carbohydrates are first converted to glucose before contributing to energy metabolism or storage as glycogen.

Glucose

Glucose is the major source of energy for most metabolic processes in the body, particularly for the brain and heart in the preterm infant. It also is a major source of carbon for de novo synthesis of fatty acids and a number of non-essential amino acids. Unless glucose is infused intravenously into the preterm infant, acute glucose production immediately after birth comes mostly from glycogenolysis, with the balance from gluconeogenesis (largely glycerol and secondarily, lactate and pyruvate [34], but also from amino acids such as alanine and glutamine) developing over the next few days. When all nutrients are plentiful, 65–70% of glucose metabolized is oxidized to carbon dioxide, mostly in the brain and heart [35].

Glucose utilization rates are about twice as high in very preterm infants as at term, consistent with the same pattern found in the fetus. The decline in whole body weight-specific glucose metabolic rate with gestational age is a result of the decreasing contribution of the brain and heart to whole body weight, with increasingly larger fractions of body weight accounted for by organs such as the gut, muscle, fat, bone, and skin that have much lower rates of glucose metabolism [36].

Several studies have documented higher steady-state weight-specific rates of glucose turnover in very preterm infants compared to term infants, primarily driven by the provision of intravenous glucose infusions in the first several days of life. Most preterm infants produce glucose after birth quite readily, often to values as high as those of term infants (4–5 mg/min/kg) from both glycogenolysis and gluconeogenesis [37, 38] (Evidence: moderate quality). Sustained rates of ~2 mg/kg/min from gluconeogenesis contribute to glycogenolysis that produce such high total rates of glucose production [39, 40], but can be augmented by intravenous lipid infusions that provide glycerol as a substrate [34]. Despite glucose infusion rates that exceed normal infant glucose turnover rates, rates of endogenous glucose production are sustained in the preterm infant. Such high rates of glucose production are important to consider in very preterm infants who are hyperglycemic and provide further support for optimizing glucose infusion rates to reduce the risk of and/or treat hyperglycemia (Evidence: moderate quality).

Whole body glucose utilization rates linearly match total glucose entry (endogenous glucose production, glucose derived from enteral feeding, and intravenous glucose infusion rates) into the preterm infant's circulation up to about 20–25 g/kg/day (about ~15–17 mg/kg/min), at which point glucose oxidation is maximized, oxidation of other substrates is minimized, and fat synthesis from glucose increasingly develops (Evidence: moderate quality). Synthesis of fat from glucose is an energy requiring process that increases CO_2 production, potentially leading to increased respiratory rate and work of breathing [41]. The lower limit of total glucose supply should exceed brain glucose requirements, allowing glucose supply to the heart. This is particularly true right after birth, before the heart develops the capacity for long-chain fatty acid oxidation. However, there also is no reason to supplement preterm infants with excessive glucose supply. Intravenous glucose infusion rates >10–11 mg/min/kg almost invariably lead to hyperglycemia, aggravated by catecholamine (endogenous or infused) suppression of insulin secretion and insulin action, as well as glycogenolysis that is augmented by glucagon and cortisol secretion (or hydrocortisone or dexamethasone treatments). Excessive glucose infusion rates have many adverse effects, including increased energy expenditure, increased oxygen consumption, increased carbon dioxide production, tachypnea (even respiratory distress) from the CO_2-induced respiratory acidosis, fatty infiltration of the heart and liver (the latter leading to steatosis), and excessive fat deposition (which possibly might lead to obesity) [42]. Thus, caution must be used when supplementing preterm infants with excessive glucose supply.

Glucose utilization rates by the brain are high compared to other organs to meet energy requirements of maintaining neuronal transmembrane potentials, axonal electrical propagation, synaptic transmission, and protein synthesis for neuronal cell replication and migration. For example, a normal-sized term neonatal brain consumes about 5–7 μmol of glucose per 100 g brain weight per min, or about 3.5–4.5 mg/min/kg body weight, which accounts for most of whole body glucose production or utilization rates [43]. Since preterm infants have larger brain/body weight ratios, they also have high glucose and energy requirements [38, 44]. In addition, alternative substrates (ketones, lactate) are low in preterm infants, making them more vulnerable to glucose deficiency and hypoglycemia (Evidence: moderate quality).

Use of insulin infusions to prevent or reduce hyperglycemia has resulted in a modest reduction in hyperglycemia but at the cost of an increase in the frequency and severity of hypoglycemic episodes, as well as a suggestion of increased mortality [32] (Evidence: high quality). Insulin infusions also have the potential to produce lactic acidosis and hypercarbia, which may compromise infants with severe lung disease and respiratory distress [45]. More effective to reduce hyperglycemia might be the infusion of higher rates of amino acids, which consistently have been shown to be associated with lower time-averaged plasma glucose concentrations and fewer episodes of marked hyperglycemia [46] (Evidence: high quality).

Glucose is readily absorbed from the gut, as well in preterm as in term infants, using a specific Na^+/glucose co-transporter [47]. D-Glucose and D-galactose released from lactose are the natural substrates for these transporters. Gut absorption of glucose is positively related to postnatal age, the duration and frequency and volume of prior feedings, and glucocorticoids (administered to the infant as well as prenatal steroids given to the mother for fetal lung maturation) [48]. Glucose is rapidly released from glucose polymers by acid hydrolysis and by salivary, pancreatic, and intestinal amylase and maltases. Such substances have been used by some to enhance energy nutrition, although beneficial effects do not appear to be independent of protein supply and there is no evidence that they promote nitrogen balance or growth on their own [49] (Evidence: moderate quality). Furthermore, if used in excess, glucose polymers can lead to hyperosmolality in the gut lumen, resulting in diarrhea.

Lactose

Lactose is the predominant carbohydrate in human milk. Intestinal lactase releases glucose and galactose from lactose in equal portions. Lactase activity in the human fetus increases during the third trimester, such that lactase activity in the very preterm infant may be only 30% of normal compared to full-term neonates [50]. Decreased lactase activity in the preterm infant might contribute to feeding intolerance [51]. For this reason, most preterm formulas reduce lactose content to 50% of that in human milk. Low lactose formulas containing essentially no lactose were reported to reduce feeding difficulties in this population, such as gastric residuals and episodes of having feedings stopped, thus enabling infants to reach full enteral feedings sooner [52] (Evidence: moderate quality). No benefit has been found to adding lactase to enteral feeds to promote growth and feeding tolerance in preterm infants [53] (Evidence: moderate quality). It is important to note, however, that intestinal lactase activity can be induced by enteral feeding, particularly by feeding human milk [54] (Evidence: moderate quality). Adding excess lactose, as with glucose polymers, should not be used in place of providing adequate protein to promote growth, particularly of lean body mass.

Non-Glucose Carbohydrates and Oligosaccharides

Non-glucose carbohydrates contained in human milk such as galactose, inositol, and mannose have specific functions in fetal and neonatal nutrition and development [55]. Human milk also contains a large variety of other oligosaccharides (prebiotics) and sugar polyol compounds (e.g. disialyllacto-N-tetraose, N-acetylglucosamine, *n*-acetylnuraminic acid, fucose, sialic acid, glycerol, erythritol, arabinose, ribose, mannitol), which may be important in reducing the incidence and/or severity of necrotizing enterocolitis (NEC) [56, 57] (Evidence: high quality). A recent systematic review that evaluated prebiotic supplementation in preterm infants, however, found enhanced pathological bacterial intestinal flora but no effect on incidence of NEC [58] (Evidence: high quality).

Galactose

Galactose is a normal component of milk lactose and thus is a natural nutrient for all newborn infants. Galactose released from lactase hydrolysis of lactose in the brush border of the intestine is readily absorbed and is almost 100% first pass cleared by the liver, where it is converted to glucose, either for storage as glycogen during feedings or released into the circulation between feedings [59].

Inositol

Inositol is a carbohydrate that plays a role in many biological functions that are particularly important to the neonate, including formation of the neural system and pulmonary surfactant phospholipid production. Though inositol is present in relatively high concentrations in human breast milk (~1,200 µmol/l) [55], it also can be produced from D-glucose at rates which are >10-fold higher than the amounts a breast-fed infant typically ingests [60]. Plasma inositol concentrations are higher in preterm infants compared to term infants and in both populations can be increased by supplementing inositol in the diet. In a randomized controlled trial, supplementation of inositol to preterm infants was shown to reduce surfactant deficiency associated respiratory distress syndrome, but primarily in infants who did not receive exogenous surfactant [61]. In the same study, it also was found that inositol supplementation reduced the incidence and severity of retinopathy of prematurity (Evidence: moderate quality). Benefits of routinely supplementing preterm infant nutrition with inositol are currently being investigated.

Mannose

Mannose is another carbohydrate that is essential for protein glycosylation and normal neurodevelopment [62]. Like glucose, the fetus during late gestation is dependent on a maternal supply of mannose [63]. Free mannose is present in very low concentrations in breast milk (~40 µmol/l), although there may be even more mannose available in milk in the form of oligosaccharides, which contribute to the establishment of non-pathogenic colonic flora [64]. Mannose is present in even higher concentrations in term and especially preterm formulas. However, full-term infants are able to produce mannose at rates that exceed nutritional intakes [60]. Further studies are needed to examine the biological role of non-glucose carbohydrates such as inositol and mannose in order to determine their specific contributions to nutritional management of the preterm infant.

Conclusions and Recommendations

Preterm infants have minimum energy requirements for basal metabolism and growth (table 2), but also have requirements for unique physiology and metabolism that influence energy expenditure. These include body size, postnatal age, physical activity, dietary intake, environmental temperatures, energy losses in the stool and urine, and clinical conditions and diseases, as well as changes in body composition. Both energy and protein are necessary to produce normal rates of growth. Carbohydrates (primarily glucose) are principle sources of energy for the brain and heart until lipid oxidation develops over several days to weeks after birth. A higher protein/energy ratio is necessary in most preterm infants to approximate normal intrauterine growth rates. Lean tissue is predominantly produced during early gestation, which continues through to term. During later gestation, fat accretion in adipose tissue adds increasingly large caloric requirements to the lean tissue growth. Once protein intake is sufficient to promote net lean body accretion, additional energy primarily produces more body fat, which increases almost linearly at energy intakes >80–90 kcal/kg/day in normal, healthy preterm infants. Rapid gains in adiposity have the potential to produce later life obesity, an increasingly recognized risk of excessive energy intake. In addition to fundamental requirements for glucose, protein, and fat, a variety of non-glucose carbohydrates found in human milk may have important roles in promoting growth and development, as well as production of a gut microbiome that could protect against NEC.

Preterm infants need relatively high amounts of energy to support growth and development. Estimates of such caloric requirements for stable, reasonably health VLBW infants are provided below. There is little evidence to support specific energy requirements for infants who are sick or infants who are growth-restricted. Total energy intake post-discharge should approach 100–120 kcal/kg/day.

Such infants need further research to define optimal feeding strategies, including energy requirements. Other research needs are listed below, noting that there currently is considerable lack of evidence for some of the most basic information needed to optimize energy nutrition of preterm infants.

Energy and Carbohydrates: Nutritional Recommendations

(1) Total energy intake for VLBW infants must be sufficient to support basal metabolism and net protein/fat balance (plus minor heat and stool losses) – 110–130 kcal/kg/day for enterally fed preterm infants (85–95 kcal/kg/day for parenterally fed infants) (Level of evidence: moderate quality).

(2) There is no evidence that energy intake above this level enhances neurological development or is required to achieve appropriate growth and body composition. High energy intakes in preterm infants results in greater fat accumulation compared to their normal fetal counterparts (Level of evidence: moderate quality).

(3) High infusion rates of glucose often results in hyperglycemia and may contribute to inflammatory injuries and fatty infiltration of liver and heart and other organs. Routine use of insulin to prevent hyperglycemia or promote growth is not beneficial and may be harmful (Level of evidence: moderate quality).

Research Recommendations

(1) Body composition studies, baseline and serial, and focusing on specific organs, are essential to define the growth of individual tissues in response to different amounts (absolute and relative to each other) of amino acids/protein, glucose and lipids, and total energy.

(2) Selected energy nutrients (essential amino acids, essential fatty acids) need more study for their individual contributions (benefits and risks) to metabolism, growth, and development.

(3) Further studies are needed to examine the biological role of non-glucose carbohydrates such as inositol and mannose and oligosaccharides and sugar polyol compounds found in human milk in order to determine their specific contributions to nutritional management of the preterm infant.

References

1 Leitch CA, Denne SC: Nutrition of the preterm infant; in Tsang RC, Uauy R, Koletzko B, Zlotkin SH (eds): Nutrition of the Preterm Infant: Scientific Basis and Practical Guidelines, ed 2. Cincinnati, Digital Educational Publishing Inc, 2005, pp 23–44.

2 Kashyap S, Schulze KF: Energy requirements and protein-energy metabolism and balance in preterm and term infants; in Thureen PJ, Hay WW Jr (eds): Neonatal Nutrition and Metabolism, ed 2. Cambridge, Cambridge University Press, 2006, pp 134–146.

3 Hay WW Jr: Fetal requirements and placental transfer of nitrogenous compounds; in Polin RA, Fox WW, Abman SH (eds): Fetal and Neonatal Physiology. Philadelphia, Elsevier Saunders, 2011, pp 1585–1602.

4 Ziegler EE, O'Donnell AM, Nelson SE, Fomon SJ: Body composition of the reference fetus. Growth 1976;40:329–341.

5 Taroni F, Liotto N, Morlacchi L, Orsi A, Giannì M, Roggero P, Mosca F: Body composition in small for gestational age newborns. Pediatr Med Chir 2008;30:296–301.

6 Johnson MJ, Wootton SA, Leaf AA, Jackson AA: Preterm birth and body composition at term equivalent age: a systematic review and meta-analysis. Pediatrics 2012;130:e640–e649.

7 Weintraub V, Francis B, Mimouni FB, Dollberg S: Effect of birth weight and postnatal age upon resting energy expenditure in preterm infants. Am J Perinatol 2009;26:173–178.

8 DeMarie MP, Hoffenberg A, Biggerstaff SL, Jeffers BW, Hay WW Jr, Thureen PJ: Determinants of energy expenditure in ventilated preterm infants. J Perinat Med 1999;27:465–472.

9 Bauer J, Werner C, Gerss J: Metabolic rate analysis of healthy preterm and full-term infants during the first weeks of life. Am J Clin Nutr 2009;90:1517–1524.

10 Thureen PJ, Phillips RE, Baron KA, DeMarie M, Hay WW Jr: Direct measurement of the energy expenditure of physical activity in preterm infants. J App Physiol 1998;85:223–230.

11 Rubecz I, Mestyan J: Postprandial thermogenesis in human milk-fed very low birth weight infants. Biol Neonate 1986;49:301–306.

12 Chong A, Murphy N, Matthews T: Effect of prone sleeping on circulatory control in infants. Arch Dis Child 2000;82:253–256.

13 Picaud JC, Putet G, Rigo J, Salle BL, Senterre J: Metabolic and energy balance in small- and appropriate-for-gestational-age, very low-birth-weight infants. Acta Paediatr Suppl 1994;405:54–59.

14 Wahlig TM, Georgieff MK: The effects of illness on neonatal metabolism and nutritional management. Clin Perinatol 1995;22:77–96.

15 Wahlig TM, Gatto CW, Boros SJ, Mamme MC, Mills MM, Georgieff MK: Metabolic response of preterm infants to variable degrees of respiratory illness. J Pediatr 1994;124:283–288.

16 Lai NM, Rajadurai SV, Tan K: Increased energy intake for preterm infants with (or developing) bronchopulmonary dysplasia/chronic lung disease. Cochrane Database Syst Rev 2006;3:CD005093.

17 Bauer J, Maier K, Linderkamp O, Hentschel R: Effect of caffeine on oxygen consumption and metabolic rate in very low birth weight infants with idiopathic apnea. Pediatrics 2001;107:660–663.

18 Fjeld CR, Cole FS, Bier DM: Energy expenditure, lipolysis, and glucose production in preterm infants treated with theophylline. Pediatr Res 1992;32:693–698.

19 Tudehope D, Fewtrell M, Kashyap S, Udaeta E: Nutritional needs of the micropreterm infant. J Pediatr 2013;162(suppl):S72–S80.

20 Bhatia J, Mena P, Denne S, Garcia C: Evaluation of adequacy of protein and energy. J Pediatr 2013;162:S31–S36.

21 Poindexter BB, Langer JC, Dusick AM, Ehrenkranz RA: Early provision of parenteral amino acids in extremely low birth weight infants: relation to growth and neurodevelopmental outcome. J Pediatr 2006;148:300–305.

22 Sjöström ES, Öhlund I, Ahlsson F, Engström E, Fellman V, Hellström A, Källén K, Norman M, Olhager E, Serenius F, Domellöf M: Nutrient intakes independently affect growth in extremely preterm infants: results from a population-based study. Unpubl data, 2013.

23 Towers HM, Schulze KF, Ramakrishnan R, Kashyap S: Energy expended by low birth weight infants in the deposition of protein and fat. Pediatr Res 1997;41:584–589.

24 Kashyap S, Forsyth M, Zucker C, Ramakrishnan R, Dell RB, Heird WC: Effects of varying protein and energy intakes on growth and metabolic response in low birth weight infants. J Pediatr 1986;108:955–963.

25 Brown LD, Hay WW Jr: Effect of hyperinsulinemia on amino acid utilization and oxidation independent of glucose metabolism in the ovine fetus. Am J Physiol Endocrinol Metab 2006;291:E1333–E1340.

26 Van Goudoever JB, Sulkers EJ, Lafeber HN, Sauer PJJ: Short-term growth and substrate use in very-low-birth-weight infants fed formulas with different energy contents. Am J Clin Nutr 2000;71:816–821.

27 Rochow N, Fusch G, Choi A, Chessell L, Elliott L, McDonald K, Kuiper E, Purcha M, Turner S, Chan E, Yang Xia M, Fusch C: Target fortification of breast milk with fat, protein, and carbohydrates for preterm infants. Unpubl data, 2013.

28 Belfort MB, Gillman MW, Buka SL, Casey PH, Mc-Cormick MC: Preterm infant linear growth and adiposity gain: trade-offs for later weight status, and IQ. J Pediatr 2013;163:1564–1569.e2.

29 Vlaardingerbroek H, Vermeulen MJ, Rook D, van den Akker CH, Dorst K, Wattimena JL, Vermes A, Schierbeek H, van Goudoever JB: Safety and efficacy of early parenteral lipid and high-dose amino acid administration to very low birth weight infants. J Pediatr 2013;163:638–644.e1–e5.

30 Van Aerde JE, Sauer PJ, Pencharz PB, Smith JM, Swyer PR: Effect of replacing glucose with lipid on the energy metabolism of newborn infants. Clin Sci (Lond) 1989;76:581–588.

31 Van Aerde JE, Sauer PJ, Pencharz PB, Smith JM, Heim T, Swyer PR: Metabolic consequences of increasing energy intake by adding lipid to parenteral nutrition in full-term infants. Am J Clin Nutr 1994; 59:659–662.

32 Beardsall K, Vanhaesebrouck S, Ogilvy-Stuart AL, Vanhole C, Palmer CR, van Weissenbruch M, Midgley P, Thompson M, Thio M, Cornette L, Ossuetta I, Iglesias I, Theyskens C, de Jong M, Ahluwalia JS, de Zegher F, Dunger DB: Early insulin therapy in very-low-birth-weight infants. N Engl J Med 2008;359: 1873–1884.

33 Helms RA, Mauer EC, Hay WW Jr, Christensen ML, Storm MC: Effect of intravenous L-carnitine on growth and fat metabolism parameters during parenteral nutrition in neonates. J Parenter Enteral Nutr 1990;14:448–453.

34 Sunehag AL: Parenteral glycerol enhances gluconeogenesis in very premature infants. Pediatr Res 2003; 53:635–641.

35 Parimi P, Kalhan SC: Carbohydrates including oligosaccharides and inositol; in Tsang RC, Uauy R, Koletzko B, Zlotkin SH (eds): Nutrition of the Preterm Infant: Scientific Basis and Practical Guidelines, ed 2. Cincinnati, Digital Education Publishing Inc, 2005, pp 81–95.

36 Thorn SR, Rozance PJ, Brown LD, Hay WW Jr: The intrauterine growth restriction phenotype: fetal adaptations and potential implications for later life insulin resistance and diabetes. Semin Reprod Med 2011;29:225–236.

37 Sunehag A, Ewald U, Larsson A, Gustafsson J: Glucose production rate in extremely immature neonates (<28 weeks) studied by use of deuterated glucose. Pediatr Res 1993;33:97–100.

38 Sunehag AL, Haymond MW, Schanler RJ, Reeds PJ, Bier DM: Gluconeogenesis in very low birth weight infants receiving total parenteral nutrition. Diabetes 1999;48:791–800.

39 Chacko SK, Ordonez J, Sauer PJ, Sunehag AL: Gluconeogenesis is not regulated by either glucose or insulin in extremely low birth weight infants receiving total parenteral nutrition. J Pediatr 2011;158:891–896.

40 Chacko SK, Sunehag AL: Gluconeogenesis continues in premature infants receiving total parenteral nutrition. Arch Dis Child Fetal Neonatal Ed 2010;95: F413–F418.

41 Thureen PJ, Hay WW Jr: Nutritional requirements of the very low birth weight infant; in Neu J (ed): Gastroenterology and Nutrition, ed 2. Philadelphia, Elsevier Saunders, 2012, pp 107–128.

42 Brown LD, Hay WW Jr: Nutritional dilemma in the preterm infant: how to promote neurocognitive development and linear growth, but reduce the risk of obesity. J Pediatr 2013;163:1543–1545.

43 Kalhan SC, Parimi P, Van BR, Gilfillan C, Saker F, Gruca L, et al: Estimation of gluconeogenesis in newborn infants. Am J Physiol Endocrinol Metab 2001; 281:E991–E997.

44 Bier DM, Leake RD, Haymond MW, Arnold KJ, Gruenke LD, Sperling MA, Kipnis DM: Measurement of 'true' glucose production rates in infancy and childhood with 6,6-dideuteroglucose. Diabetes 1977;26:1016–1023.

45 Bottino M, Cowett RM, Sinclair JC: Interventions for treatment of neonatal hyperglycemia in very low birth weight infants. Cochrane Database Syst Rev 2011;10:CD007453.

46 Burattini I, Bellagamba MP, Spagnoli C, D'Ascenzo R, Mazzoni N, Peretti A, Cogo PE, Carnielli P; Marche Neonatal Network: Targeting 2.5 versus 4 g/kg/day of amino acids for extremely low birth weight infants: a randomized clinical trial. J Pediatr 2013;163:1278–1282.e1.

47 Wright EM: The intestinal Na$^+$/glucose cotransporter. Annu Rev Physiol 1993;55:575–589.

48 Shulman RJ: In vivo measurements of glucose absorption in preterm infants. Biol Neonate 1999;76: 10–18.

49 Shulman RJ, Feste A, Ou C: Absorption of lactose, glucose polymers, or combination in premature infants. J Pediatr 1995;127:626–631.

50 Antonowicz I, Lebenthal E: Developmental pattern of small intestinal enterokinase and disaccharidase activities in the human fetus. Gastroenterology 1977; 72:1299–1303.

51 Shulman RJ, Schanler RJ, Lau C, Heitkemper M, Ou CN, Smith EO: Early feeding, feeding tolerance, and lactase activity in preterm infants. J Pediatr 1998;133: 645–649.

52 Griffin MP, Hansen JW: Can the elimination of lactose from formula improve feeding tolerance in premature infants? J Pediatr 1999;135:587–592.

53 Tan-Dy CR, Ohlsson A: Lactase-treated feeds to promote growth and feeding tolerance in preterm infants. Cochrane Database Syst Rev 2013;3:CD004591.

54 Shulman RJ, Wong WW, Smith EO: Influence of changes in lactase activity and small-intestinal mucosal growth on lactose digestion and absorption in preterm infants. Am J Clin Nutr 2005;81:472–479.

55 Cavalli C, Teng C, Battaglia FC, Bevilacqua G: Free sugar and sugar alcohol concentrations in human breast milk. J Pediatr Gastroenterol Nutr 2006;42: 215–221.

56 Kunz C, Rodriguez-Palmero M, Koletzko B, Jensen R: Nutritional and biochemical properties of human milk. Part I: General aspects, proteins, and carbohydrates. Clin Perinatol 1999;26:307–333.

57 Quigley MA, Henderson G, Anthony MY, McGuire W: Formula milk versus donor breast milk for feeding preterm or low birth weight infants. Cochrane Database Syst Rev 2007;4:CD002971.

58 Srinivasjois R, Rao S, Patole S: Prebiotic supplementation in preterm neonates: updated systematic review and meta-analysis of randomised controlled trials. Clin Nutr 2013;32:958–965.

59 Kliegman RM, Sparks JW: Perinatal galactose metabolism. J Pediatr 1985;107:831–841.

60 Brown LD, Cheung A, Harwood JE, Battaglia FC: Inositol and mannose utilization rates in term and late-preterm infants exceed nutritional intakes. J Nutr 2009;139:1648–1652.

61 Hallman M, Bry K, Hoppu K, Lappi M, Pohjavuori M: Inositol supplementation in premature infants with respiratory distress syndrome. N Engl J Med 1992;326:1233–1239.

62 Davis JA, Freeze HH: Studies of mannose metabolism and effects of long-term mannose ingestion in the mouse. Biochim Biophys Acta 2001;1528:116–126.

63 Brusati V, Józwik M, Józwik M, Teng C, Paolini C, Marconi AM, Battaglia FC: Fetal and maternal non-glucose carbohydrates and polyols concentrations in normal human pregnancies at term. Pediatr Res 2005;58:700–704.

64 Coppa GV, Pierani P, Zampini L, Bruni S, Carloni I, Gabrielli O: Characterization of oligosaccharides in milk and feces of breast-fed infants by high-performance anion-exchange chromatography. Adv Exp Med Biol 2001;501:307–314.

65 American Academy of the Pediatric (AAP) Committee on Nutrition: Nutritional needs of the preterm infant; in Kleinman RE (ed): Pediatric Nutrition Handbook, ed 6. Elk Grove Village/IL, AAP, 2009, pp 79–112.

66 Agostini C, Buonocore G, Carnielli VP, et al: Enteral nutrient supply for preterm infants: commentary from the European Society for Pediatric Gastroenterology, Hepatology, and Nutrition Committee on Nutrition. J Pediatr Gastroenterol Nutr 2010;50:85–91.

William W. Hay, Jr., MD
Anschutz Medical Campus F441
University of Colorado School of Medicine, Perinatal Research Center
13243 East 23rd Avenue, Aurora, CO 80045 (USA)
E-Mail bill.hay@ucdenver.edu

Koletzko B, Poindexter B, Uauy R (eds): Nutritional Care of Preterm Infants: Scientific Basis and Practical Guidelines.
World Rev Nutr Diet. Basel, Karger, 2014, vol 110, pp 82–98 (DOI: 10.1159/000358460)

Enteral and Parenteral Lipid Requirements of Preterm Infants

Alexandre Lapillonne

Paris Descartes University, APHP Necker Hospital, Paris, France, and CNRC, Baylor College of Medicine, Houston, Tex., USA

Reviewed by Berthold Koletzko, Dr. von Hauner Children's Hospital, University of Munich Medical Center, Munich, Germany; Hester Vlaardingerbroek, Department of Pediatrics, Academic Medical Center-Emma Children's Hospital, Amsterdam, The Netherlands

Abstract

Lipids provide infants with most of their energy needs. The major portion of the fat in human milk is found in the form of triglycerides, the phospholipids and cholesterol contributing for only a small proportion of the total fat. Long-chain polyunsaturated fatty acids (LC-PUFAs) are crucial for normal development of the central nervous system and have potential for long-lasting effects that extend beyond the period of dietary insufficiency. Given the limited and highly variable formation of docosahexaenoic acid (DHA) from α-linolenic acid, and because DHA is critical for normal retinal and brain development in the human, DHA should be considered to be conditionally essential during early development. In early enteral studies, the amount of LC-PUFAs administered in formula was chosen to produce the same concentration of arachidonic acid and DHA as in term breast milk. Recent studies report outcome data in preterm infants fed formula with DHA content 2–3 times higher than the current concentration. Overall, these studies show that providing larger amounts of DHA supplements is associated with better neurological outcomes and may provide other health benefits. One study further suggests that the smallest babies are the most vulnerable to DHA deficiency and likely to reap the greatest benefit from high-dose DHA supplementation. Current nutritional management may not provide sufficient amounts of preformed DHA during the parenteral and enteral nutrition periods and in very preterm/very low birth weight infants until due date and higher amounts than those routinely used are likely to be necessary to compensate for intestinal malabsorption, DHA oxidation, and early deficit. Recommendations for the healthcare provider are made in order to prevent lipid and more specifically LC-PUFA deficit. Research should be continued to fill the gaps in knowledge and to further refine the adequate intake for each group of preterm infants.

© 2014 S. Karger AG, Basel

Lipids provide infants with most of their energy needs; additionally, fat stores constitute the major energy reserve at the time of birth. However, very low birth weight (VLBW) infants and extremely low birth weight (ELBW) infants have very limited fat stores and thus depend on what is provided by enteral and parenteral nutrition [1].

Recent interest has focused on the quality of dietary lipid supply in early life as a major determinant of growth, infant development, and long-term health. Long-chain polyunsaturated fatty acids (LC-PUFAs) are of special interest since n–3 and n–6 LC-PUFAs are critical for neurodevelopment and especially the retina and visual cortical maturation. Altered neurodevelopment may lead to long-lasting effects that extend beyond the period of dietary insufficiency [1]. Furthermore, LC-PUFAs also have potentially significant modulatory effects on developmental processes that affect short- and long-term health outcomes related to growth, body composition, immune and allergic responses, and the prevalence of nutrition-related chronic diseases in later life [1]. LC-PUFA status of preterm infants depends on the amount of LC-PUFAs supplied exogenously, intestinal absorption, and, finally, the capacity of the preterm infant to synthesize the C:20 and C:22 elongated products of the parent fatty acids, α-linolenic (C18:3 n–3) and linoleic (C18:2 n–6) acid.

The aim of the present work is to review the recent literature and current recommendations regarding lipids as they pertain to preterm infant nutrition. Particularly, findings that relate to fetal accretion, intestinal absorption, metabolism, effects on development, and current practices and recommendations will be used to update recommendations for healthcare providers.

Total Dietary Lipid Intake, Cholesterol, Saturated Fats, Medium-Chain Triglycerides

Fat is the major source of energy in human milk (i.e. 40–55% of the total energy provided). The average fat content is about 3.8 g/100 ml and provides a high energy density per unit volume of the feed [1]. The variability of the fat content of human milk is very large and although milk fat content increases with duration of lactation, there appears to be little difference between milk from mothers of term and preterm babies. To date there are insufficient data to determine if addition of supplemental fat to human milk may affect short- or long-term growth outcomes and neurodevelopmental outcomes [2]. The major portion of the fat in human milk is found in the form of triglycerides (98% by weight of the total milk fat), the phospholipids (0.7%) and cholesterol (0.5%) contributing for only a small proportion of the total fat. Because of their non-polar nature, the lipids are mainly present in breast milk in the form of milk fat globules.

Intestinal fat digestion and absorption is reduced in preterm infants and as much as 20–30% of the dietary lipids are excreted in the stools [3]. The possible reasons are numerous and include low enzyme secretion (gastric, pancreatic colipase-dependent triglyceride lipase, bile-salt-stimulated lipase (BSSL), pancreatic phospholipase A_2) and low luminal bile salt concentration [3]. Furthermore, pasteurization (62.5°C for 30 min), used to provide microbiological safety of human milk, alters the nutritional and biological quality of human milk compared to fresh milk by activating the milk BSSL and changing the structure of milk fat globules.

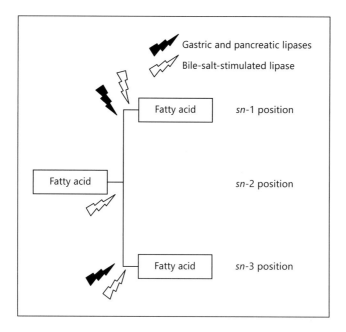

Fig. 1. Stereospecificity and chain lengths of fatty acids at the *sn*-1, *sn*-2 and *sn*-3 positions in triglycerides determine the metabolic fate of dietary fat during digestion and absorption. The enzymatic hydrolysis of dietary triglycerides is a major activity of digestion, largely occurring in the duodenum. Preferential hydrolysis by pancreatic and lipoprotein lipases target the fatty acids in the *sn*-1 and *sn*-3 positions resulting in two free fatty acids and one *sn*-2 monoglyceride which has a water solubility and is absorbed well. In human milk, palmitic acid and myristic acid are found in high proportions at the *sn*-2 position of triglycerides and is therefore well absorbed. The BSSL has no stereospecificity and equally cleaves the three fatty acids from the triglyceride.

Considerable amounts of cholesterol are deposited in tissues, including brain, during growth and dietary cholesterol contributes to the cholesterol pool in plasma and tissues. However, the major proportion of deposited cholesterol appears to be derived from endogenous synthesis and there is yet no evidence that the dietary supply of cholesterol affects nervous system development [1]. Whether or not the preterm infant would benefit from a dietary supply of cholesterol similar to that provided by the human milk (i.e. 10–20 mg/dl) is not known.

In breast milk, long-chain saturated fatty acids such as palmitic acid and myristic acid are found in high proportions (70 and 60% respectively) at the *sn*-2 position of triglycerides. The *sn*-1 and *sn*-3 positions are mainly occupied by unsaturated fatty acids such as oleic acid. The position of the fatty acid in triglycerides can affect digestibility and the metabolism because, during digestion, the gastric and pancreatic lipases prefer to release the fatty acids at the *sn*-1 and *sn*-3 positions in the proximal intestine (fig. 1). The fatty acid present at position *sn*-2 thus remains within a monoglyceride, which can then be more easily absorbed. Since the palmitic acid as free fatty acid in the lumen can form insoluble and unabsorbed calcium soaps, the *sn*-2

Lapillonne

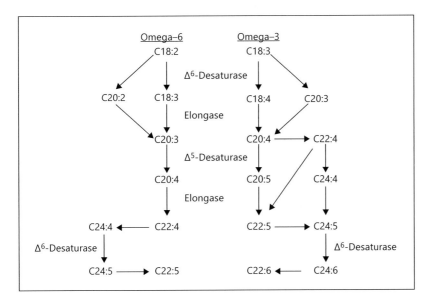

Fig. 2. Synthesis of omega–6 and omega–3 long-chain fatty acids from the parent essential fatty acids.

position of palmitic acid in breast milk ensures a maximum intestinal absorption co-efficient. The use of structured lipids (synthetic β-palmitate) increases fat and mineral absorption of preterm infants [4] and may offer health benefits (improved growth, modulation of microbiota and possible immune benefits).

Since the coefficient of fat absorption decreases with increasing chain length and increases with increasing number of double bonds of the fatty acid, high concentrations of medium-chain triglycerides (MCTs) have been used in some preterm formulas to increase the coefficient of fat absorption of preterm infants [3]. Beside their good absorption even in the presence of low intraluminal bile salts and pancreatic lipases, further arguments for the use of MCTs include are their carnitine-independent transport into the mitochondria and subsequent oxidation that is more rapid that for longer-chain fatty acids. Therefore, other substrates such as glucose and essential fatty acids (EFAs) can be spared from oxidation. Finally, there was no evidence of difference in short-term growth parameters when high and low MCT formulas were compared [5].

Overall, there are only few relevant new data compared to the previous edition [1] and the recent ESPGHAN recommendations for enteral nutrition of the preterm infant [6] that would support a significant modification of current recommendations.

PUFA Fetal Accretion Rate and Metabolism

LC-PUFA of the omega–6 (n–6) and omega-3 (n–3) series are derived from the EFA precursors linoleic acid (n–6) and α-linolenic acid (n–3) by consecutive enzymatic desaturation and chain elongation (fig. 2). LC-PUFAs are incorporated in practically all tissues of the fetus and infant, and they are the predominant PUFA in mammalian brain and neuronal tissues. In humans, most brain LC-PUFAs are accumulated during the phase of rapid brain growth in the last trimester of gestation and the first 2 years after birth.

Lipids are transferred across the placenta to meet fetal demands, including the EFAs linoleic acid (LA, C18:2 n–6) and α-linolenic acid (ALA, C18:3 n–3), as well as LC-PUFA. The placenta selectively favors the transfer of the fatty acids arachidonic acid (ARA) and docosahexaenoic acid (DHA) at all stages during pregnancy. Analyses of fetal autopsy tissue yield estimates of intrauterine accretion of LC-PUFAs and show that the accumulation of LC-PUFAs is not linear during the last trimester [7]. Recent estimates suggest that the fetal accretion rates are lower than previously estimated; transfer for ARA and DHA respectively was estimated at 26.4 and 9.5 mg/kg/day between 25 and 35 weeks of gestation and 31.6 and 13.8 mg/kg/day respectively between 35 and 40 weeks of gestation [7]. In term infants, most ARAs and DHAs are stored in adipose tissue (44 and 50%, respectively), substantial amounts of ARA are in skeletal muscle (40%) and brain (11%); for DHA, brain (23%) and skeletal muscle (21%) represent the most relevant tissue pools [7].

Evidence from stable isotope studies in premature infants demonstrates that ARA and DHA synthesis occurs to some degree at an early age when the infant would mostly depend on placental transfer [8]. Using the 'stable isotope natural abundance' approach in formula-fed preterm infants, mean endogenous synthesis of ARA has been estimated to be 27 and 12 mg/kg/day at 1 and 7 months of age, respectively, and that of DHA to be 13 and 2 mg/kg/day, respectively [9]. Whether conversion in human milk-fed preterm infants is similar to that in formula-fed preterm infants or if conversion is affected by the supply of dietary EFAs or LC-PUFAs remains to be established but this study demonstrates that endogenously synthesized LC-PUFAs are likely insufficient to meet requirements based on the fetal accretion rate.

Recent studies also suggest that variability in biochemical and functional central nervous system responses to changes in diet are partly explained by single nucleotide polymorphisms in genes responsible for EFA desaturation. This adds complexity to defining LC-PUFA needs and to establish the effect of other nutrients (i.e. LC-PUFA precursors, n–3/n–6 fatty acid ratio), which affect endogenous LC-PUFA synthesis [10].

Essential PUFA can be converted into long-chain derivatives (LC-PUFAs) or stored in tissues in the form of triglycerides or phospholipids, but they can also undergo total or partial β-oxidation, and hence supply energy or acetate units for the neosynthesis of saturated or monounsaturated fatty acids (fig. 3). ALA, and LA to a much lower extent, is particularly sensitive to oxidation and it is estimated that 75% of ingested ALA is either partially or completely oxidized. To date, none of the estimated accretion estimates have considered the balance between DHA oxidation and endogenous biosynthesis. Present evidence has shown that human adults oxidize DHA to a greater extent than previously thought [11]. DHA oxidation is likely to also occur in preterm infants, especially when energy intake does not meet requirements.

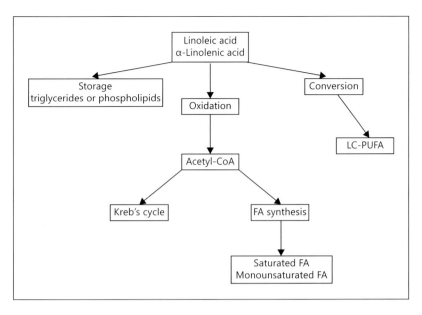

Fig. 3. Metabolic pathways of the essential fattys, linoleic acid and alpha-linolenic acid.

Overall these data demonstrate that exogenous supply of DHA, and to a lesser extent that of ARA, is critical in preterm infants and that both fatty acids are conditional essential nutrients in preterm infants.

Digestion and Absorption of LC-PUFAs

Human milk fat is provided in the form of milk fat globules mainly consisting of triglycerides (98%), phospholipids (1%), and cholesterol and cholesterol esters (0.5%). Breast milk supplies the two EFAs, LA and ALA, as well as their long-chain derivatives, ARA and DHA (table 1). In breast milk, LC-PUFAs are mainly triglycerides esterified at the *sn*-2 and *sn*-3 positions and can be part of the phospholipid fraction [12]. Human milk contains BSSL and palmitic acid in the β position of the triglycerides molecule. These unique components increase bioavailability of human milk fat by improving absorption and digestion. Heat inactivates BSSL and changes the structure of milk fat globules. These actions may be the reason why feeding pasteurized milk is associated with a 30% reduction in fat absorption and growth rate [13]. Fortification of human milk, particularly with calcium, may further impair LC-PUFA absorption. Overall, only 70–80% of ARA and DHA from pasteurized breast milk are absorbed by very preterm infants [14].

LC-PUFAs from fish oils or from single-cell algae are added as triglycerides to the fat blend of preterm formulas. DHA in algal oils has a weak positional specificity and contains equal amounts of DHA in the *sn*-1, *sn*-2, and *sn*-3 positions, unlike the DHA

Table 1. Composition of LC-PUFA in milk from mothers of preterm infants

Ref.	Site	Age, weeks	n	% total fatty acids		Sample time point(s)
				DHA	ARA	
[50]	USA	26–36	46	0.22	0.56	M (day of life 42)
[21]	Australia	<33	61	0.3	0.5	Pooled; 2-week intervals; 26–40 weeks
[51]	Netherlands	27–33	20	0.26	0.48	M (day of life 28)
[52]	Hungary	23–33	8	0.27	0.66	Mean 5 sample times over 3 weeks
[53]	Canada	28–34	25	0.3	0.54	<42 days of life
[54]	Netherlands	26–36	65	0.32	0.49	Mean C, T & M
[55]	Germany	24–33	19	0.32	0.59	Mean 4 sample times over 1 month
[56]	Netherlands	30–35	5	0.4	0.6	M (3rd week of life)
[57]	Finland	25–33	23	0.4	0.44	Mean 5 sample times over 3 months
[58]	Spain	33–36	6	0.55	0.69	Mean C, T & M
[19]	Norway	26–30	141	0.7	0.5	M (4 weeks of life)
[21]	Australia	<33	60[a]	1	0.5	Pooled; 2-week intervals; 26–40 weeks

C = Colostrum (week 1); T = transitional (week 2); M = mature (>2 weeks).
[a] Mothers were supplemented with 3 g of tuna oil per day.

triglycerides present in breast milk. These chemical differences may reduce absorption of DHA derived from algal sources. In contrast, fish oils provide DHA with a bond located in the *sn*-2 position which improves absorption; it also contains eicosapentaenoic acid (EPA), which is well absorbed but has not yet been proven to be safe in preterm infants when provided at a high amount [14].

Timing and Amount of Enteral Lipid Administration

The possible effects of enteral LC-PUFA supplementation which include improving neurological and visual development altering growth and modulation of immune functions and are extensively reviewed elsewhere [14–16]. In experimental studies, LC-PUFAs have been shown to play important roles in central nervous system development. Poor accumulation of retinal and brain DHA leads to abnormal retinal physiology, poor visual acuity, increased duration of visual fixation, and increased stereotyped behaviors and locomotor activity. The evidence most relevant to the issue of causality showed that control performance levels were restored when DHA was added to the diets of animals in which brain DHA concentration had been severely reduced. Nevertheless, the magnitude of these effects is not large, despite the fact that the studies were conducted under profound dietary restriction. The relevance of these findings to human development is unclear.

Studies in preterm humans indicate possible benefits for retinal and cognitive development, as suggested by greater retinal sensitivity to photic stimulation assessed by electroretinography, more mature visual acuity, and short-term effects on global

Lapillonne

developmental outcomes at 6–18 months after DHA supplementation of preterm infant formula in controlled clinical studies. With regard to neurodevelopment in preterm infants, recent meta-analyses suggest that benefits of formula supplementation with LC-PUFA are less clear [17]. This is somewhat surprising because many studies indicate that LC-PUFAs play an important role during development. Among many possible explanations for the difficulty in demonstrating clinical benefits of LC-PUFA supplementation in preterm formulas by meta-analysis are the extreme variability in study design of studies and the selection of relatively mature and healthy preterm infants which are likely less DHA-deficient than VLBW infants [14].

Interestingly, the amount of LC-PUFAs used in early studies was chosen to produce the same concentration of ARA and DHA in formula as in term breast milk (i.e. 0.2–0.4% fatty acids). This may not be a wise approach for preterm infants and, particularly, for very and extremely preterm infants because the amount of DHA provided by ingesting breast milk is below the in utero accretion rate. Three studies report outcome data in preterm infants fed milk with a higher DHA content of 0.5–1.7% of total fatty acids [18–22]. The first study, which examined the effect of providing DHA supplementation (0.50% of total fatty acids) for up to 9 months after term, showed that DHA improved growth in the whole cohort of preterm infants and improved mental development in boys [18].

In a more recent study, the effects of the supplementation of human milk with oils that provided an extra 32 mg of DHA and ARA per 100 ml was assessed [19]. This intervention started when 100 ml/kg of enteral feeding was tolerated and lasted until hospital discharge. Combined with the LC-PUFAs in human milk, the supplementation provided infants with a mean intake of 59 mg/kg/day of DHA and 48 mg mg/kg/day of ARA [17]. At the 6-month follow-up evaluation, the intervention group performed better than the control group in the problem-solving subscore of the Ages and Stages Questionnaire, and in the electrophysiologic assessment of event-related potentials suggesting better recognition memory. At 20 months' postnatal age, no differences in the mental and motor development scores of the Ages and Stages Questionnaire or in the Mental Development Index (MDI) score of the Bayley Scales of Infant Development were observed, but the intervention group had better results at 20 months at the free-play sessions, suggesting positive effects from supplementation on functions related to attention. Finally, plasma DHA concentration at discharge was positively correlated with the Bayley MDI and with 'sustained attention' [23].

The third study was designed to compare the effects of a high versus standard DHA intake (i.e. 1 vs. 0.35% total fatty acids as DHA) while ARA intake was kept constant (0.5% total fatty acids). This study included both breast-fed and formula-fed infants. Mothers who provided breast milk took capsules containing 3 g of either tuna oil (900 mg DHA) or soy oil (no DHA), which resulted in milk with either high or standard DHA content. A formula with matching high versus standard DHA concentrations was used for infants who required supplementary feeds. The feeding regimen was

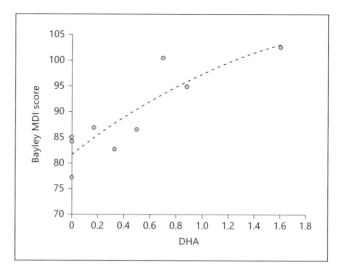

Fig. 4. Relationship of DHA intake (expressed as % of total fatty acid in milk during hospitalization) and Bayley MDI score at 18–20 months' corrected age of preterm infants [adapted from 12, 15, 34].

started between days 2 and 5 after birth and maintained until expected term. All infants received a standard term formula with DHA after the expected term. Visual acuity was improved significantly at 4 months' corrected age [22]. At 18 months there were no overall differences in MDI or in the Psychomotor Developmental Index (PDI) of the Bayley Scales, but fewer infants were classified as having an MDI score <70 [20]. Infants who weighed <1,250 g and were fed the high-DHA diet had a higher MDI score than controls (mean difference 4.6; 5% CI 0.1, 9.0; p < 0.05), but the difference was not significant when gestational age at delivery, sex, maternal education, and birth order were taken into account. Girls, but not boys, fed a high-DHA diet had higher MDI scores and were less likely to have mild or significant developmental delay than control girls. Finally, the early advantage seen on visual and cognitive functions did not translate into any clinically meaningful change in language development or behavior when assessed in early childhood [24]. Supplementation of VLBW infants with larger doses of DHA may be beneficial for functions beyond development since this trial did demonstrate a reduction in the incidence of oxygen treatment at 36 weeks (boys or infants with a birth weight of <1,250 g only) fed the high versus standard DHA intake, and a lower incidence of hay fever (boys only) at either 12 and 18 months [20, 25].

Overall, these studies show that providing larger amounts of DHA supplements is associated with better neurological outcomes (fig. 4) and possibly better respiratory outcomes. One study suggested that the smallest babies are the most vulnerable to DHA deficiency and likely to reap the greatest benefit from high-dose DHA supplementation [20]. The observation that a non-significant difference in mean MDI translated to fewer infants with a low MDI score suggests that a high dose of DHA is more efficient, or is only efficient, in certain subgroups of infants, probably those at high risk of DHA deficiency. It should also be noted that none of the studies prevented the

Lapillonne

early DHA deficit due to parenteral nutrition [26]. This early DHA deficit may explain, at least in part, why development assessed at 18 months remained below the normal range observed in term infants.

Practical Consideration with Regard to Enteral LC-PUFA Supplementation

The fat and fatty acid content of human milk is known to be highly variable. For example, fatty acid composition varies among countries, between specific women, by length of gestation and stage of lactation, throughout the day, and within a feeding. Variability is greater for ALA and DHA than for LA and ARA [27, 28]. The worldwide mean (±SD) concentration of DHA in breast milk (by weight) is 0.32 ± 0.22% (range 0.06–1.4%) and of ARA is 0.47 ± 0.13% (range 0.24–1%) [29]. When viewed as a percentage contribution to total fatty acids, DHA is often slightly higher in preterm than full-term milk [30]. The LC-PUFA content of banked human milk appears to be similar to mature milk [14].

Preterm infant formulas are currently supplemented routinely with commercially available sources of LC-PUFA so that the fatty acid composition resembles that of human milk. Most of the LC-PUFA oils added to infant formulas are derived from microorganisms. Some, however, are derived from a combination of low-EPA fish oil as a source of DHA and oil from microorganisms as a source of ARA. The usual DHA content of preterm formulas ranges between 0.2 and 0.4% of total fatty acids but the infants fed these formulas have constantly exhibited a reduced DHA status at time of discharge of hospital or expected term [14] (table 2).

Human milk responds to changes in the maternal diet, and LC-PUFA supplementation of mother increases DHA concentration in milk. Mothers who live in coastal areas or on islands produce milk with the highest DHA levels. At milk DHA contents above 0.8% of fatty acids (~45 mg/kg/day), none of the infants have an erythrocyte DHA concentration below 6% at expected term, but at milk DHA content of 1% (~55 mg/kg/day), the erythrocyte DHA concentration ranges between 6.5 and 9%, which are values expected to be seen in term infants at birth (table 2). Preterm infants receiving 59 mg DHA/kg/day exhibit increased plasma DHA concentration by 12% during time from study inclusion to hospital discharge [19].

Three of the six reports of preterm infants fed preterm formula supplemented with omega–3, but not omega–6 LC-PUFAs showed some indices of lower growth [31]. Since then, all trials have investigated the effects of omega–3 LC-PUFA supplementation in preterm formulas together with ARA supplementation and none have demonstrated a negative effect of supplementation on indices of growth [31]. Furthermore, supplementing lactating mothers with fish oil to increase the DHA content of human milk to approximately 1% dietary fatty acids had no effect on weight or head circumference up to 18 months' corrected age compared with standard feeding practice (0.2–0.3% DHA) [20]. In fact, preterm infants fed higher DHA were 0.7 cm longer at 18

Table 2. One approach, when feeding preterm infants, would be to match the concentrations of DHA in the fetal blood in utero. In that case, the DHA status of preterm infants should increase during hospitalization in order to reach, at expected term, a level comparable to that of term infants at birth [34]. Many studies have used LC-PUFA concentrations in plasma (PPL) or red blood cell (RBC) phospholipids in an attempt to describe the LC-PUFA status at expected term. DHA status of preterm infants fed current preterm formulas containing 0.2–0.37% fatty acids as DHA, which translates into 14 to 30 mg/kg/day, or breast milk exhibit a decline in their DHA status between birth and expected term (or hospital discharge). Those fed a DHA dose >45 mg/kg/day exhibit a DHA status that either increases during hospitalization or reach a level comparable to that of term infants

Reference	DHA, mg/kg/day	Effects on DHA status
Current DHA intake, see [14]	14–30	Decline in DHA status
[19]	32	Decline in DHA status (PPL)
[21]	45[a]	RBC DHA at expected term <6%[d]
[21]	54[b]	RBC DHA at expected term = 6.5–9%[d]
[19]	59[c]	Increase in DHA status by 12% (PPL)

[a] Human milk from Danish mothers likely consuming fish.
[b] Human milk supplemented with a DHA supplement.
[c] Mother's milk of women receiving 3 g of tuna oil per day.
[d] Values observed for RBC DHA in term infants at birth is ~8%.

months' corrected age despite a decline in preterm infant ARA status was observed [20]. It should be noted that the diet received by the preterm was not deprived in preformed ARA since the supplementation of the mother with fish oil did not alter the milk ARA content (i.e. 0.5 ± 0.1% of total fatty acids).

Strategies to increase DHA intake of preterm infants by supplementing lactating mothers with fish oil is very efficient to induce changes in milk DHA content but it leads to a large variation in the DHA content of the human milk with values as low as 0.3% and as high as 2.5% [21]. Therefore, adding DHA ± ARA directly into the feeding is likely the most reliable method for delivering adequate amount of LC-PUFAs to preterm infants [19].

Recommendations

- We strongly endorse human milk feeding as the preferred method of feeding preterm infants. Because of the variation of its DHA content due to the mother's diet, nutritional counseling during the lactation period is recommended.
- Nutrient recommendations for LC-PUFAs should be expressed as absolute amount per kg/day, not as a proportion of total fatty acids because the latter applies only if full enteral feeding is reached.
- DHA and ARA should be considered conditionally essential during early development and both should be provided during enteral feeding of preterm infants.
- A reasonable range of intake for DHA is to 18–60 mg/kg/day (approx. 0.3–1.0% of fatty acids). Intakes of 55–60 mg/kg/day (approx. 1.0%) of DHA from the

time of preterm birth to expected term have been tested, appear to be safe, promote normal DHA status, and appear to improve visual and neurocognitive functions and, therefore, are likely to be the estimated average requirement for very preterm infants.

- A reasonable range of intake for ARA is to 18–45 mg/kg/day. ARA should be provided during the DHA supplementation period but limited data are available to define the optimal dose of ARA. When a dose of DHA of 55–60 mg/kg/day is provided, the estimated average requirement for ARA is 35–45 mg/kg/day as this level has been shown to support growth.
- Limited data are available to define if there is any benefit for including EPA in the diet of preterm infants. Therefore, we recommend not exceeding 20 mg/kg/day of EPA, which is the mean amount of EPA provided daily by human milk + 1 SD when fed at 180 ml/kg/day.
- Limited data are available to define requirements of LC-PUFAs in subgroups of preterm infants, but it is likely that the infants with a birth weight <1,250 g will benefit the most of the higher intake.
- The recommendations for DHA, ARA, and EPA specified above should be continued until the infant reaches expected due date. After the expected due date, recommendations for term infants should be applied [32].

Timing and Amount of Parenteral Lipid Administration

Lipid emulsions are used in pediatric parenteral nutrition as a non-carbohydrate source of energy in a low volume and with low osmolarity. They also provide EFAs to prevent EFA deficiency [8]. Evidence has accumulated that in addition to their nutritional role as a source of energy and EFAs, lipid emulsions can influence numerous physiopathological processes including oxidative stress, immune responses and inflammation [33]. It has also become clear that preterm infants have special nutritional needs in early life and there is now a considerable body of evidence to suggest that lipids administered at this age may determine various outcomes in later life, including both physical growth and intellectual development [34].

Lipid emulsions contain various oils with egg yolk phospholipids as the emulsifier and glycerol to make the emulsion isotonic. For pediatric patients including preterm infants, the use of the standard 20% emulsions, which contain a lower ratio of phospholipid emulsifier/triglycerides than standard 10% lipid emulsions, is recommended since it allows more efficient triglyceride clearance, even at a higher triglyceride intake [8].

The initiation of lipids within the first 2 days of life in very preterm infants appears to be safe and well tolerated but few data support the early initiation of parenteral administration of lipids as a means to improve growth or decrease long-term morbidity [35, 36]. In contrast, a positive effect of early parenteral lipids on nitrogen balance has been shown in two separated studies [37, 38]. In the larger one, the efficacy of the introduction of a high dose of parenteral lipids (i.e. 2–3 g/kg/day) combined with 2.4 g/kg/day of amino acids (AA) from birth onwards was compared to a group receiving a similar amount of AA but no lipids [38]. The nitrogen balance on day 2 was significantly greater and plasma urea levels were significantly lower, suggesting that administration of parenteral lipids combined with AA from birth onwards improves conditions for anabolism. On the other hand, triglycerides and glucose concentrations were significantly greater in the AA + lipid group compared with the control group and more infants required insulin therapy. There were no benefits on growth, hospital clinical outcomes or total duration of hospital stay and, therefore, the clinical benefits of such a strategy remain to be proven.

Despite the limited available data, there are concerns that lipid emulsions might have potential adverse effects, including chronic lung disease, increases in pulmonary vascular resistance, impaired pulmonary gas exchange, bilirubin toxicity, sepsis and free radical stress [8]. Furthermore, it is a matter of debate as to what extent lipid emulsions are involved in the development of cholestasis [8, 39]. Also, questions arise on long-term detrimental effects of lipid emulsion since aortic stiffness and myocardial function in young adulthood has been shown to be associated with the fact of being exposed to soybean lipid emulsion during neonatal life [40]. Guidelines with regard to side effects or use in special disease conditions are therefore prudent and it is recommended to avoid the supply of lipid emulsions in high dosages and to adjust the delivery of intravenous lipids to plasma triglyceride concentrations [8].

Practical Implication with Regard to Parenteral LC-PUFA Administration

The adequacy of historical soybean lipid emulsions for the nutritional needs of newborn and premature infants might be questioned. Although an intake of PUFA is required to prevent any EFA deficiency, it is known that excessive intake, particularly of LA, has detrimental effects which include a decrease in the formation of DHA acid from its parent precursor. A reduction in the amounts of potentially pro-inflammatory n–6 fatty acids from soybean oil may be indicated, for example in premature infants with compromised lung function given their influence on pulmonary vasculature [41, 42].

The provision of alternative emulsions containing oil mixtures which are less inflammatory, such as those rich in n–9 fatty acids, may be better for redox status. Despite a lower PUFA content in olive oil/soybean oil emulsion, higher levels of n–6 PUFA intermediates were observed, suggesting a higher degree of endogenous LA conversion [43].

The MCT-containing lipid emulsions contain equal proportions of long- and medium-chain triglycerides. These emulsions are of possible interest since they may, to some extent, protect LC-PUFAs from β-oxidation, confer some benefit with regard to fat oxidation in preterm infants, and increase the incorporation of EFAs and LC-PUFAs into circulating lipids [39].

Whether carnitine supplementation of parenterally fed neonates is required to improve long-chain fatty acid oxidation, lipid tolerance and ketogenesis are still a matter of debate, but to date, there is no evidence to support the routine supplementation of parenterally fed neonates with carnitine [44].

Finally, the use of fish oil in lipid emulsions, which has specific anti-inflammatory effects via n–3 fatty acids, might offer additional benefits. There is a theoretical advantage to use lipid emulsions containing fish oil to maintain adequate DHA status. Since it has been shown that cord plasma and red blood cell DHA content increases with gestational age, it may expected that infants receiving parenteral lipids exhibit similar pattern of circulating DHA. The few data published to date show that providing lipid emulsion containing 10% fish oil at a dose of ≤2 g/kg/day fail to demonstrate an increase in circulating DHA [45] whereas providing a target dose of 3–3.5 g/kg/day of a lipid emulsion containing 15% of fish oil beneficially modulates the DHA profile [46].

Although these alternative lipid emulsions appear promising, the clinical benefits of lipid emulsions that are not purely soybean-based (e.g. MCT-soybean, olive-soybean, and soybean-MCT-olive-fish emulsions) remain to be demonstrated. In a recent meta-analysis, only a weak association of such lipid emulsions with fewer episodes of sepsis has been demonstrated, with no beneficial effects on bronchopulmonary dysplasia, necrotizing enterocolitis, retinopathy of prematurity, patent ductus arteriosus, intraventricular hemorrhage, significant jaundice, hypertriacylglycerolemia, or hyperglycemia [36]. Other studies demonstrated that lipid emulsions containing fish oil lower plasma lipids [45], bilirubinemia [46] or plasma γ-glutamyl transferase [47] but have no preventive effect on cholestasis [48]. Finally, a randomized but not blinded study suggests that emulsions containing fish oil may reduce the risk of severe retinopathy [49, 59–61]. Overall, lipid emulsion containing fish oil appears to have potential beneficial effects in preterm infants. However, these lipid emulsions, primarily designed for adult care, provide as much EPA as DHA and no ARA, and it remains to be demonstrated that such intakes are safe in preterm infants.

Recommendations
- The initiation of lipids within the first 2 days of life in very preterm infants appears to be safe and well tolerated. When infused at a similar amount (g/kg/day) than that of amino acid, a dose of 2–3 g/kg/day of parenteral lipids can safely be used from birth onwards.
- Lipid emulsions that are not purely soybean-based should be preferred over the soybean or soybean/sunflower-based emulsion since they reduce the risk of sepsis and promote more favorable LC-PUFA profile.

- Lipid emulsions containing fish oil are potentially useful to favor better DHA status and improve various health outcomes. Their routine use is not recommended since their clinical benefits and safety have not yet been fully demonstrated in preterm infants.

Disclosure Statement

The author has no conflicts of interest to disclose.

References

1 Koletzko B, Innis SM: Lipids; in Tsang RC, Uauy R, Koletzko B, Zlotkin SH (eds): Nutrition of the Preterm Infant, Scientific Basis and Practical Guidelines. Cincinnati, Digital Educational Publishing, Inc, 2005, pp 97–140.
2 Kuschel CA, Harding JE: Fat supplementation of human milk for promoting growth in preterm infants. Cochrane Database Syst Rev 2000;2:CD000341.
3 Lindquist S, Hernell O: Lipid digestion and absorption in early life: an update. Curr Opin Clin Nutr Metab Care 2010;13:314–320.
4 Carnielli VP, Luijendijk IH, van Goudoever JB, Sulkers EJ, Boerlage AA, Degenhart HJ, et al: Feeding premature newborn infants palmitic acid in amounts and stereoisomeric position similar to that of human milk: effects on fat and mineral balance. Am J Clin Nutr 1995;61:1037–1042.
5 Klenoff-Brumberg HL, Genen LH: High versus low medium chain triglyceride content of formula for promoting short term growth of preterm infants. Cochrane Database Syst Rev 2003;1:CD002777.
6 Agostoni C, Buonocore G, Carnielli VP, De Curtis M, Darmaun D, Decsi T, et al: Enteral nutrient supply for preterm infants: commentary from the European Society of Paediatric Gastroenterology, Hepatology and Nutrition Committee on Nutrition. J Pediatr Gastroenterol Nutr 2010;50:85–91.
7 Kuipers RS, Luxwolda MF, Offringa PJ, Boersma ER, Dijck-Brouwer DA, Muskiet FA: Fetal intrauterine whole body linoleic, arachidonic and docosahexaenoic acid contents and accretion rates. Prostaglandins Leukot Essent Fatty Acids 2012;86:13–20.
8 Koletzko B, Goulet O, Hunt J, Krohn K, Shamir R: 1. Guidelines on Paediatric Parenteral Nutrition of the European Society of Paediatric Gastroenterology, Hepatology and Nutrition (ESPGHAN) and the European Society for Clinical Nutrition and Metabolism (ESPEN), Supported by the European Society of Paediatric Research (ESPR). J Pediatr Gastroenterol Nutr 2005;41(suppl 2):S1–S87.

9 Carnielli VP, Simonato M, Verlato G, Luijendijk I, De Curtis M, Sauer PJ, et al: Synthesis of long-chain polyunsaturated fatty acids in preterm newborns fed formula with long-chain polyunsaturated fatty acids. Am J Clin Nutr 2007;86:1323–1330.
10 Lattka E, Illig T, Heinrich J, Koletzko B: Do FADS genotypes enhance our knowledge about fatty acid related phenotypes? Clin Nutr 2010;29:277–287.
11 Plourde M, Chouinard-Watkins R, Vandal M, Zhang Y, Lawrence P, Brenna JT, et al: Plasma incorporation, apparent retroconversion and β-oxidation of ^{13}C-docosahexaenoic acid in the elderly. Nutr Metab (Lond) 2011;8:5.
12 Straarup EM, Lauritzen L, Faerk J, Hoy Deceased CE, Michaelsen KF: The stereospecific triacylglycerol structures and fatty acid profiles of human milk and infant formulas. J Pediatr Gastroenterol Nutr 2006;42:293–299.
13 Andersson Y, Savman K, Blackberg L, Hernell O: Pasteurization of mother's own milk reduces fat absorption and growth in preterm infants. Acta Paediatr 2007;96:1445–1449.
14 Lapillonne A, Groh-Wargo S, Gonzalez CH, Uauy R: Lipid needs of preterm infants: updated recommendations. J Pediatr 2013;162:S37–S47.
15 Atwell K, Collins CT, Sullivan TR, Ryan P, Gibson RA, Makrides M, et al: Respiratory hospitalisation of infants supplemented with docosahexaenoic acid as preterm neonates. J Paediatr Child Health 2013;49:E17–E22.
16 Molloy C, Doyle LW, Makrides M, Anderson PJ: Docosahexaenoic acid and visual functioning in preterm infants: a review. Neuropsychol Rev 2012;22:425–437.
17 Schulzke SM, Patole SK, Simmer K: Long-chain polyunsaturated fatty acid supplementation in preterm infants. Cochrane Database Syst Rev 2011;2:CD000375.

18 Fewtrell MS, Abbott RA, Kennedy K, Singhal A, Morley R, Caine E, et al: Randomized, double-blind trial of long-chain polyunsaturated fatty acid supplementation with fish oil and borage oil in preterm infants. J Pediatr 2004;144:471–479.

19 Henriksen C, Haugholt K, Lindgren M, Aurvag AK, Ronnestad A, Gronn M, et al: Improved cognitive development among preterm infants attributable to early supplementation of human milk with docosahexaenoic acid and arachidonic acid. Pediatrics 2008;121:1137–1145.

20 Makrides M, Gibson RA, McPhee AJ, Collins CT, Davis PG, Doyle LW, et al: Neurodevelopmental outcomes of preterm infants fed high-dose docosahexaenoic acid: a randomized controlled trial. JAMA 2009;301:175–182.

21 Smithers LG, Gibson RA, McPhee A, Makrides M: Effect of two doses of docosahexaenoic acid in the diet of preterm infants on infant fatty acid status: results from the DINO trial. Prostaglandins Leukot Essent Fatty Acids 2008;79:141–146.

22 Smithers LG, Gibson RA, McPhee A, Makrides M: Higher dose of docosahexaenoic acid in the neonatal period improves visual acuity of preterm infants: results of a randomized controlled trial. Am J Clin Nutr 2008;88:1049–1056.

23 Westerberg AC, Schei R, Henriksen C, Smith L, Veierod MB, Drevon CA, et al: Attention among very low birth weight infants following early supplementation with docosahexaenoic and arachidonic acid. Acta Paediatr 2011;100:47–52.

24 Smithers LG, Collins CT, Simmonds LA, Gibson RA, McPhee A, Makrides M: Feeding preterm infants milk with a higher dose of docosahexaenoic acid than that used in current practice does not influence language or behavior in early childhood: a follow-up study of a randomized controlled trial. Am J Clin Nutr 2010;91:628–634.

25 Manley BJ, Makrides M, Collins CT, McPhee AJ, Gibson RA, Ryan P, et al: High-dose docosahexaenoic acid supplementation of preterm infants: respiratory and allergy outcomes. Pediatrics 2011;128:e71–e77.

26 Lapillonne A, Eleni dit Trolli SE, Kermorvant-Duchemin E: Postnatal docosahexaenoic acid deficiency is an inevitable consequence of current recommendations and practice in preterm infants. Neonatology 2010;98:397–403.

27 Brenna JT, Lapillonne A: Background paper on fat and fatty acid requirements during pregnancy and lactation. Ann Nutr Metab 2009;55:97–122.

28 Yuhas R, Pramuk K, Lien EL: Human milk fatty acid composition from nine countries varies most in DHA. Lipids 2006;41:851–858.

29 Brenna JT, Varamini B, Jensen RG, Diersen-Schade DA, Boettcher JA, Arterburn LM: Docosahexaenoic and arachidonic acid concentrations in human breast milk worldwide. Am J Clin Nutr 2007;85:1457–1464.

30 Bokor S, Koletzko B, Decsi T: Systematic review of fatty acid composition of human milk from mothers of preterm compared to full-term infants. Ann Nutr Metab 2007;51:550–556.

31 Lapillonne A, Carlson SE: Polyunsaturated fatty acids and infant growth. Lipids 2001;36:901–911.

32 Nations FaAOotU (ed): Fat and Fatty Acids in Human Nutrition. Report of an Expert Consultation. FAO Food and Nutrition Reports. Rome, FAO 2010.

33 Calder PC, Jensen GL, Koletzko BV, Singer P, Wanten GJ: Lipid emulsions in parenteral nutrition of intensive care patients: current thinking and future directions. Intensive Care Med 2010;36:735–749.

34 Eleni dit Trolli SE, Kermorvant-Duchemin E, Huon C, Bremond-Gignac D, Lapillonne A: Early lipid supply and neurological development at one year in very low birth weight preterm infants. Early Hum Dev 2012;88(suppl 1):S25–S29.

35 Simmer K, Rao SC: Early introduction of lipids to parenterally-fed preterm infants. Cochrane Database Syst Rev 2005;2:CD005256.

36 Vlaardingerbroek H, Veldhorst MA, Spronk S, van den Akker CH, van Goudoever JB: Parenteral lipid administration to very-low-birth-weight infants – early introduction of lipids and use of new lipid emulsions: a systematic review and meta-analysis. Am J Clin Nutr 2012;96:255–268.

37 Ibrahim HM, Jeroudi MA, Baier RJ, Dhanireddy R, Krouskop RW: Aggressive early total parental nutrition in low-birth-weight infants. J Perinatol 2004;24:482–486.

38 Vlaardingerbroek H, Vermeulen MJ, Rook D, van den Akker CH, Dorst K, Wattimena JL, et al: Safety and efficacy of early parenteral lipid and high-dose amino acid administration to very low birth weight infants. J Pediatr 2013;163:638–644.e1–e5.

39 Krohn K, Koletzko B: Parenteral lipid emulsions in paediatrics. Curr Opin Clin Nutr Metab Care 2006;9:319–323.

40 Lewandowski AJ, Lazdam M, Davis E, Kylintireas I, Diesch J, Francis J, et al: Short-term exposure to exogenous lipids in premature infants and long-term changes in aortic and cardiac function. Arterioscler Thromb Vasc Biol 2011;31:2125–2135.

41 Driscoll DF, Bistrian BR, Demmelmair H, Koletzko B: Pharmaceutical and clinical aspects of parenteral lipid emulsions in neonatology. Clin Nutr 2008;27:497–503.

42 Houeijeh A, Aubry E, Coridon H, Montaigne K, Sfeir R, Deruelle P, et al: Effects of n–3 polyunsaturated fatty acids in the fetal pulmonary circulation. Crit Care Med 2011;39:1431–1438.

43 Gobel Y, Koletzko B, Bohles HJ, Engelsberger I, Forget D, Le Brun A, et al: Parenteral fat emulsions based on olive and soybean oils: a randomized clinical trial in preterm infants. J Pediatr Gastroenterol Nutr 2003;37:161–167.

44 Cairns PA, Stalker DJ: Carnitine supplementation of parenterally fed neonates. Cochrane Database Syst Rev 2000;4:CD000950.

45 D'Ascenzo R, D'Egidio S, Angelini L, Bellagamba MP, Manna M, Pompilio A, et al: Parenteral nutrition of preterm infants with a lipid emulsion containing 10% fish oil: effect on plasma lipids and long-chain polyunsaturated fatty acids. J Pediatr 2011; 159:33–38.e1.

46 Rayyan M, Devlieger H, Jochum F, Allegaert K: Short-term use of parenteral nutrition with a lipid emulsion containing a mixture of soybean oil, olive oil, medium-chain triglycerides, and fish oil: a randomized double-blind study in preterm infants. JPEN J Parenter Enteral Nutr 2012;36:81S–94S.

47 Tomsits E, Pataki M, Tolgyesi A, Fekete G, Rischak K, Szollar L: Safety and efficacy of a lipid emulsion containing a mixture of soybean oil, medium-chain triglycerides, olive oil, and fish oil: a randomised, double-blind clinical trial in premature infants requiring parenteral nutrition. J Pediatr Gastroenterol Nutr 2010;51:514–521.

48 Savini S, D'Ascenzo R, Biagetti C, Serpentini G, Pompilio A, Bartoli A, et al: The effect of five intravenous lipid emulsions on plasma phytosterols in preterm infants receiving parenteral nutrition: a randomized clinical trial. Am J Clin Nutr 2013;98:312–318.

49 Pawlik D, Lauterbach R, Walczak M, Hurkala J, Sherman MP: Fish-oil fat emulsion supplementation reduces the risk of retinopathy in very low birth weight infants: a prospective, randomized study. JPEN J Parenter Enteral Nutr 2013, Epub ahead of print.

50 Bitman J, Wood L, Hamosh M, Hamosh P, Mehta NR: Comparison of the lipid composition of breast milk from mothers of term and preterm infants. Am J Clin Nutr 1983;38:300–312.

51 Carnielli VP, Verlato G, Pederzini F, Luijendijk I, Boerlage A, Pedrotti D, et al: Intestinal absorption of long-chain polyunsaturated fatty acids in preterm infants fed breast milk or formula. Am J Clin Nutr 1998;67:97–103.

52 Kovács A, Funke S, Marosvölgyi T, Burus I, Decsi T: Fatty acids in early human milk after preterm and full-term delivery. J Pediatr Gastroenterol Nutr 2005;41:454–459.

53 Clandinin MT, Van Aerde JE, Parrott A, Field CJ, Euler AR, Lien EL: Assessment of the efficacious dose of arachidonic and docosahexaenoic acids in preterm infant formulas: fatty acid composition of erythrocyte membrane lipids. Pediatr Res 1997;42:819–825.

54 Beijers RJ, Schaafsma A: Long-chain polyunsaturated fatty acid content in Dutch preterm breast milk; differences in the concentrations of docosahexaenoic acid and arachidonic acid due to length of gestation. Early Hum Dev 1996;44:215–223.

55 Genzel-Boroviczény O, Wahle J, Koletzko B: Fatty acid composition of human milk during the first month after term and preterm delivery. Eur J Pediatr 1997;156:142–147.

56 Jacobs NJ, van Zoeren-Grobben D, Drejer GF, Bindels JG, Berger HM: Influence of long-chain unsaturated fatty acids in formula feeds on lipid peroxidation and antioxidants in preterm infants. Pediatr Res 1996;40:680–686.

57 Luukkainen P, Salo MK, Nikkari T: The fatty acid composition of banked human milk and infant formulas: the choices of milk for feeding preterm infants. Eur J Pediatr 1995;154:316–319.

58 Rueda R, Ramírez M, García-Salmerón JL, Maldonado J, Gil A: Gestational age and origin of human milk influence total lipid and fatty acid contents. Ann Nutr Metab 1998;42:12–22.

59 Lapillonne A, Jensen CL: Reevaluation of the DHA requirement for the premature infant. Prostaglandins Leukot Essent Fatty Acids 2009;81:143–150.

60 Klein CJ: Nutrient requirements for preterm infant formulas. J Nutr 2002;132:1395S–1577S.

61 Tsang RC, Uauy R, Koletzko B, Zlotkin SH: Nutrition of the Preterm Infant: Scientific Basis and Practical Guidelines. Cincinnati, Digital Educating Publishing, Inc, 2005, p 427.

Prof. Alexandre Lapillonne, MD, PhD
Department of Neonatology
Necker-Enfants Malades Hospital
149 rue de Sevres, FR–75015 Paris (France)
E-Mail alexandre.lapillonne@nck.aphp.fr

Koletzko B, Poindexter B, Uauy R (eds): Nutritional Care of Preterm Infants: Scientific Basis and Practical Guidelines.
World Rev Nutr Diet. Basel, Karger, 2014, vol 110, pp 99–120 (DOI: 10.1159/000358461)

Water, Sodium, Potassium and Chloride

Christoph Fusch[a] · Frank Jochum[b]

[a]Department of Pediatrics, McMaster University & Hamilton Health Sciences, Hamilton, Ont., Canada;
[b]Department of Pediatrics, Evangelisches Waldkrankenhaus Spandau, Berlin, Germany

Reviewed by Brenda Poindexter, Riley Hospital for Children at Indiana University Health, Indianapolis, Ind., USA;
Ricardo Uauy, National Institute of Nutrition and Food Technology, University of Chile, Santiago de Chile, Chile

Abstract

The sudden disruption of excessive placental supply with fluids and electrolytes is challenging for
neonatal physiology during the period of postnatal adaptation. Different from many other nutrients,
the body experiences large changes in daily requirements during the first 7–14 postnatal days, and
on the other hand does not tolerate conditions of excess and deficiency very well. Imbalances of
fluid and electrolytes are common in neonates, which – in addition – might be further aggravated
by NICU treatment procedures. Therefore, fluid and electrolyte management can be one of the most
challenging aspects of neonatal care of the premature infant. An understanding of the physiological
adaptation process to extrauterine life – and how immaturity effects that transition – is the basis
which is needed to understand and manage fluid and electrolyte balance in premature infants. This
chapter addresses the physiology of postnatal adaptation and other aspects of fluid and electrolyte
management (concerning potassium, sodium and chloride) of the preterm infant.

© 2014 S. Karger AG, Basel

'Water – the major nutrient' is the title of a review published in 1982 by Bent Friis-Hansen in the *Journal of Pediatrics* [1]. This title illustrates that water represents the major component of the human body as well as of enteral and parenteral nutrition [2]. The homeostasis of a mammalian organism depends on intact water metabolism. Water is integral to all of life's functions. It carries nutrients to cells, removes waste, and makes up the physicochemical milieu that allows cellular work to occur. Different from most nutrients, the human body has no water stores and needs a continuous 'short interval' supply to assure basal metabolic processes.

Water physiology and homeostasis show the highest inter- and intraindividual variation when compared to all other nutrients. This is caused by individual differences in body size, proportion, body surface, skin properties as well as conditions occurring during the period of postnatal transition in relation to immaturity, postnatal age and intensity of support needed.

Physiology

Knowledge about the physiology of water and electrolyte metabolism is needed for safe administration of fluids and electrolytes, and to become competent to adjust these to actual needs of a newborn in order to avoid harm. Too low intake may compromise circulation and metabolism, while inappropriate high intake of fluid or electrolytes may lead to or promote conditions like patent ductus arteriosus (PDA), chronic lung disease (CLD), etc.

Water is not equally distributed within the different body compartments. Fat mass is the energy store of the body and shows the highest inter- and intraindividual variability of all body compartments. Energy metabolism occurs only in the cytoplasma of the adipocyte, mostly to maintain intracellular homeostasis, to store and release triglycerides as well as to produce hormones like leptin. The major part of the adipocyte is the triglyceride-containing vacuole which is assumed to be free of water.

Lean mass represents a metabolically active cell mass. It consumes most of the body's energy by substrate oxidation and protein synthesis. Water is found only in lean tissue, thus metabolism of water and electrolytes is correlated closer with lean than with total body mass – of importance when subjects with different body composition are compared. Body water decreases remarkably during early life – from 90% at 24 gestational weeks to 75% at term [3, 4], mostly because fat mass is accumulated during the third trimester [5]. The time course of the water content of the human body during the entire lifespan is given in figure 1.

Body Water Compartments

Within lean mass body water is separated in different compartments, each playing a different physiological role and experiencing different physiological conditions and regulatory mechanisms.

Intracellular Fluid (ICF) and Extracellular Fluid (ECF): The ICF is located within the cytoplasm, enveloped by the double-lipid cellular membrane. Its leading ion is potassium. ECF represents water volume outside the cell membrane. Its leading ion is sodium. ECF is subdivided into intravascular (IVC) and extravascular (EVC) compartments as well as a 'third space' which characterizes free fluid in preformed cavities under physiological (e.g. urine, CSF) and pathological conditions (e.g. ascites, pleural effusions). ECF and IVC decrease during childhood. In preterm and term infants, total blood volume is 85–100 ml/kg compared to 60–70 ml/kg in adults [6–8].

The sizes of water compartments in healthy term infants on day 1 of life are (% of body weight) 75 ± 5% for body water, 31 ± 6% for ECF, 44 ± 8% for ICF and 10 ± 1% for IVC [9]. In ELBW infants ECF is 48 ± 11% [10].

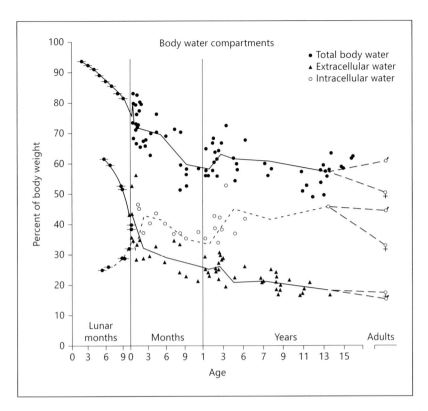

Fig. 1. Age-related changes of total body water and its compartments, the intracellular and extracellular volume, from fetal life until adolescence [2].

Mechanisms That Regulate Body Fluids (fig. 2)

Control of Body Water: Whole-body water homeostasis is regulated via ECF, it serves as an interface with the environment. ECF regulation (intake, absorption, excretion) is effected via IVC volume. The amount of water and sodium is independently regulated – within certain limits. The regulatory response must (1) maintain adequate circulation and blood pressure and (2) keep osmolality of the ECF compartment within 3% of the set point (280–290 mosm) [11–13]. Regulation is achieved through changes in intake via (i) thirst (except for newborns when intake is controlled by others), (ii) vascular tone, heart rate and contractility, and (iii) renal excretion of water and electrolytes. The system is modulated through hormonal action on renal excretion of water and solutes, including the renin-angiotensin-aldosterone system, arginine vasopressin, and atrial natriuretic peptide.

The ECF control mechanism functions as follows: ECF increase leads to an increase in IVC volume and blood pressure. Increased vascular pressure increases urinary flow until the ECF volume returns to baseline. Hypotonicity suppresses antidi-

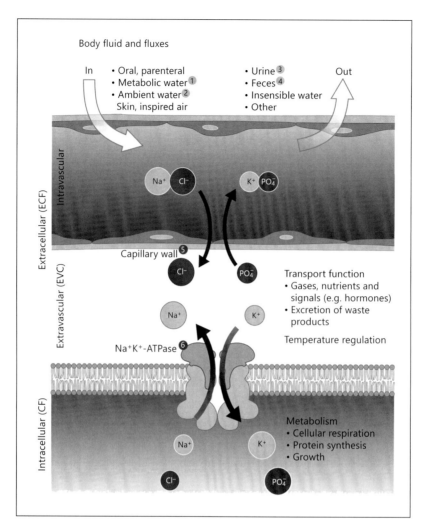

Fig. 2. Water and electrolyte fluxes between body water compartments. Remarks: 1) metabolic water production depending on exact intake of carbohydrates, protein and fat (approx. 15 ml/kg/day), 2) input via skin and inspired air (see fig. 3), 3) volume depending upon need for excretion of fixed acids and urea and desired urine osmolarity, 4) fecal water losses: quantities are negligibly small in healthy subjects, but considerable in diarrhea and/or in presence of ileostoma (e.g. NEC surgery), 5) oncotic pressure, 6) activity of Na^+/K^+-ATPase defines the long-term ratio of ECF/ICF; short-term changes are subject to short-term variation of ECV; content of water and electro-/osmolytes: any change in either ICV or ECV osmolarity will result in movement of water into the compartment with the higher osmolarity.

uretic hormone secretion, thus diluting urinary osmotic load [13, 14]. Conversely, a decrease in ECF volume results in decreased cardiac output and glomerular filtration pressure, leading to decreased urinary flow that lasts until intake replenishes the lost volume. Hypertonicity, which accompanies many low-volume states, stimulates thirst and renal resorption of water [15].

Fusch · Jochum

Regulation of ICF and ECF: The different electrolyte concentrations of ICF and ECF are achieved by energy-dependent active transport of Na^+/K^+-ATPase. It also establishes the transmembranal Na^+/K^+ gradient by continuously shuffling Na^+ ions out of, and K^+ ions into the cell. Cellular membranes thus appear to be relatively impermeable to sodium. The Na^+/K^+-ATPase pump is the most important regulator of the ICF:ECF ratio [16, 17]. As a consequence, ICF is shielded from direct interface with the external environment preventing most tissues from sudden and large changes of solute or water concentration. Studies in endothelial cells show that Na^+/K^+-ATPase consumes about 5–15% of resting energy expenditure [18]. Like other enzymes, the Na^+/K^+-ATPase pump depends on pH and temperature optima and is disturbed in cases when the supply of oxygen and energy is insufficient. Other regulatory mechanisms of this enzyme are poorly understood. Dysfunction of the Na^+/K^+-ATPase leads to an osmotic sodium shift from ECF to the ICF. This can produce intracellular edema compromising cell integrity.

Regulation of IVF and EVF: Under normal conditions (intact capillary wall) the EVF:IVF ratio is mainly dependent on blood pressure and oncotic-hydrostatic pressure as well as from the permeability of the capillary wall. Compared to term infants and adults, the EVF:IVF ratio is elevated in preterm infants [2]. Permeability of the capillary wall does not seem to be higher in neonates when compared to later life [19]. However, plasma oncotic pressure has been proven to be lower in term neonates and preterm infants compared to adults. This is especially the case in respiratory distress syndrome (RDS) and may therefore explain changes in the EVF:IVF ratio [20–24].

An increased EVF:IVF ratio in sepsis is due to cytokine-induced 'leaky' capillary walls. Depending on the degree of capillary leakage, fluid and proteins may migrate from IVF to EVF thereby aggravating the loss of IVF [25].

Fetal Water and Electrolyte Metabolism: During fetal life there is transplacental net transfer of water to the fetus. Sodium and other electrolytes are actively (co-)transported via different mechanisms [26–28], such that an equilibrium between mother and fetus is established. Maternal plasma electrolyte concentrations determine fetal levels. Under normal conditions the exchange is not rate-limited.

Urine production starts at 5 weeks' gestation [29]. At 20 and 32 weeks' gestation, 4.5 and 6 ml/kg/h are produced, respectively. Urinary production at term is 8–15 ml/kg/h and up to 8 mmol Na/kg/day are excreted, which is considerably higher than after completed postnatal adaptation [26–30].

Fetal urine osmolarity is low, usually not exceeding serum levels. Thus, fractional urinary Na excretion of the human fetus is very high (i.e. 8–18%) compared to later postnatal life (<1%) [30]. Because of excessive maternal donation of fluid and electrolytes, fetal kidneys are not forced and/or able to produce concentrated urine of high osmolarity which is also accompanied by the anatomic and physiological immaturity of fetal kidneys.

Factors Influencing Water Input (fig. 3): Water influx occurs via metabolic water, oral and parenteral intake. Oxidation of carbohydrates and fat generates 0.6 ml

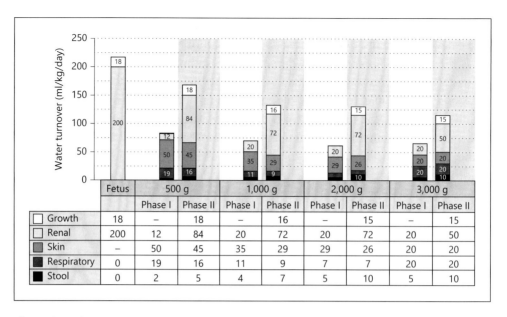

	Fetus	500 g		1,000 g		2,000 g		3,000 g	
		Phase I	Phase II	Phase I	Phase II	Phase I	Phase II	Phase I	Phase II
☐ Growth	18	–	18	–	16	–	15	–	15
☐ Renal	200	12	84	20	72	20	72	20	50
▨ Skin	–	50	45	35	29	29	26	20	20
▩ Respiratory	0	19	16	11	9	7	7	20	20
■ Stool	0	2	5	4	7	5	10	5	10

Fig. 3. Contributions to water turnover (ml/kg/day) as related to gestational and postnatal age. Phase I represents day 1 of life; phase II the period of stable growth. Remarks: 1) for infants with birth weights <2,000 g thermoneutral incubator treatment at 80–90% relative humidity was assumed, 2) figures for AGA term infants are measured data, averaged from different studies (for references see text), corresponding figures for preterm infants are estimated (for references see text), 3) figures for fetal period reflect last trimester conditions.

H_2O/g CHO and 1.0 ml H_2O/g fat. Oxidation of proteins – an unwanted pathway – generates 0.4 ml H_2O/g protein oxidized [31]. Thus, production of metabolic water is 5–15 ml/kg/day, provided that the infant is adequately supplied with nutrients. Increased metabolism due to environmental stress or disease enhances metabolic water up to 20 ml/kg/day [32, 33]. In older subjects, enteral intake is usually regulated by thirst or regulated by social factors. These control mechanisms do not apply in premature and term infants because intake is controlled by parents, nurses, or doctors.

Factors Influencing Water Output (fig. 3): Water output occurs by insensible water loss via skin and respiration, by urine production, fecal losses, and growth. Transcutaneous losses depend from gestational and postnatal age and from environment. Small infants have higher losses due to an unfavorable body surface:body mass ratio [34–44]. The amount of insensible water loss mainly determines the need for fluid administration during the first postnatal days.

Evaporation of water from the upper respiratory tract accounts for one third of net insensible water loss [45]. Higher respiratory rates in premature infants cause larger losses (0.8–0.9 ml/kg/h) when compared with term neonates (0.5 ml/kg/h) [45, 46]. Water losses can be considerably reduced (near zero) when infants are cared in 85–100% relative humidity and 37°C air.

Minimum urine volume of newborns may be calculated from the potential renal solute load (PRSL) of the diet provided and from their ability to concentrate urine. PRSL refers to solutes of dietary origin that need to be excreted in urine if none was diverted into formation of new tissue and none was lost through non-renal routes. Excretion of these solutes requires water and the capacity of neonatal kidneys to concentrate solutes is limited, therefore renal solute load exerts a major effect on water balance [47]. The maximum urinary concentration is dependent on gestational age: it may be up to 700 mosm/l in term, but <500 mosm/l in preterm infants [48–50]. On the other hand, preterm infants may achieve a maximum water diuresis of 6.0 ml/kg/h of free water in the presence of a total urine production of 9.8 ml/kg/h [51]. The premature infant may be placed at risk for volume depletion when a mismatch occurs between renal solute load and ability to produce concentrated urine.

Water losses via stool are negligible in early life of premature infants prior to establishing enteral feeds [52]. When full enteral feeding is achieved, fecal losses amount to 5–10 ml/kg/day [52].

Water is also needed for growth. A growth rate of 15 g/kg/day results in a net storage of about 12 ml water and 1.0–1.5 mmol Na/kg/day.

Metabolism of Na, K and Cl

Factors Influencing Intake: There is no endogenous production or release of electrolytes into the human body, making it completely dependent on enteral or parenteral intake. Enteral absorption is actively regulated within certain limits. Electrolyte homeostasis is a major factor for body homeostasis and effective regulatory mechanisms for intake exist: salt depletion results in specific 'hunger' for salty nutrients. However, in newborns, intake is completely affected by others and is dependent on the preparation of the diet used.

Factors Influencing Output: Electrolytes leave the body via feces, sweat, and urine. The authors are not aware of published data on electrolyte content of neonatal sweat or insensible perspiration. Urinary output is the only way that is actively regulated. Urinary excretion depends on intake, but there are physiological limits of preterm excretory function dependent on gestational and postnatal age. Typical urinary concentrations during normohydration are 20–40 mmol/l for Na^+ and 10–30 mmol/l for K^+ [data calculated from 53, 54].

Under physiological conditions daily urinary electrolyte excretion is fairly constant, indicating that water and electrolytes are regulated independently – within physiological conditions. However, in special situations, a high urinary volume may contain high amounts of electrolytes: diuretics lead to urinary Na^+ concentrations up to 70 mmol/l [data recalculated using 54, 55] frequently causing hyponatremia and arterial hypotension. Inappropriate Na losses may also occur after recovery from renal failure because regulation of electrolyte excretion in the distal/proximal tubule is impaired.

Fecal Na$^+$ losses were found to be dependent on gestational and postnatal age: immature infants lose more sodium (0.1 mmol/kg/day) than term infants (0.02 mmol/kg/day), and, with increasing postnatal age, stool losses decrease to 30% of initial values. Fecal potassium losses are twice as high as sodium losses, but show no relation with gestational age [56].

Additional losses may occur under conditions like bowel obstruction, ileostoma, pleural effusions, peritoneal drainage, and repeated CSF drainage. In clinical routine it is a good advice to measure electrolyte concentrations of such fluid losses.

Electrolytes are also needed for growth. The amount is determined by the rate of formation of lean tissue. A mean growth rate of 15 g/kg/day results in a net storage of about 1.0–1.5 mmol Na/kg/day. Insufficient sodium intake impairs longitudinal growth and weight gain in otherwise healthy preterm infants [57, 58]. It is reasonable to assume corresponding figures for K and Cl.

Postnatal Adaptation of Fluid and Electrolyte Homeostasis in VLBW Infants

General Aspects: Several postnatal physiological changes and adaptive processes affect metabolism of water and electrolytes. Stop of placental supply with fluids, electrolytes and nutrients, of placental clearance, onset of insensible water loss and thermoregulation have a sudden impact whereas oral intake and renal regulation of fluid and electrolyte follow later. Postnatal adaptation may be divided into the period of transition with loss of body weight (phase I), the intermediate period introducing full fluids/nutrition (phase II) and the period of stable growth with regular weight gain (phase III). Besides the postnatal regulation of water balance, adaptive processes occur simultaneously also in other organs (e.g. respiratory or metabolic adaptation).

Phase I: Rearrangement of Fluid Compartments: The immediate postnatal phase is characterized by a fall in urinary output caused by a fall in glomerular filtration rate. The first urine formed postnatally is hypertonic to plasma with an increased concentration of urea, potassium and phosphate, but not of sodium and chloride [29]. Changes in urine volume thus appear to be brought about by a decrease in free water clearance. This may be mediated by increased arginine vasopressin plasma levels present in the neonate around delivery [59]. This relative oliguria may last for a variable period (hours to days) and is mainly determined by underlying conditions and diseases like respiratory distress. It is followed by a diuretic phase: body fluid compartments are rearranged by isotonic or hypertonic (i.e. hypernatremic and hyperchloremic) contraction of ECF during the first postnatal days. These changes are caused by evaporative water loss via the immature skin and by continuing natriuresis (as present during fetal life) [60]. Both processes adapt to extrauterine conditions at different rates: the epidermal layer of the skin cornifies during the first days of life, while the kidneys increase glomerular filtration rate and their ability to concentrate urine over 5–10 days. It is unknown whether this continuing natriuresis reflects a delayed adaptation of renal regulation after birth or if it occurs as part of an active regulation of ICF contraction until a certain signal is received that ICF has sufficiently contracted.

The end of this transitional period is usually characterized by (i) urine volume <2.0 ml/kg/h, (ii) urine osmolarity > serum osmolarity, (iii) fractioned sodium excretion is diminishing from >3 to ≤1%, and (iv) urine specific gravity above >1.012. In healthy preterm infants, the transitional period is usually completed after 3–5 days. In VLBW infants, the length of phase I seems to be additionally modulated by the degree of respiratory insufficiency and may take up to 8 days [53, 54, 61–70]. Phase I starts at birth and ends usually with maximum weight loss.

Clinical goals for fluid and electrolyte administration during this period are to (i) allow ECF contraction without compromising IVF volume and cardiovascular function, (ii) allow a negative balance of 2–5 mmol Na/kg/day, (iii) maintain normal serum electrolyte levels, (iv) allow sufficient urinary output to excrete waste (like urea, acid equivalents etc.) and to avoid oliguria (<0.5–1.0 ml/kg/h) for longer than 12 h, (v) ensure regulation of body temperature by providing sufficient fluid for transepidermal evaporation, and (vi) to give sufficient calories to meet maintenance needs during this period equal to non-growth energy expenditure (approx. 40–60 kcal/kg/day).

Phase II: the Intermediate Phase – Establishment of Oral Feeding: This phase is characterized by decreasing transcutaneous water loss, falling urine volume to <1–2 ml/kg/h, and a low sodium excretion. If electrolyte supplements are not started, low serum electrolyte concentrations will develop due to ongoing renal electrolyte and water losses. During this phase, intestinal ability to digest oral feedings increases.

Clinical goals for fluid and electrolyte administration during this period are to (i) replete the body for electrolyte losses that may have inadvertently occurred during the first phase of ECF contraction, (ii) replace actual water and electrolytes losses in order to maintain water and electrolyte homeostasis, and (iii) increase oral feedings until sufficient calorie, protein and fluid intake is established.

Postnatal Adaptation Phase III – Stable Growth: This phase is dominated by continuous weight gain and a positive sodium balance as well as accretion of newly formed body tissue mass – ideally at a rate comparable to intrauterine growth (approx. 15–20 g/kg/day). Neonatal epidermis is completely cornified, and kidney function has fully adapted to extrauterine conditions.

Ideally, full enteral intake of fluids and other nutrients has been achieved. Consequently, a balance between caloric and protein supply, potential renal solute load (PRSL, total fluid volume to respect limited IVC capacity of VLBW preterm infants due to conditions like PDA) and renal concentrating ability must be found.

Clinical goals for fluid and electrolyte administration during this period are to (i) replace ongoing losses of water and electrolytes in order to maintain homeostasis, and (ii) provide extra water and electrolytes to allow tissue accumulation at intrauterine rates.

Data from Clinical Trials

Phase I

Transition without Major Problems/Complications: No randomized clinical trials were identified assessing needs for fluid and sodium in healthy VLBW infants without RDS. Unfortunately, the major question of postnatal physiology has not yet been answered: What is the normal weight loss that should be achieved after birth? What is the optimal weight loss for minimal overall morbidity? Though perinatal care has reduced the incidence of RDS in VLBW infants, most of these infants still experience problems linked to pulmonary immaturity. This might explain the lack of data in healthy VLBW or ELBW infants.

Transition Complicated by Respiratory Distress Syndrome: Postnatal ECF contraction is delayed in immature infants suffering from RDS [29, 71] and usually appears together with respiratory stabilization. The exact reason for this delay is unclear, but it is possibly related to pulmonary edema [72–76]. On the one hand, improved oxygenation [77, 78] was shown not to be the initial step in respiratory stabilization, but that diuresis precedes respiratory improvement [79–82]. On the other hand, Modi and Hutton [60] found that – prior to improvement in respiratory function – infants continued to exhibit a net stimulus to retain sodium and that diuresis and renal sodium handling improve as a consequence of respiratory improvement. It was speculated that the postnatal fall in pulmonary vascular resistance and increased left atrial return will lead to release of atrial natriuretic peptide. Respiratory improvement goes along with a fall in pulmonary vascular resistance which increases left atrial pressure and thus atrial natriuretic peptide release. This rise results in responses markedly different from those in utero.

Clinical Trials on Fluid and Sodium Intake

Phase I

The initial regimen of fluid and sodium administration during postnatal adaptation is linked to later outcome of infants with RDS (i.e. CLD and PDA) [58, 60, 69, 83–90]. Currently, there is evidence that preterm infants benefit from a restrictive fluid regimen. It is of interest to note that since 2000 no new clinical trials have been published.

Fluids: In two randomized trials, Lorenz et al. [91] and Kavvadia et al. [92, 93] found no adverse effects on short-term outcome comparing a restricted versus a standard fluid regimen. Lorenz et al. [91] controlled fluid intake in 88 VLBW infants to allow either a 5–7 or 10–12% weight loss but found no differences for intraventricular hemorrhage, PDA, bronchopulmonary dysplasia, necrotizing enterocolitis (NEC), dehydration, or metabolism. Kavvadia et al. [92] conducted one trial (n = 168) comparing a standard fluid regimen (starting at 60 ml/kg/day then stepwise incrementing over 1 week to 150 ml/kg/day) with a regimen that supplied 20% less fluid. They published two papers about the same trial reporting different primary outcomes. The first paper defined the study aim as to compare the effect of two levels of fluid intake on postnatal fluid balance, electrolyte and metabolic disturbances and sample size was calculated to detect a difference in the rate of jaundice. Besides higher urinary osmolarities and lower urine volumes in the restricted group, no significant differences on jaundice, hypotension, hypoglycemia, and hyponatremia were noted. In the second paper, the authors defined the primary outcome of the same trial as survival without CLD and acute renal failure which was also used for samples size calculation [93]. These time differences for postnatal steroids or oxygen dependency were described and contributed to the use of colloid solutions but not to crystalloid ones. It was concluded that fluid restriction to <90% of maintenance fluid does not increase adverse effects. The authors suggested that fluid input in VLBW infants can be handled flexibly to allow gradual loss of 5–15% of birth weight during the first week of life without short- and long-term effects. The CLD rate was found to be linked to fluid volume on day 2 of life. Each increment of 10 ml/kg/day increased the risk of CLD to 6%.

Stonestreet et al. [94] compared two groups of VLBW infants (n = 36) receiving a regimen of 'normal' maintenance or a surplus of +20 ml/kg/day during days 1–10 of life. Renal function and inulin space were measured. On average, group 1 received 126 and group 2 received 162 ml/kg/day and 4.5 and 3.1 mmol/kg/day for Na and K, respectively. The group on high fluid and sodium intake lost less weight on day 8 (11 vs. 16%) and did not show contraction of ECF volume as did those receiving lower fluid and sodium intakes. Clinical outcomes were not assessed.

In a retrospective study in 1,382 ELBW neonates, Poindexter and colleagues [95] found that a higher fluid intake and less weight loss until day 10 of life were associated with an increased risk of BPD. They suggest that careful attention to fluid balance might be an important factor to reduce BPD rates.

Four Cochrane meta-analyses (1998, 2001, 2008, 2010) have been published, all reviewing an identical set of four randomized clinical studies comparing different levels of fluid intake during the first week of life [96]. A benefit of fluid restriction for outcome (PDA, NEC, death) was proven. Trends but not statistically significant differences were found for a higher risk of dehydration (fluid restriction) and CLD (liberal fluids). There are eight published reviews, all give comparable conclusions, however none of these add more supporting information from recent clinical trials [97–103]. In summary, there seems to be sufficient evidence to recommend careful restriction of fluid intake so that physiological needs are met, benefitting cardiovascular and intestinal function without significant dehydration [67, 91, 92, 96].

Sodium: Costarino et al. [104] compared two regimens of sodium intake in a randomized controlled trial with 17 VLBW infants. In the restricted group (no sodium during days 1–5), serum osmolarity was more likely to be normal and the incidence of BPD was significantly lower compared to the maintenance group (3–4 mmol Na/kg/day).

Sodium restriction revealed a 25% incidence of hyponatremia compared to 25% of hypernatremic infants in the maintenance group.

A higher incidence of hyponatremia in unsupplemented infants (38 vs. 14% in supplemented; n = 46) was also reported by Al-Dahhan et al. [53, 56, 105]. They recommend 5 mmol Na/kg/day to infants <30 weeks and 4 mmol/kg/day for infants between 30 and 35 weeks. Outcome parameters focused on short-term fluid and sodium homeostasis, but not major morbidity. The follow-up study assessed the long-term effect on neurodevelopment of this early intervention at the age of 10–13 years: whereas lower Na intake seems to be beneficial during the initial phase of adaptation to prevent BPD, a higher sodium intake during the phase of stable growth (5 vs. 2 mmol/kg/day during 4–14 days of life) was related to better brain function [106].

Hartnoll et al. [107] pointed out that postnatal sodium supplementation should be individually tailored and delayed until onset of postnatal ECF contraction or marked clinical weight loss.

Considering all published data there seems to be sufficient evidence to restrict sodium intake in VLBW infants during the period of ECF contraction until a weight loss of approximately 6% has occurred [65, 96, 104]. The rate of infants needing supplemental oxygen and developing BPD was considerably lower in those with restricted intake. However, infants with sodium restriction seem to lose more body weight (delta of 5%) than infants. This difference does not seem to be caused by differences in fluid intake [65]. There is also evidence that infants on sodium restriction have a higher risk of developing hyponatremia.

Diuretics: No recent data are available concerning the early use of diuretics. Furosemide may reduce body water load and promote closure of PDA, but its effect on prostaglandin may keep it open. A routine use of furosemide must be weighed against the risk of developing a symptomatic PDA [108]. Studies were all done before the era of prenatal steroids, surfactant and indomethacin [109–111]. No benefit of furosemide on the clinical course and outcome of RDS could be found. Elective administration of diuretics should be carefully weighed against the risk of precipitating hypovolemia and electrolyte imbalances.

Capillary Leak (Sepsis) and HIE: Inflammatory mediators increase capillary permeability. Subsequently, high molecular substances shift from the IVC to the EVC compartment lowering IVC oncotic pressure. This condition presents clinically as edema or free fluid in the third space. Symptomatic treatment of capillary leak can be achieved by administration of high molecular substances exceeding the size of capillary leaks [112]. Intravenous human albumin with a low or medium molecular weight might have only a short-term effect. By potentially escaping from IVF they increase oncotic pressure in the EVF and deteriorate the situation.

With respect to HIE, the authors are not aware of any published randomized trials investigating fluid and electrolyte regimens that improve outcome of preterm infants suffering from intrauterine asphyxia.

Phase II and III

General Aspects: In this phase, renal and cardiovascular conditions are stabilized and parenteral fluid administration is stepwise replaced by oral feeding. The authors are not aware of randomized, controlled clinical studies investigating appropriate fluid and electrolyte regimens during this period of enteral/parenteral supply. Therefore, recommendations for fluid and electrolytes can only be made on the basis of physiological studies, observations and case reports.

Water: Coulthard and Hey [113] showed that healthy preterm infants (29–34 weeks) were able to cope with water intakes ranging from 96–200 ml/kg/day from the third day of life. These figures may reflect the range of fluid load neonates can deal with, and they may serve as lower and upper limits for reasonable daily allowances. In another study [114], 100 infants (<1,750 g) were randomized into 'dry' (50, 60, 70, 80, 90, 100 and 120 ml/kg/day during the first week, 150 ml/kg/day until 4 weeks) and a control group (80, 100, 120 and 150 ml/kg/day during the first week, 200 ml/kg afterwards). 27 (dry) and 15 (control) neonates survived without BPD at the age of 28 days ($p < 0.05$). The result suggests that fluid restriction during phase II and III can reduce mortality and morbidity in low-birth-weight infants.

Sodium: Because of insufficient data, recommendations for Na^+ can only be estimated. In balance studies, term breast-fed infants required only 0.4–0.7 mmol Na/kg/day during the first 4 months to achieve adequate growth [115]. The authors recommend 1.0–2.0 mmol Na/kg/day as a safe daily intake to cover incidental cutaneous or gastrointestinal losses. The published data show a slightly better outcome and a lower incidence for complications with a low initial Na^+Cl^- (1 mmol/kg/day) and fluid administration. The individual variability of newborns with different birth weight, disease, needs and losses requires to adjust fluid and electrolyte intake to the individual situation.

Potassium: Data on neonatal K^+ supplementation is rare. Controversy about providing potassium to infants is often a matter of anxiety rather than related to data from controlled trials. Most neonatal episodes of moderate hyperkalemia have no clinical consequences. In fact, upper limits for neonatal K^+ plasma levels given in standard references exceed those for all other age groups. Whether this is due to more hemolysed blood samples, blood sampling in a hypoperfused extremity, or a greater tolerance to extracellular K^+ is uncertain. Hyperkalemia varies inversely with urinary output, but not with K^+ intake, arterial pH, asphyxia, respiratory distress, gestational age, or birth weight [116].

Causes for non-oliguric hyperkalemia in VLBW infants are not understood. Urinary K^+ excretion seems to be correlated with renal aldosterone excretion [117]. It was speculated that rising plasma K^+ levels following birth stimulate the neonatal renin-angiotensin-aldosterone axis, just as K^+ loading does in rats [118]. Prevention of hyperkalemia should aim more at keeping K^+ intracellular than providing the daily requirement recommended for stable and growing infants. Also, early intravenous protein administration seems to lower plasma potassium levels similar to insulin therapy. If those measures fail, urinary K^+ excretion can be increased by furosemide which stimulates PGE_2 synthesis. This was shown in one neonate by Engle and Arant [117].

It is common practice to start potassium supplementation once plasma K levels remain or return to within normal range. Different balance studies [51, 56, 105, 119, 120] show that growing preterm infants retain about 1.0–1.5 mmol K/kg/day similar to intrauterine growth. The recommended amount of 2–3 mmol K/kg/day is similar to that achieved with human milk [121]. Milk formulas which contained higher K^+ levels did not have negative effects on the infant, as long as renal function is normal and there is no mineralocorticoid deficiency. Recommendations do not differentiate between enteral and parenteral electrolyte intake because electrolytes are almost completely absorbed from the intestine under healthy conditions. No data are available about electrolyte absorption in preterm or term neonates.

Stabilization without Problems

Fluid Volume and Sodium Intake: Different authors showed a relationship between fluid intake and sodium requirements. The following paragraph groups representative studies on the basis of fluid volume.

If neonatal fluid intake is 170 ml/kg/day or above, urinary Na^+ excretion is high and sodium balance is usually negative. Even a Na^+ intake of 10 mmol/kg/day did not compensate renal losses, and half of the infants developed hyponatremia [122]. When fluid volumes exceed 200 ml/kg/day, most ELBW infants will not be able to maintain Na^+Cl^- balance, regardless of the amount of Na^+Cl^- provided.

The effect of different sodium intake (1.1–3.0 mmol/kg/day) in combination with different fluid intakes (between 140 and 170 ml/kg/day) was investigated in different studies [123–126]. Physiological Na^+ concentrations were found in the investigated neonates. In all studies the growth rate was not related to sodium intake.

With a moderate fluid volume (<140 ml/kg/day), a Na^+ intake of 1 mmol/kg/day is adequate to maintain Na^+ balance in ELBW neonates [69, 75, 91, 104, 127–129]. There was no increase in morbidity among infants given less Na^+ and less fluid; ELBW infants did well on a Na^+ intake <2 mmol/kg/day. There was a trend to a higher incidence of PDA and CLD in infants given more Na^+ and a higher fluid intake [85, 104, 130]. If more fluid is administered, even to replace higher insensible water loss, additional Na^+Cl^- must be prescribed.

Stabilization with Problems (e.g. BPD/CLD)

Effect of Fluid Restriction: Fluid restriction is widely used during the phase of stable growth because it is thought to diminish pulmonary edema in BPD. However, its benefit for the clinical course of BPD has never been proven in clinical trials during the phase of stable growth [131]. Unjustified fluid restriction will lead to insufficient nutrient intake. This will jeopardize appropriate postnatal growth, the main goal during this period, because it is the only causal treatment of BPD/CLD. A randomized trial in preterm infants with CLD comparing standard versus concentrated ready-to-feed formula containing 30 kcal/oz found that the enriched formula achieved a postnatal growth pattern comparable to that in utero [132].

Effect of Diuretics: BPD in preterm infants is considered to be aggravated by lung edema. Therefore, diuretics are often prescribed. From all diuretics (enteral loop, distal loop or aerosolized) [108, 133–136] there is only sufficient published data for thiazide and furosemide to perform a systematic review. The most recent Cochrane analysis confirmed that thiazide with spironolactone significantly reduces the risk for death before discharge in infants with CLD [135], but increases the risk for hyponatremia and hypokalemia thus requiring supplementation. There was no difference between thiazide and spironolactone or thiazide alone. Infants >3 weeks of age with CLD showed improved lung compliance and oxygenation under long-term use of furosemide. There was no clear benefit for adding either spironolactone or metolazone [135, 137]. In view of lack of data from randomized trials concerning long-term clinical outcomes, the use of diuretics including furosemide was not recommended.

Effect of Postnatal Steroids: Though steroids are used to treat infants with prolonged need for oxygen, only little is studied about their impact on water and electrolyte homeostasis. A major side effect is the increase of blood pressure [138–141]. It possibly is a consequence of increased renal sodium retention [142]. The increased blood pressure itself leads to a higher glomerular filtration rate and therefore increases diuresis which then may affect body weight and electrolyte metabolism [143, 144]. Application of steroids at the age of 9–27 days of life led to pressure diuresis, weight loss and increased osmolar load to the kidney. There are no published data available about sodium losses or balances after steroid treatment.

Effect of Xanthines: Methylxanthines are sometimes used to treat infants with BPD because of their bronchodilatory effect. Besides central stimulation, xanthines are known to increase diuresis, urinary volume and sodium excretion. In premature infants xanthines inhibit solute reabsorption and increase fractional excretion of sodium and potassium. These effects are transient and disappeared after 24 h despite continuing xanthine maintenance therapy [145].

Effect of Prenatal Steroids: Prenatal steroids may affect neonatal fluid balance via maturational processes of skin, kidneys and circulation. They potentially enhance epithelial cell maturation, improve skin barrier [146, 147] and maturation of lung Na^+/K^+-ATPase leads to earlier postnatal reabsorption of fetal lung fluid. Omar et al. [148] measured lower insensible water loss, a decreased incidence of hyponatremia, and an earlier diuresis and natriuresis in ELBW neonates. In a randomized animal study on lambs the prenatal betamethasone group compared to the controls were found to have a more mature renal and cardiovascular system [149]. These effects stabilize fluid and electrolyte balance during postnatal adaptation [148–152]. There are no adverse or harmful effects on fluid balance reported.

Conditions of Excess and Deficiency

Inadequate intake of fluids and/or electrolytes may lead to pathological conditions that can immediately affect body homeostasis, metabolism and cellular function. However, a healthy preterm infant will be able to handle conditions of excess and deficiencies across a range that is wider than our recommended values. For example, a healthy preterm infant with normal renal function might well be able to maintain homeostasis despite a short-term intake exceeding 7 mmol/kg/day or as little as 1 mmol/kg/day. The same holds true for fluid intake <110 or >200 ml/kg/day.

However, the less precisely a regimen meets actual needs of an individual, the more effort is required to keep body homeostasis to avoid that a point is reached where the system will decompensate. It is important to note that there are no serum levels established (like for water) or of sufficient reliability (sodium, potassium) to reflect body stores. The correct picture is only captured if the whole spectrum of laboratory values and clinical conditions is taken into account. There is obviously a high potential for misinterpretation. A comprehensive review of this topic is given by Lorenz [153].

Obviously the potential to compensate for inadequate intake/provision of water and electrolytes is significantly more limited in extremely premature infants or those with further acute or chronic pathologies. Maintenance of homeostasis is an energy-consuming process and the exposure of compromised infants to additional deviations of the internal milieu will increase metabolic stress and the risk for further complications. Restriction of manuscript length unfortunately do not allow to discuss further details. The interested reader may be referred to the previous edition of this book [154].

Conclusions
- There is evidence that careful restriction of fluid and sodium intake during the first postnatal days reduces the risk for CLD.
- This fluid restriction is associated with an increased risk for hyponatremia.
- A higher sodium intake after the first week of life may be beneficial for growth and mental development.

Considerations for Future Research
- The available evidence has been created largely by studies performed between 1980 and 2000, and is based mostly on data obtained from more mature preterm infants (>28 weeks of gestation). Since 2000, little new evidence has become available.
- In more recent years, the population of preterm has changed particularly with respect to the following aspects:
- more immature babies are being taken care of from 23 weeks of gestation onwards,
- less invasive respiratory support (nCPAP, INSURE, LISA, NIPPV, NHFOV) is now provided which impacted not only the clinical course, but also pulmonary and cardiovascular physiology,

- fetal health state tends to have improved, i.e. babies seem to be born in a more healthy condition, especially the incidence of inflammatory reactions with edema/capillary leak seems to have decreased.
- Therefore, new clinical trials are needed to assess fluid and electrolyte needs of these more immature infants under the current conditions of care, which should aim to also assess later neurodevelopmental outcomes.

References

1 Friis-Hansen B: Water – the major nutrient. Acta Paediatr Scand Suppl 1982;299:11–16.
2 Friis-Hansen B: Body water compartments in children: changes during growth and related changes in body composition. Pediatrics 1961;28:169–174.
3 Fomon SJ, Haschke F, Ziegler EE, Nemeth M: Body composition of reference children from birth to age 10 years. Am J Clin Nutr 1982;35:1169–1175.
4 Widdowson E: Changes of body composition during growth; in Davis J, Dobbing J (eds): Scientific Foundations of Paediatrics. London, Heinemann, 1981, pp 330–342.
5 Fusch C, Slotboom J, Fuehrer U, Schumacher R, Keisker A, Zimmermann W, Moessinger AC, Boesch C, Blum J: Neonatal body composition: dual-energy X-ray absorptiometry, magnetic resonance imaging, and three-dimensional chemical shift imaging versus chemical analysis in piglets. Pediatr Res 1999;46: 465–473.
6 Nicholson J, Pesce M: Laboratory testing and reference values in infants and children; in Nelson W, Behrman R, Kliegman R, Arvin A (eds): Textbook of Pediatrics, ed 15. Philadelphia, Saunders, 2002, pp 2031–2084.
7 Raubenstine DA, Ballantine TV, Greecher CP, Webb SL: Neonatal serum protein levels as indicators of nutritional status: normal values and correlation with anthropometric data. J Pediatr Gastroenterol Nutr 1990;10:53–61.
8 Roithmaier A, Arlettaz R, Bauer K, Bucher HU, Krieger M, Duc G, Versmold HT: Randomized controlled trial of Ringer solution versus serum for partial exchange transfusion in neonatal polycythaemia. Eur J Pediatr 1995;154:53–56.
9 Offringa PJ, Boersma ER, Brunsting JR, Meeuwsen WP, Velvis H: Weight loss in full-term Negroid infants: relationship to body water compartments at birth? Early Hum Dev 1990;21:73–81.
10 Shaffer SG, Ekblad H, Brans YW: Estimation of extracellular fluid volume by bromide dilution in infants less than 1,000 grams birth weight. Early Hum Dev 1991;27:19–24.
11 Andersson B: Regulation of body fluids. Annu Rev Physiol 1977;39:185–200.

12 Boehles H: Ernährungsstörungen im Kindesalter. Stuttgart, Wissenschaftliche Verlagsgesellschaft, 1991, p 26.
13 Robertson G, Berl T: Water metabolism; in Brenner BM, Rector F (eds): The Kidney. Philadelphia, Saunders, 1986, pp 385–431.
14 Guyton A, Scanlon L, Armstrong G: Effects of pressoreceptor reflex and Cushing reflex on urinary output. Fed Proc 1952;11:61–62.
15 Mann JF, Johnson AK, Ganten D, Ritz E: Thirst and the renin-angiotensin system. Kidney Int Suppl 1987;21(suppl):27–34.
16 Linshaw MA: Selected aspects of cell volume control in renal cortical and medullary tissue. Pediatr Nephrol 1991;5:653–665.
17 Macknight AD, Leaf A: Regulation of cellular volume. Physiol Rev 1977;57:510–573.
18 Gruwel ML, Alves C, Schrader J: Na^+/K^+-ATPase in endothelial cell energetics: ^{23}Na nuclear magnetic resonance and calorimetry study. Am J Physiol 1995; 268:H351–H358.
19 Carlton DP, Cummings JJ, Scheerer RG, Bland RD: Lung vascular protein permeability in preterm fetal and mature newborn sheep. J Appl Physiol 1994;77: 782–788.
20 Bhat R, Malalis L, Shukla A, Vidyasagar D: Colloid osmotic pressure in infants with hyaline membrane disease. Chest 1983;83:776–779.
21 Ekblad H: Postnatal changes in colloid osmotic pressure in premature infants: in healthy infants, in infants with respiratory distress syndrome, and in infants born to mothers with premature rupture of membranes. Gynecol Obstet Invest 1987;24:95–100.
22 Kero P, Korvenranta H, Alamaakala P, Selanne P, Kiilholma P, Valimaki I: Colloid osmotic pressure of cord blood in relation to neonatal outcome and mode of delivery. Acta Paediatr Scand Suppl 1983; 305:88–91.
23 Sola A, Gregory GA: Colloid osmotic pressure of normal newborns and premature infants. Crit Care Med 1981;9:568–572.
24 Wu PY, Udani V, Chan L, Miller FC, Henneman CE: Colloid osmotic pressure: variations in normal pregnancy. J Perinat Med 1983;11:193–199.

25 Jobe A, Jacobs H, Ikegami M, Berry D: Lung protein leaks in ventilated lambs: effects of gestational age. J Appl Physiol 1985;58:1246–1251.

26 Brunette MG, Leclerc M, Claveau D: Na$^+$ transport by human placental brush border membranes: are there several mechanisms? J Cell Physiol 1996;167:72–80.

27 Smith CH, Moe AJ, Ganapathy V: Nutrient transport pathways across the epithelium of the placenta. Annu Rev Nutr 1992;12:183–206.

28 Spitzer A: Renal physiology and function development; in Edelmann CM (ed): The Kidney and Urinary Tract. Boston, Little Brown, 1978, pp 25–128.

29 Modi N: Development of renal function. Br Med Bull 1988;44:935–956.

30 Haycock GB: Development of glomerular filtration and tubular sodium reabsorption in the human fetus and newborn. Br J Urol 1998;81(suppl 2):33–38.

31 Martin D: Wasser und anorganische Elemente; in Harpner H, Martin D, Mayes P, Rodwell V (eds): Medizinische Biochemie, ed 19. Berlin, Springer, 1983, pp 657–671.

32 Kurzner SI, Garg M, Bautista DB, Sargent CW, Bowman CM, Keens TG: Growth failure in bronchopulmonary dysplasia: elevated metabolic rates and pulmonary mechanics. J Pediatr 1988;112:73–80.

33 Weinstein MR, Oh W: Oxygen consumption in infants with bronchopulmonary dysplasia. J Pediatr 1981;99:958–961.

34 Baumgart S: Radiant energy and insensible water loss in the premature newborn infant nursed under a radiant warmer. Clin Perinatol 1982;9:483–503.

35 Baumgart S: Partitioning of heat losses and gains in premature newborn infants under radiant warmers. Pediatrics 1985;75:89–99.

36 Wheldon AE, Rutter N: The heat balance of small babies nursed in incubators and under radiant warmers. Early Hum Dev 1982;6:131–143.

37 Baumgart S, Engle WD, Fox WW, Polin RA: Radiant warmer power and body size as determinants of insensible water loss in the critically ill neonate. Pediatr Res 1981;15:1495–1499.

38 Brück K: Neonatal thermal regulation; in Polin RA, Fox WW (eds): Fetal and Neonatal Physiology. Philadelphia, Saunders, 1992, pp 488–514.

39 Hammarlund K, Sedin G, Stromberg B: Transepidermal water loss in newborn infants. VIII. Relation to gestational age and post-natal age in appropriate and small for gestational age infants. Acta Paediatr Scand 1983;72:721–728.

40 Hey EN, Katz G: Evaporative water loss in the newborn baby. J Physiol 1969;200:605–619.

41 Sedin G, Hammarlund K, Nilsson GE, Stromberg B, Oberg PA: Measurements of transepidermal water loss in newborn infants. Clin Perinatol 1985;12:79–99.

42 Williams PR, Oh W: Effects of radiant warmer on insensible water loss in newborn infants. Am J Dis Child 1974;128:511–514.

43 Wu PY, Hodgman JE: Insensible water loss in preterm infants: changes with postnatal development and non-ionizing radiant energy. Pediatrics 1974;54:704–712.

44 Brück K: Heat production and temperature regulation; in Stave U (ed): Perinatal Physiology. New York, Plenum Medical, 1987, p 455.

45 Sulyok E, Jequier E, Prod'hom LS: Respiratory contribution to the thermal balance of the newborn infant under various ambient conditions. Pediatrics 1973;51:641–650.

46 Sinclair JC: Metabolic rate and temperature control; in Smith CA, Nelson N (eds): The Physiology of the Newborn Infant, ed 4. Springfield, Thomas, 1976, pp 354–415.

47 Ziegler EE, Fomon SJ: Fluid intake, renal solute load, and water balance in infancy. J Pediatr 1971;78:561–568.

48 Chevalier RL: Developmental renal physiology of the low birth weight pre-term newborn. J Urol 1996;156:714–719.

49 Rees L, Brook CG, Shaw JC, Forsling ML: Hyponatraemia in the first week of life in preterm infants. Part I. Arginine vasopressin secretion. Arch Dis Child 1984;59:414–422.

50 Svenningsen NW, Aronson AS: Postnatal development of renal concentration capacity as estimated by DDAVP test in normal and asphyxiated neonates. Biol Neonate 1974;25:230–241.

51 Leake RD, Zakauddin S, Trygstad CW, Fu P, Oh W: The effects of large volume intravenous fluid infusion on neonatal renal function. J Pediatr 1976;89:968–972.

52 Jhaveri MK, Kumar SP: Passage of the first stool in very low birth weight infants. Pediatrics 1987;79:1005–1007.

53 Al-Dahhan J, Haycock GB, Chantler C, Stimmler L: Sodium homeostasis in term and preterm neonates. I. Renal aspects. Arch Dis Child 1983;58:335–342.

54 Rees L, Shaw JC, Brook CG, Forsling ML: Hyponatraemia in the first week of life in preterm infants. Part II. Sodium and water balance. Arch Dis Child 1984;59:423–429.

55 Reiter PD, Makhlouf R, Stiles AD: Comparison of 6-hour infusion versus bolus furosemide in premature infants. Pharmacotherapy 1998;18:63–68.

56 Al-Dahhan J, Haycock GB, Chantler C, Stimmler L: Sodium homeostasis in term and preterm neonates. II. Gastrointestinal aspects. Arch Dis Child 1983;58:343–345.

57 Bower TR, Pringle KC, Soper RT: Sodium deficit causing decreased weight gain and metabolic acidosis in infants with ileostomy. J Pediatr Surg 1988;23:567–572.

58 Haycock GB: The influence of sodium on growth in infancy. Pediatr Nephrol 1993;7:871–875.

59 Leung AK, McArthur RG, McMillan DD, Ko D, Deacon JS, Parboosingh JT, Lederis KP: Circulating antidiuretic hormone during labour and in the newborn. Acta Paediatr Scand 1980;69:505–510.

60 Modi N, Hutton JL: The influence of postnatal respiratory adaptation on sodium handling in preterm neonates. Early Hum Dev 1990;21:11–20.

61 Bauer K, Bovermann G, Roithmaier A, Gotz M, Proiss A, Versmold HT: Body composition, nutrition, and fluid balance during the first two weeks of life in preterm neonates weighing less than 1,500 grams. J Pediatr 1991;118:615–620.

62 Bauer K, Buschkamp S, Marcinkowski M, Kossel H, Thome U, Versmold HT: Postnatal changes of extracellular volume, atrial natriuretic factor, and diuresis in a randomized controlled trial of high-frequency oscillatory ventilation versus intermittent positive-pressure ventilation in premature infants <30 weeks' gestation. Crit Care Med 2000;28:2064–2068.

63 Bauer K, Versmold H: Postnatal weight loss in preterm neonates less than 1,500 g is due to isotonic dehydration of the extracellular volume. Acta Paediatr Scand Suppl 1989;360:37–42.

64 Bauer K, Versmold H, Prolss A, De-Graaf SS, Meeuwsen-Van-der-Roest WP, Zijlstra WG: Estimation of extracellular volume in preterm infants less than 1,500 g, children, and adults by sucrose dilution. Pediatr Res 1990;27:256–259.

65 Hartnoll G, Betremieux P, Modi N: Randomised controlled trial of postnatal sodium supplementation on body composition in 25 to 30 week gestational age infants. Arch Dis Child Fetal Neonatal Ed 2000;82:F24–F28.

66 Maclaurin JC: Changes in body water distribution during the first two weeks of life. Arch Dis Child 1966;41:286–291.

67 Modi N: Adaptation to extrauterine life. Br J Obstet Gynaecol 1994;101:369–370.

68 Shaffer SG, Bradt SK, Hall RT: Postnatal changes in total body water and extracellular volume in the preterm infant with respiratory distress syndrome. J Pediatr 1986;109:509–514.

69 Shaffer SG, Meade VM: Sodium balance and extracellular volume regulation in very low birth weight infants. J Pediatr 1989;115:285–290.

70 Lorenz JM, Kleinman LI, Ahmed G, Markarian K: Phases of fluid and electrolyte homeostasis in the extremely low birth weight infant. Pediatrics 1995;96:484–489.

71 Tang W, Ridout D, Modi N: Influence of respiratory distress syndrome on body composition after preterm birth. Arch Dis Child Fetal Neonatal Ed 1997;77:F28–F31.

72 Bland RD: Edema formation in the newborn lung. Clin Perinatol 1982;9:593–611.

73 Bland RD: Edema formation in the lungs and its relationship to neonatal respiratory distress. Acta Paediatr Scand Suppl 1983;305:92–99.

74 Brown ER, Stark A, Sosenko I, Lawson EE, Avery ME: Bronchopulmonary dysplasia: possible relationship to pulmonary edema. J Pediatr 1978;92:982–984.

75 Ertl T, Sulyok E, Bodis J, Csaba IF: Plasma prolactin levels in full-term newborn infants with idiopathic edema: response to furosemide. Biol Neonate 1986;49:15–20.

76 Jefferies AL, Coates G, O'Brodovich H: Pulmonary epithelial permeability in hyaline-membrane disease. N Engl J Med 1984;311:1075–1080.

77 Cort R: Renal function in the respiratory distress syndrome. Acta Paediatr Scand 1962;51:313–323.

78 Guignard JP, Torrado A, Mazouni SM, Gautier E: Renal function in respiratory distress syndrome. J Pediatr 1976;88:845–850.

79 Costarino AT, Baumgart S, Norman ME, Polin RA: Renal adaptation to extrauterine life in patients with respiratory distress syndrome. Am J Dis Child 1985;139:1060–1063.

80 Engle WD, Arant BS, Wiriyathian S, Rosenfeld CR: Diuresis and respiratory distress syndrome: physiologic mechanisms and therapeutic implications. J Pediatr 1983;102:912–917.

81 Heaf DP, Belik J, Spitzer AR, Gewitz MH, Fox WW: Changes in pulmonary function during the diuretic phase of respiratory distress syndrome. J Pediatr 1982;101:103–107.

82 Langman CB, Engle WD, Baumgart S, Fox WW, Polin RA: The diuretic phase of respiratory distress syndrome and its relationship to oxygenation. J Pediatr 1981;98:462–466.

83 Bell EF: Fluid therapy; in Sinclair JC, Bracken M (eds): Effective Care of the Newborn. Oxford, Oxford University Press, 1992, pp 59–71.

84 Bell EF, Warburton D, Stonestreet BS, Oh W: High-volume fluid intake predisposes premature infants to necrotising enterocolitis. Lancet 1979;2:90.

85 Bell EF, Warburton D, Stonestreet BS, Oh W: Effect of fluid administration on the development of symptomatic patent ductus arteriosus and congestive heart failure in premature infants. N Engl J Med 1980;302:598–604.

86 Haycock GB, Aperia A: Salt and the newborn kidney. Pediatr Nephrol 1991;5:65–70.

87 Modi N: Sodium intake and preterm babies. Arch Dis Child 1993;69:87–91.

88 Stevenson JG: Fluid administration in the association of patent ductus arteriosus complicating respiratory distress syndrome. J Pediatr 1977;90:257–261.

89 Van Marter LJ, Allred EN, Leviton A, Pagano M, Parad R, Moore M: Antenatal glucocorticoid treatment does not reduce chronic lung disease among surviving preterm infants. J Pediatr 2001;138:198–204.

90 Van Marter LJ, Leviton A, Allred EN, Pagano M, Kuban KC: Hydration during the first days of life and the risk of bronchopulmonary dysplasia in low birth weight infants. J Pediatr 1990;116:942–949.

91 Lorenz JM, Kleinman LI, Kotagal UR, Reller MD: Water balance in very low-birth-weight infants: relationship to water and sodium intake and effect on outcome. J Pediatr 1982;101:423–432.

92 Kavvadia V, Greenough A, Dimitriou G, Forsling ML: Randomized trial of two levels of fluid input in the perinatal period – effect on fluid balance, electrolyte and metabolic disturbances in ventilated VLBW infants. Acta Paediatr 2000;89:237–241.

93 Kavvadia V, Greenough A, Dimitriou G, Hooper R: Randomised trial of fluid restriction in ventilated very low birth weight infants. Arch Dis Child Fetal Neonatal Ed 2000;83:F91–F96.

94 Stonestreet BS, Bell EF, Warburton D, Oh W: Renal response in low-birth-weight neonates. Results of prolonged intake of two different amounts of fluid and sodium. Am J Dis Child 1983;137:215–219.

95 Oh W, Poindexter BB, Perritt R, Lemons JA, Bauer CR, Ehrenkranz RA, Stoll BJ, Poole K, Wright LL: Association between fluid intake and weight loss during the first ten days of life and risk of bronchopulmonary dysplasia in extremely low birth weight infants. J Pediatr 2005;147:786–790.

96 Bell EF, Acarregui MJ: Restricted versus liberal water intake for preventing morbidity and mortality in preterm infants. Cochrane Database Syst Rev 2008;1:CD000503.

97 Aggarwal R, Deorari AK, Paul VK: Fluid and electrolyte management in term and preterm neonates. Indian J Pediatr 2001;68:1139–1142.

98 Chow JM, Douglas D: Fluid and electrolyte management in the premature infant. Neonatal Netw 2008;27:379–386.

99 Murat I, Humblot A, Girault L, Piana F: Neonatal fluid management. Best Pract Res Clin Anaesthesiol 2010;24:365–374.

100 Modi N: Management of fluid balance in the very immature neonate. Arch Dis Child Fetal Neonatal Ed 2004;89:F108–F111.

101 Oh W: Fluid and electrolyte management of very low birth weight infants. Pediatr Neonatol 2012;53:329–333.

102 Lorenz JM: Fluid and electrolyte therapy and chronic lung disease. Curr Opin Pediatr 2004;16:152–156.

103 Hartnoll G: Basic principles and practical steps in the management of fluid balance in the newborn. Semin Neonatol 2003;8:307–313.

104 Costarino AT, Gruskay JA, Corcoran L, Polin RA, Baumgart S: Sodium restriction versus daily maintenance replacement in very low birth weight premature neonates: a randomized, blind therapeutic trial. J Pediatr 1992;120:99–106.

105 Al-Dahhan J, Haycock GB, Nichol B, Chantler C, Stimmler L: Sodium homeostasis in term and preterm neonates. III. Effect of salt supplementation. Arch Dis Child 1984;59:945–950.

106 Al-Dahhan J, Jannoun L, Haycock GB: Effects of salt supplementation of newborn premature infants on neurodevelopmental outcome at 10–13 years of age. Arch Dis Child Fetal Neonatal Ed 2002;86:F120–F123.

107 Hartnoll G, Betremieux P, Modi N: Randomised controlled trial of postnatal sodium supplementation in infants of 25–30 weeks gestational age: effects on cardiopulmonary adaptation. Arch Dis Child Fetal Neonatal Ed 2001;85:F29–F32.

108 Brion LP, Soll RF: Diuretics for respiratory distress syndrome in preterm infants. Cochrane Database Syst Rev 2000;2:CD001454.

109 Marks KH, Berman W, Friedman Z, Whiteman V, Lee C, Maisels MJ: Furosemide in hyaline membrane disease. Pediatrics 1978;62:785–788.

110 Savage MD, Wilkinson AR, Baum JD, Roberton NRC: Furosemide in respiratory distress syndrome. Arch Dis Child 1975;50:709–713.

111 Yeh TF, Shibli A, Leu ST, Ravel D, Pildes RD: Early furosemide therapy in premature infants (2,000 g) with respiratory distress syndrome: a randomised controlled trial. J Pediatr 1984;105:603–609.

112 Salmon JB, Mythen MG: Pharmacology and physiology of colloids. Blood Rev 1993;7:114–120.

113 Coulthard MG, Hey EN: Effect of varying water intake on renal function in healthy preterm babies. Arch Dis Child 1985;60:614–620.

114 Tammela OK, Koivisto ME: Fluid restriction for preventing bronchopulmonary dysplasia? Reduced fluid intake during the first weeks of life improves the outcome of low-birth-weight infants. Acta Paediatr 1992;81:207–212.

115 Ziegler EE, Fomon SJ: Major minerals; in Fomon SJ (ed): Infant Nutrition, ed 2. Philadelphia, Saunders, 1974, pp 267–297.

116 Leslie GI, Carman G, Arnold JD: Early neonatal hyperkalaemia in the extremely premature newborn infant. J Paediatr Child Health 1990;26:58–61.

117 Engle WD, Arant BS: Urinary potassium excretion in the critically ill neonate. Pediatrics 1984;74:259–264.

118 Nakamaru M, Misono KS, Naruse M, Workman RJ, Inagami T: A role for the adrenal renin-angiotensin system in the regulation of potassium-stimulated aldosterone production. Endocrinology 1985;117:1772–1778.

119 Arant BS, Seikaly MG: Intrarenal angiotensin II may regulate developmental changes in renal blood flow. Pediatr Nephrol 1989;3:C142.

120 Butterfield J, Lubchenco L, Bergstedt J, O'Brien D: Patterns in electrolyte and nitrogen balance in the newborn premature infant. Pediatrics 1960;26: 777–791.

121 Gross SJ: Growth and biochemical response of preterm infants fed human milk or modified infant formula. N Engl J Med 1983;308:237–241.

122 Engelke SC, Shah BL, Vasan U, Raye JR: Sodium balance in very low-birth-weight infants. J Pediatr 1978;93:837–841.

123 Babson SG, Bramhall JL: Diet and growth in the premature infant. The effect of different dietary intakes of ash-electrolyte and protein on weight gain and linear growth. J Pediatr 1969;74:890–900.

124 Raiha NC, Heinonen K, Rassin DK, Gaull GE: Milk protein quantity and quality in low-birth-weight infants. I. Metabolic responses and effects on growth. Pediatrics 1976;57:659–684.

125 Polberger SK, Axelsson IA, Raiha NC: Growth of very low birth weight infants on varying amounts of human milk protein. Pediatr Res 1989;25:414–419.

126 Day GM, Radde IC, Balfe JW, Chance GW: Electrolyte abnormalities in very low birth weight infants. Pediatr Res 1976;10:522–526.

127 Asano H, Taki M, Igarashi Y: Sodium homeostasis in premature infants during the early postnatal period: results of relative low volume of fluid and sodium intake (abstract). Pediatr Nephrol 1987; 1:C38.

128 Ekblad H, Kero P, Takala J, Korvenranta H, Valimaki I: Water, sodium and acid-base balance in premature infants: therapeutical aspects. Acta Paediatr Scand 1987;76:47–53.

129 Kojima T, Fukuda Y, Hirata Y, Matsuzaki S, Kobayashi Y: Effects of aldosterone and atrial natriuretic peptide on water and electrolyte homeostasis of sick neonates. Pediatr Res 1989;25:591–594.

130 Brown ER, Stark A, Sosenko I, Lawson EE, Avery ME: Bronchopulmonary dysplasia: possible relationship to pulmonary edema. J Pediatr 1978;92: 982–984.

131 Tammela OK: Appropriate fluid regimens to prevent bronchopulmonary dysplasia. Eur J Pediatr 1995;154:S15–S18.

132 Puangco MA, Schanler RJ: Clinical experience in enteral nutrition support for premature infants with bronchopulmonary dysplasia. J Perinatol 2000;20:87–91.

133 Brion LP, Primhak RA: Intravenous or enteral loop diuretics for preterm infants with (or developing) chronic lung disease. Cochrane Database Syst Rev 2000;4:CD001453.

134 Brion LP, Primhak RA, Yong W: Aerosolized diuretics for preterm infants with (or developing) chronic lung disease. Cochrane Database Syst Rev 2000;2:CD001694.

135 Brion LP, Yong SC, Perez IA, Primhak R: Diuretics and chronic lung disease of prematurity. J Perinatol 2001;21:269–271.

136 Stewart A, Brion LP, Ambrosio-Perez I: Diuretics acting on the distal renal tubule for preterm infants with (or developing) chronic lung disease. Cochrane Database Syst Rev 2011;9:CD001817.

137 Hoffman DJ, Gerdes JS, Abbasi S: Pulmonary function and electrolyte balance following spironolactone treatment in preterm infants with chronic lung disease: a double-blind, placebo-controlled, randomized trial. J Perinatol 2000;20:41–45.

138 Cummings JJ, D'Eugenio DB, Gross SJ: A controlled trial of dexamethasone in preterm infants at high risk for bronchopulmonary dysplasia. N Engl J Med 1989;320:1505–1510.

139 Durand M, Sardesai S, McEvoy C: Effects of early dexamethasone therapy on pulmonary mechanics and chronic lung disease in very low birth weight infants: a randomized, controlled trial. Pediatrics 1995;95:584–590.

140 Kari MA, Heinonen K, Ikonen RS, Koivisto M, Raivio KO: Dexamethasone treatment in preterm infants at risk for bronchopulmonary dysplasia. Arch Dis Child 1993;68:566–569.

141 Merritt TA, Hallman M, Berry C, Pohjavuori M, Edwards DK, Jaaskelainen J, Grafe MR, Vaucher Y, Wozniak P, Heldt G, et al: Randomized, placebo-controlled trial of human surfactant given at birth versus rescue administration in very low birth weight infants with lung immaturity. J Pediatr 1991;118:581–594.

142 Brem AS: Insights into glucocorticoid-associated hypertension. Am J Kidney Dis 2001;37:1–10.

143 Bos AF, van-Asselt WA, Okken A: Dexamethasone treatment and fluid balance in preterm infants at risk for chronic lung disease. Acta Paediatr 2000;89: 562–565.

144 Gladstone IM, Ehrenkranz RA, Jacobs HC: Pulmonary function tests and fluid balance in neonates with chronic lung disease during dexamethasone treatment. Pediatrics 1989;84:1072–1076.

145 Mazkereth R, Laufer J, Jordan S, Pomerance JJ, Boichis H, Reichman B: Effects of theophylline on renal function in premature infants. Am J Perinatol 1997;14:45–49.

146 Aszterbaum M, Feingold KR, Menon GK, Williams ML: Glucocorticoids accelerate fetal maturation of the epidermal permeability barrier in the rat. J Clin Invest 1993;91:2703–2708.

147 Okah FA, Pickens WL, Hoath SB: Effect of prenatal steroids on skin surface hydrophobicity in the premature rat. Pediatr Res 1995;37:402–408.

148 Omar SA, DeCristofaro JD, Agarwal BI, La-Gamma EF: Effects of prenatal steroids on water and sodium homeostasis in extremely low birth weight neonates. Pediatrics 1999;104:482–488.

149 Smith LM, Ervin MG, Wada N, Ikegami M, Polk DH, Jobe AH: Antenatal glucocorticoids alter postnatal preterm lamb renal and cardiovascular responses to intravascular volume expansion. Pediatr Res 2000;47:622–627.

150 Berry LM, Polk DH, Ikegami M, Jobe AH, Padbury JF, Ervin MG: Preterm newborn lamb renal and cardiovascular responses after fetal or maternal antenatal betamethasone. Am J Physiol 1997;272: R1972–R1979.

151 Ervin MG, Berry LM, Ikegami M, Jobe AH, Padbury JF, Polk DH: Single dose fetal betamethasone administration stabilizes postnatal glomerular filtration rate and alters endocrine function in premature lambs. Pediatr Res 1996;40:645–651.

152 Ervin MG, Seidner SR, Leland MM, Ikegami M, Jobe AH: Direct fetal glucocorticoid treatment alters postnatal adaptation in premature newborn baboons. Am J Physiol 1998;274:R1169–R1176.

153 Lorenz JM: Assessing fluid and electrolyte status in the newborn. National Academy of Clinical Biochemistry. Clin Chem 1997;43:205–210.

154 Fusch C, Jochum F: Water, sodium, potassium and chloride; in Tsang RC, Uauy R, Koletzko B, Zlotkin S (eds): Nutrition of the Preterm Infant. Cincinnati, Digital Educational Publishing, Inc, 2005, pp 201–245.

Prof. Christoph Fusch, MD, PhD, FRCPC
Department of Pediatrics
McMaster University & Hamilton Health Sciences
1280 Main Street West, Hamilton, ON L8S 4KB (Canada)
E-Mail fusch@mcmaster.ca

Koletzko B, Poindexter B, Uauy R (eds): Nutritional Care of Preterm Infants: Scientific Basis and Practical Guidelines.
World Rev Nutr Diet. Basel, Karger, 2014, vol 110, pp 121–139 (DOI: 10.1159/000358462)

Nutritional Care of Premature Infants: Microminerals

Magnus Domellöf

Division of Pediatrics, Department of Clinical Sciences, Umea University, Umea, Sweden

Reviewed by Christoph Fusch, Department of Pediatrics, McMaster University, Hamilton, Ont., Canada;
Alexandre Lapillonne, Paris Descartes University, APHP Necker Hospital, Paris, France

Abstract

Microminerals, including iron, zinc, copper, selenium, manganese, iodine, chromium and molybdenum, are essential for a remarkable array of critical functions and need to be supplied in adequate amounts to preterm infants. Very low birth weight (VLBW) infants carry a very high risk of developing iron deficiency which can adversely affect neurodevelopment. However, a too high iron supply in iron-replete VLBW infants may induce adverse effects such as increased infection risks and impaired growth. Iron needs are influenced by birth weight, growth rates, blood losses (phlebotomy) and blood transfusions. An enteral iron intake of 2 mg/kg/day for infants with a birth weight of 1,500–2,500 g and 2–3 mg/kg/day for VLBW infants is recommended. Higher doses up to 6 mg/kg/day are needed in infants receiving erythropoietin treatment. Regular monitoring of serum ferritin during the hospital stay is advisable. Routine provision of iron with parenteral nutrition for VLBW infants is not recommended. Less certainty exists for the advisable intakes of other microminerals. It appears prudent to provide enterally fed VLBW infants with daily amounts per kilogram body weight of 1.4–2.5 mg zinc, 100–230 µg copper, 5–10 µg selenium, 1–15 µg manganese, 10–55 µg iodine, 0.03–2.25 µg chromium, and 0.3–5 µg molybdenum. Future scientific findings may justify deviations from these suggested ranges.   © 2014 S. Karger AG, Basel

Microminerals, including iron, zinc, copper, selenium, manganese, iodine, chromium and molybdenum, are essential for a remarkable array of critical functions in humans. On the other hand, several of these elements can also be toxic at high concentrations. Therefore, it is important to carefully define requirements in order to avoid both deficiencies and adverse effects.

Iron

Preterm infants are at high risk of iron deficiency (ID), which may have adverse effects on brain development and function. However, in contrast to most other nutrients, there is no mechanism for excretion of iron from the human body and iron is a high-

Table 1. Recommended cut-offs for the diagnosis of iron overload, iron deficiency and anemia in VLBW infants at different ages

	Newborn	2 months	4 months	6–24 months
Iron overload: S-ferritin, µg/l	>300	>300	>250	>200
Iron deficiency: S-ferritin, µg/l	<35	<40	<20	<10–12
Anemia: Hb, g/l	<135	<90	<105	<105

ly reactive prooxidant, so excessive iron supplementation of infants may have adverse effects.

The combination of hemoglobin (Hb) and ferritin is considered the most sensitive measure of the effects of iron interventions in children and adults. Age-specific cut-offs for iron status indicators, including Hb and ferritin, should be used for young children since there are large physiological changes in iron status and red cell morphology occurring during the first year of life (table 1) [1].

The main public health problem associated with ID in childhood is the risk of poor neurodevelopment. Animal studies have shown that iron is essential for normal brain development. Several well-performed case-control studies in children have shown a consistent association between ID anemia in infancy and long-lasting poor cognitive and behavioral performance. A meta-analysis of 17 randomized clinical trials in children (newborn to adolescent) showed that iron supplementation had a positive effect on mental development indices [2]. A recent meta-analysis has suggested that preventive iron supplements in infancy (starting at 0–6 months of life) have a positive effect on motor development [3].

Unnecessary iron supplementation of iron-replete infants may have adverse effects, including increased risk of infections and impaired growth [4]. In preterm infants, non-protein-bound iron has been suggested to cause formation of reactive oxygen species and possibly increase the risk for oxidative disorders, e.g. retinopathy of prematurity, especially when given in high doses as a component of blood transfusions or as an adjunct to erythropoietin therapy [5].

Since iron cannot be excreted from the body, intestinal absorption of iron is strictly regulated. Preterm infants show a higher fractional iron absorption compared to term infants: 25–40% from iron supplements given between feedings [6, 7] and 11–27% from iron-fortified formula [8, 9]. Studies are lacking on iron bioavailability from multinutrient-fortified human milk but it may be higher than from preterm formula since, in term infants, iron absorption is significantly higher from human milk compared to formula [10]. However, the iron content in unfortified human milk is very low (about 0.3 mg/l) [11].

Using a factorial approach, Griffin and Cooke [9] estimated the iron requirements of a preterm infant with a birth weight of 1 kg to reach a maximum of 0.37 mg/kg/day at around term age. This corresponds to an enteral intake of 1.4–2 mg/kg/day assuming 20–27% absorption. However, such estimations of iron requirements have not considered blood losses and blood transfusions. In very low birth weight (VLBW) infants, iron losses due to phlebotomy amount to about 6 mg/kg per week and each red blood cell transfusion typically adds 8 mg/kg of iron. Hepatic iron stores as well as serum ferritin concentrations in preterm infants are highly correlated to the number of blood transfusions received [12]. Furthermore, the timing of umbilical cord clamping is of great importance for the amount of blood transfused from the placenta to the newborn. A 3-min delay, compared to immediate cord clamping, has been shown to increase the newborn's blood volume on average by 32%, corresponding to 14 mg/kg of iron. A recent Cochrane review concluded that delayed cord clamping (30–120 s) of preterm infants seems to be associated with less need for blood transfusion, less intraventricular hemorrhage and less necrotizing enterocolitis [13]. Erythropoietin treatment results in greatly increased iron requirements and high doses of supplemental iron are recommended as an adjunct to this therapy. Thus, local practice regarding umbilical cord clamping, blood sampling, blood transfusions and erythropoietin treatment will greatly influence iron requirements of preterm infants.

Enteral Iron
The risk for preterm infants to develop ID anemia during the first 6 months of life is as high as 77% [14]. Placebo-controlled trials demonstrated that an enteral iron intake of 2 mg/kg/day from iron supplements or iron-fortified formula effectively prevents ID anemia in preterm or low birth weight infants without observed adverse effects [15]. In a recent trial, iron supplements were also shown to reduce the risk of behavioral problems at 3 years of age in low birth weight infants [16].

The effects of higher doses of iron have been investigated only in very few randomized trials. Friel et al. [17] found no benefit with regard to anemia or neurodevelopment of giving 3–6 mg/kg/day of iron compared to 2–3 mg/kg/day up to 9 months of age to preterms with an average birth weight of 1.5 kg. However, the high iron group had higher glutathione peroxidase concentrations (a marker of oxidative stress), lower plasma zinc and copper levels and a higher number of respiratory tract infections, suggesting possible adverse effects with the higher concentrations of iron. Similarly, Barclay et al. [18] found no effect on Hb of an iron intake of 3.6–6.8 mg/kg/day as compared to 1.0–1.6 mg/kg/day from 2 to 30 weeks postnatal age in infants with an average birth weight of 2,000 g. However, there was a lower erythrocyte superoxide dismutase activity in the high iron group, suggesting altered copper metabolism – a possible adverse effect of iron. In a recent study, Taylor and Kennedy [19] randomized 150 VLBW infants to receive 2 mg/kg/day (from fortified breast milk or preterm formula) or 4 mg/kg/day (with additional 2 mg/kg/day supplementation) of iron from 2 to 3 weeks of age until 36 weeks' postmenstrual age or discharge. There was no significant effect on the main outcome which was hematocrit at 36 weeks or the number of transfusions, nor was there any difference in neonatal morbidity, reticulocyte count or weight at 36 weeks. Unfortunately, this study did not include measurements of ferritin or follow-up after discharge from the neonatal unit.

Two randomized studies in VLBW infants have suggested that early (2 weeks of age) as compared to late (6–8 weeks) start of iron supplementation results in less need for blood transfusions [20, 21]. It is generally not recommended to give iron before 2 weeks of age to newborns since there is data suggesting that antioxidant systems are not fully active until that age [22].

Parenteral Iron

Theoretically, according to factorial calculations, parenteral iron requirements would be 0.2–0.37 mg/kg/day in VLBW infants [9]. Parenteral iron has been given in much higher doses (up to 3 mg/kg/day) in erythropoietin trials for prevention of anemia of prematurity. Only few of those studies have evaluated different doses or modalities of iron intake, but they suggest that enteral iron up to 6 mg/kg/day is as effective as parenteral iron in reducing the number of blood transfusions [23]. There is insufficient data on safety of high parenteral doses of iron but a Cochrane meta-analysis has shown that early erythropoietin treatment, which includes supplemental iron, increases the risk of retinopathy of prematurity [5].

Except for the aforementioned erythropoietin studies, there has been only one published clinical trial of parenteral iron in preterms: Friel et al. [24] randomized 26 VLBW infants to receive parenteral nutrition with iron dextran (0.2–0.25 mg/kg/day) or no iron from 1 to 5 weeks of age. No differences were observed in Hb concentrations, need for blood transfusions, growth or infections. All infants in that study had a low enteral iron intake and a negative iron balance due to blood sampling.

In contrast to iron dextran, iron saccharate (iron sucrose) has not been associated with the risk of anaphylactic reactions. However, there are no studies of iron saccharate in preterms. Iron can be added to non-lipid-containing parenteral nutrition solutions immediately prior to infusion or it can be given as separate bolus infusions on a daily or weekly basis. It is not recommended to add iron compounds to lipid-containing parenteral nutrition solutions due to the risk of destabilization of lipid droplets and increased lipid peroxidation.

Recommendations

We recommend a dietary iron intake of 2 mg/kg/day for infants with a birth weight of 1,500–2,500 g and 2–3 mg/kg/day for infants with a birth weight of <1,500 g (table 2). Prophylactic iron (given as iron drops, preterm formula or fortified human milk) should be started at 2–6 weeks of age (at 2 weeks in VLBW infants). Infants who receive erythropoietin treatment will need a higher dose (up to 6 mg/kg/day) during the treatment period.

Domellöf

Table 2. Enteral and parenteral recommendations (per kg/day) for ELBW and VLBW infants

Nutrient	Enteral recommendation	Parenteral recommendation	Content in 2 ml Peditrace®
Iron, mg	2–3	0–0.25	–
Zinc, mg	1.4–2.5	0.4*	0.5
Copper, µg	100–230	40*	40
Selenium, µg	5–10	5–7*	4
Manganese, µg	1–15	1*	2
Iodine, µg	10–55	10*	2
Chromium, µg	0.03–2.25	0.05–0.3*	–
Molybdenum, µg	0.35	0.25*	–

* Approximate values. Iodine recommendation assumes no use of iodine containing antiseptics.

Since iron status is highly variable between individuals, depending mainly on phlebotomy losses and blood transfusions, we recommend to follow all VLBW infants with (e.g. weekly) measurements of serum ferritin during the hospital stay (using a low blood volume laboratory method). The normal range of ferritin in preterms is 35–300 µg/l (table 1). If ferritin is <35 µg/l, the iron dose should be increased and a dose of 3 to 4–6 mg/kg/day may be required during a limited period. If ferritin is >300 µg/l, which is common in infants who have received multiple blood transfusions, iron supplementation and fortification should be discontinued until ferritin falls below this level. In case of ongoing infection with increased CRP concentrations, serum ferritin may be falsely elevated. There is no evidence that enteral iron supplementation or fortification needs to be discontinued during an ongoing infection if the infant tolerates enteral feeds.

Hb measurements are less useful than ferritin for routine monitoring of iron status in VLBW infants since it does not indicate iron overload and has a lower sensitivity and specificity for detecting ID. The combination of Hb, ferritin and reticulocytes is useful for differentiating between ID anemia and anemia of prematurity.

Due to safety concerns and practical difficulties with regard to compounding and stability, we do not recommend the routine provision of iron in parenteral nutrition for preterms. Most preterms will tolerate enteral feeds within a few weeks after birth and enteral iron supplements will then be sufficient to cover the requirements. However, for those preterms with prolonged need of total parenteral nutrition, we recommend 0.2–0.25 mg/kg/day of parenteral iron.

Iron supplements or intake of iron-fortified formula in the recommended doses should be continued also after discharge, at least until 6–12 months of age, depending on diet. Hb and serum ferritin should be checked at follow-up visits (table 1).

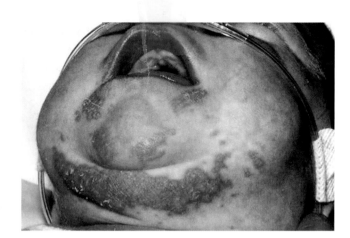

Fig. 1. Typical skin rash in an infant with zinc deficiency (photograph with courtesy of Nicholas Embleton).

Zinc

Zinc is essential for many enzymes and plays an important role in growth and tissue differentiation. Zinc deficiency is a common and well-described problem in infants and children, not least in preterms, and leads to stunted growth, increased risk for infections, skin rash (fig. 1), and possibly poor neurodevelopment [25].

In contrast to iron and copper, zinc does not have a prooxidant effect and adverse effects of excess zinc intakes are rarely reported. There is one described case in which long-term oral zinc supplementation at a dose of 3.6 mg/kg/day resulted in symptomatic copper deficiency in a young child, likely due to inhibition of copper absorption [26].

Zinc homeostasis is maintained by regulation of absorption and endogenous excretion to the gastrointestinal tract and this regulation seems to be functional to some extent also in moderately preterm infants [27]. The fractional absorption in preterm infants is about 30–40% but it is higher from breast milk than from formula [28].

Marginal zinc deficiency is difficult to diagnose due to the lack of a reliable biomarker. Even though serum or plasma zinc is most commonly used, it is not a sensitive indicator of marginal zinc deficiency.

Klein [28] estimated zinc requirements in preterm infants using a factorial method. The requirement for retained zinc (i.e. the amount that absorbed zinc must exceed zinc losses) was estimated to be approximately 400 μg/kg at 30–32 weeks of gestation. Based on data from 14 metabolic balance studies, it has been calculated that an enteral zinc intake of 2.0–2.25 mg/kg/day is required to achieve this zinc retention [29].

The concentration of zinc in colostrum is high (5.4 mg/l, decreasing to 1.1 mg/l at 3 months). The high concentration of zinc in early breast milk in combination with the release of stored zinc from hepatic metallothionein helps protect the infant from zinc deficiency during early infancy. However, these mechanisms are insufficient in infants with a birth weight <1,500–2,000 g.

There have been few clinical trials of different zinc intakes in preterm infants. Díaz-Gómez et al. [30] randomized 37 preterm infants with an average birth weight of 1.7 kg to receive a post-discharge formula with a zinc concentration of 0.5 or 1.0 mg/100 ml (0.7 vs. 1.5 mg/100 kcal). At 3 months post-term, dietary zinc intake was 0.7 vs. 1.4 mg/kg/day in the low and high zinc groups respectively. Infants in the high zinc group had significantly higher serum zinc concentrations at 3 months corrected age and significantly higher linear growth, suggesting that infants in the low zinc group had an insufficient intake.

Friel et al. [31] randomized 52 preterm infants with an average birth weight of 1.1 kg to receive a regular term formula with or without an added zinc supplement from 1 month before discharge (average baseline weight 1.9 kg) to 6 months. The two formulas had zinc concentrations of 6.7 and 11 mg/l, respectively, and energy content of 66 kcal/100 ml. Assuming an energy intake of 120 kcal/kg/day, this corresponds to zinc intakes of 1.2 and 2.0 mg/kg/day. 36 infants completed the study to 6 months. The high zinc group had higher plasma zinc concentrations at 3 months and showed improved linear growth and higher motor development scores at 6 months.

These clinical trials suggest that an intake of at least 1.4–2 mg/kg/day is needed in order to achieve optimal growth in preterm infants. Current recommendations for enteral zinc intake in preterms is 1–2 mg/kg/day [32, 33] or as high as 1–3 mg/kg/day [34].

Recommendation
We recommend an enteral intake of 1.4–2.5 mg/kg/day and a parenteral intake around 400 μg/kg/day (table 2). In patients with significant enterostomy fluid losses, plasma zinc should be followed, since they have high risk of zinc deficiency.

Copper

Copper is an essential nutrient. Its main function in the organism is being a component of different enzymes, e.g. in the electron transport chain, in collagen formation, and in neuropeptide synthesis. It is also a component of antioxidant enzymes, e.g. copper/zinc superoxide dismutase (CuZn-SOD).

Severe copper deficiency is a rare condition associated with anemia, neutropenia, thrombocytopenia and osteoporosis [35]. Little is known about the prevalence and possible health impact of marginal copper deficiency. Risk factors for copper deficiency include low birth weight, inappropriate diet in infancy (e.g. unmodified cow's milk which has a low copper concentration), prolonged diarrhea and intestinal malabsorption [28, 35]. Copper deficiency at 1–8 months postnatally was reported relatively frequently in preterm infants in the 1970s and 1980s [36]. However, most of these case reports were of infants who received copper-free long-term parenteral nutrition and there are no similar recent reports.

Copper status can be assessed by the measurement of the plasma concentration of copper or ceruloplasmin, the main copper-binding protein in plasma. However, these indicators are insensitive to marginal copper deficiency. The activity of CuZn-SOD in erythrocytes is considered to be the most sensitive marker of Cu deficiency.

The intrauterine accretion rate of copper is approximately 50 µg/kg/day [37]. There is a hepatic store of copper at birth, bound to metallothionein, which is utilized during early infancy. Fractional copper absorption is about 60% from breast milk but as low as 16% from unmodified cow's milk. Copper homeostasis is maintained by regulation of both intestinal absorption as well as biliary excretion.

Using a factorial method, the required net retention of copper in preterm infants has been estimated to 30 µg/kg/day, corresponding to a parenteral requirement of 40 µg/kg/day and an enteral requirement of 100 µg/kg/day [28].

The copper content of human milk declines from 600 µg/l during the first week of lactation (800 µg/l in preterm milk) to 220 µg/l by 5 months [38]. Drinking water can be contaminated with copper from water tubings and the upper allowable limit of copper in drinking water is 2,000 µg/l.

Iron and especially zinc may, in sufficient doses, impair copper absorption. It has therefore been suggested that the zinc to copper molar ratio in infant formulas should not exceed 20 [28].

High doses of copper can damage the liver, kidneys and central nervous system [39]. A few cases have been reported where infants and young children have developed cirrhosis due to high chronic copper exposure from drinking water from copper pipes or copper utensils for preparation of foods. Infant rhesus monkeys fed infant formula with a high copper concentration (6.6 mg/l, corresponding to about 1,000 µg/100 kcal) from birth to 5 months did not show any clinical evidence of copper toxicity and there was no histologic damage to the liver [40].

There are very few clinical trials of different copper intakes in preterm infants. Enteral feeding of 41–89 µg/kg/day of copper in preterm infants has been associated with copper deficiency [41]. Tyrala [42] showed no clear benefit of a copper intake of 294 µg/kg/day compared to 121 µg/kg/day in preterm infants as assessed by copper balance, serum copper and ceruloplasmin. However, no adverse effects were observed in the high copper group. Zinc intakes in those infants were 2.0–2.3 mg/kg/day.

Estimates for enteral copper requirements have changed little over the past 25 years. The most recent recommendations are for intakes of between 120 and 150 µg/kg/day [32] or between 100 and 130 µg/kg/day [33]. However, a recent calculation, based on nine published studies of copper balance in preterm infants, has suggested that enteral copper requirements may be 210–232 µg/kg/day if zinc intake is 2–2.25 mg/kg/day, in order to achieve a net copper retention of 30 µg/kg/day [29].

Recommendations
We recommend an enteral intake of 100–230 µg/kg/day and a parenteral intake near 40 µg/kg/day (table 2). The zinc to copper molar ratio in infant formulas should not exceed 20. Parenteral copper should be avoided if cholestasis is present.

Selenium

Selenium is an essential trace element which plays an important role as a component of selenoproteins, including glutathione peroxidases, antioxidant enzymes which prevent free radical formation and oxygen toxicity, as well as deiodinases, which are required for the metabolism of thyroid hormones.

Selenium deficiency in animals leads to cardiomyopathy, muscle weakness, muscle pains, cataracts and erythrocyte macrocytosis. Selenium deficiency in humans has been suggested to be associated with a large number of conditions, including cancer, liver cirrhosis, hypertension, osteopenia and poor immune function, even though all these associations have not been proven to be causal. Selenium deficiency is endemic in some provinces of China, due to low soil levels of selenium, and is believed to be the main cause of Keshan disease, an often fatal cardiomyopathy primarily affecting children and young women. Outside of China, selenium deficiency has only rarely been described in patients with prolonged parenteral nutrition or severe malnutrition. Children receiving long-term parenteral nutrition without selenium supplementation have been reported to develop low plasma selenium, erythrocyte macrocytosis, loss of hair and skin pigmentation and muscle weakness, which respond to selenium supplementation [43].

Preterm infants are at high risk for oxidative stress-related disorders, including bronchopulmonary dysplasia, retinopathy of prematurity and cerebral white matter injury. Selenium deficiency has been associated with an increased susceptibility to oxidative lung injury in rats. Several studies have demonstrated that plasma selenium concentrations decrease during the first weeks of life in VLBW infants, suggesting possible selenium insufficiency [44]. Furthermore, several studies have shown an association between low plasma selenium levels and bronchopulmonary dysplasia in preterm infants [45].

Excessive selenium exposure in adults leads to selenosis, characterized by headache, loss of hair and nails, skin rash, discoloration of teeth, paresthesia and paralysis. There have been no reports of adverse effects caused by excessive selenium intakes in infants or preterms.

Daniels et al. [46] performed a randomized trial of selenium supplementation of parenteral nutrition at a dose of 3 μg/kg/day in 38 VLBW infants. Supplemented infants had higher plasma selenium concentrations than unsupplemented infants, but still lower than term, breast-fed infants. Tyrala et al. [47] showed in a clinical study of 17 preterm infants that selenium supplementation of formula resulting in intakes of 3.2–4.7 μg/kg/day, compared to unsupplemented formula giving 1.4–1.8 μg/kg/day, resulted in improved selenium status. Clinical outcomes were not assessed in these studies.

Darlow et al. [48] performed a randomized, controlled, blinded trial of selenium supplementation in 534 VLBW infants in New Zealand, a country in which soil and food are low in selenium. The supplemental dose was 5 μg/kg/day enterally or 7 μg/

kg/day parenterally. The lower enteral dose was chosen, allowing for additional selenium present in breast milk and formula. Supplements were given from 4 days of life and continued until 36 weeks' postmenstual age or discharge. A significant effect was observed on plasma selenium concentrations, which reached similar levels as healthy, term infants. However, no significant effect was observed on oxygen dependency at 28 days of age, which was the primary outcome. Among the secondary outcomes, no effects were observed except that selenium-supplemented infants had significantly fewer sepsis episodes. In a multivariate analysis, this effect was restricted to those infants who received antenatal steroids. No adverse effects were observed in this study.

Dietary selenium is highly bioavailable. A stable isotope study showed that 60–80% of selenium in formula was absorbed in preterm infants [49]. A balance study has shown that net absorption of selenium from breast milk was 77% in extremely low birth weight infants [44].

Selenium status is usually assessed by measuring serum or plasma concentrations of selenium or the activity of glutathione peroxidase in plasma or red blood cells. In preterm infants, glutathione peroxidase activity is not a useful marker of selenium status since it is affected also by immaturity and oxygen exposure [44].

Selenium concentrations in breast milk are significantly associated with maternal selenium intake. Selenium concentrations in breast milk most often range between 6 and 28 µg/l in the USA and Europe, with averages commonly 15–18 µg/l [28, 44]. Based on 15 µg/l in breast milk and an intake of 150 ml/kg/day, this corresponds to an intake of 2.3 µg/kg/day.

Previous recommendations for enteral intakes in preterm infants are 1.3–4.5 µg/kg/day according to Tsang et al. [32] or 5–10 µg/kg/day according to ESPGHAN 2010 [33]. Previous recommendations for parenteral intakes in preterms are 1.5–4.5 µg/kg/day according to Tsang et al. [32] and 2–3 µg/kg/day according to ESPGHAN [33].

Recommendations
We recommend an enteral intake of 5–10 µg/kg/day (table 2), similar to the dose given in the Darlow study [48] which achieved a selenium status similar to term infants. We recommend parenteral intakes similar to the enteral intakes (table 2).

Manganese

Manganese is an essential trace element which is a cofactor for many enzymes. Manganese-dependent superoxide dismutase (SOD2 or Mn-SOD) is important for cellular defense against free oxygen radicals. Reduced activity of this enzyme has been shown in manganese-deficient animals, and mice lacking SOD2 die after a few days due to massive oxidative stress. Manganese-dependent enzymes are also important for bone formation and manganese deficiency in animals leads to abnormal skeletal development.

There are very few reports of manganese deficiency in humans. The most comprehensive description is from a paper in which experimental manganese deficiency was induced in 7 adult subjects [50]. In that study, a manganese-deficient diet for 39 days resulted in negative manganese balance, biochemical evidence of bone resorption and clinical scaly dermatitis. There has been only one clinical report of manganese deficiency, in a 4-year-old girl with short bowel syndrome who, since the neonatal period, had received total parenteral nutrition which was deficient in manganese. She had short stature and brittle bones as well as a low serum manganese concentration. Bone density and longitudinal growth improved after manganese supplementation [51].

In contrast, there have been many reports of possible adverse effects of high manganese intakes. The main adverse effect of manganese is a neurotoxic effect, called manganism, which can occur with excessive occupational exposure to airborne manganese. Several studies have shown an association between dietary manganese exposure, blood magnesium concentrations and poor cognitive development in children [52]. Manganese deposition in the brain can be detected with magnetic resonance imaging and recent studies have suggested that commercially available manganese containing parenteral trace element supplements can result in pathological manganese deposits in basal ganglia. This has been described in adult patients on long-term total parenteral nutrition [53].

The main regulation of manganese homeostasis occurs at the absorption step. Intestinal absorption of manganese is usually assumed to be low. In a study performed in adults, fractional absorption of manganese was about 8% from human milk, 2% from cow's milk, 0.7% from soy formula and 2–6% from cow's milk-based infant formulas with different iron contents [54]. However, studies in rodents have shown that manganese absorption is higher in the postnatal period than later in life and it has been suggested that this is also true for humans. In rat pups, manganese absorption is 85% from preterm infant formula [55]. The actual fractional absorption of manganese in preterm infants is unknown and may be higher than usually assumed.

The main excretory route for manganese is via the bile and a small amount is lost in urine. In conditions with poor bile excretion, e.g. parenteral nutrition-associated cholestasis, manganese retention is increased.

Average manganese concentrations in breast milk range from <0.1 to 40 µg/l in different studies. In European studies, reported median concentrations vary between 2.6 and 10 µg/l. There is no clear correlation between maternal dietary manganese intake and breast milk manganese concentration. Assuming a breast milk manganese content of 6.5 µg/l and a milk intake of 150 ml/kg/day, a breast-fed infant would receive 1.0 µg/kg/day of manganese.

Manganese is sometimes added as a supplement but sometimes also present as a contaminant in preterm formulas. Current European preterm formulas contain 5–13 µg of manganese per 100 ml, corresponding to an intake of 7.5–20 µg/kg/day.

Similar to their enteral counterparts, parenteral nutrition products can be contaminated with manganese. Manganese excretion via bile is low, especially in long-term TPN with cholestasis, so retention approaches 100%.

Based on fetal tissue concentration data by Casey and Robinson [56] the intrauterine accretion rate of manganese in a 1-kg fetus would be about 7 µg/kg/day.

There are no published intervention studies or observational studies comparing different doses of enteral or parenteral manganese in preterm infants.

Previous recommendations for enteral manganese intakes in preterms range from 0.7–7.5 µg/kg/day [32] to 6.3–25 µg/kg/day [33].

Recommendations

Based on the average breast milk manganese content and the lower range of manganese in current preterm formulas, an enteral intake of manganese of 1–15 µg/kg/day can be recommended (table 2). The lower range is low compared to the estimated fetal accretion rate, but seems prudent since manganese deficiency has never been described in a preterm infant while there is legitimate concern for manganese toxicity.

There has been a long tradition of recommending 1 µg/kg/day of parenteral manganese to preterms. In the ESPEN/ESPGHAN guidelines for children, a maximum of 1 µg/kg/day is recommended [57]. Even though this is lower than the theoretical fetal accretion rate, no case of manganese deficiency has been described in preterms or children. Based on this, we suggest a parenteral intake of 1 µg/kg/day of manganese (table 2).

Since 60–80% of the manganese in blood is contained in red blood cells, it is recommended to measure manganese concentrations in erythrocytes or whole blood. It is recommended to check blood manganese concentrations regularly in patients on long-term TPN. If the patient develops cholestasis, blood concentrations of manganese should be determined and parenteral manganese should be reduced or discontinued.

Iodine

Iodine is a trace element which is an integral part of the thyroid hormones thyroxine (T_4) and triiodothyronine (T_3), which are essential for regulating and stimulating metabolism, temperature control and normal growth and development.

Iodine deficiency results in hypothyroidism, thyroid enlargement (goiter), mental retardation (cretinism), poor growth and increased neonatal and infant mortality.

In utero iodine deficiency causes irreversible damage to the developing fetal brain. Iodine deficiency in pregnant mothers, which occurs in areas where iodine deficiency is endemic, results in cretinism in the newborn. Cretinism is characterized by severe mental retardation, deafness, strabismus and motor spasticity. There is also some evidence that even moderate or mild iodine deficiency in pregnant women increases the risk of neurodevelopmental deficits in the offspring [58].

Thanks to salt iodization programs, iodine deficiency is now rare in the USA, Canada, Australia and also in many European countries. However, iodine deficiency is still relatively common in some European countries, e.g. France and Belgium, due to a low proportion of households using iodized salt [59].

Excessive iodine has a well-known inhibitory effect on thyroid hormone synthesis and release, also resulting in hypothyroidism. In hospitals where iodine is routinely used as a disinfectant, preterm infants can be exposed to high doses of topical iodine, which is absorbed through the skin and can result in mild or severe hypothyreosis [60]. Hypothyroidism has also been described in a breast-fed preterm infant whose mother was exposed to topical iodine disinfectants [61]. We therefore recommend to avoid the use of iodine-containing antiseptics during care of preterm infants and their lactating mothers.

Iodine is effectively absorbed in the intestine; in healthy adults the absorption is >90% and it is assumed to be high also in infants and preterms. Excretion of iodine occurs through the urine.

Urinary iodine in spot urine samples is the easiest method to assess iodine deficiency, but it works only at the population level due to interindividual differences in urine production and hydration status.

In the newborn, thyroid-stimulating hormone (TSH) in serum is a sensitive marker of iodine status. Serum T_4 is often used even though it is a less sensitive biomarker of iodine nutrition status. It is well documented that many preterm infants have low serum T_4 concentrations, especially those with a very low gestational age at birth and severe illness. It is unclear whether this transient hypothyreosis is caused by developmental changes or related to iodine nutritional status [62].

The average iodine concentration in European mothers' breast milk is 70–90 µg/l, corresponding to an intake of 12 µg/kg/day, assuming an intake of 150 ml/kg/day. Breast milk iodine concentrations in the USA have previously been about twice as high but a recent, small study showed an iodine content in USA breast milk of 33–117 µg/l [63].

Based on urinary iodine in healthy, iodine-sufficient newborns, it has been estimated that the mean daily iodine intake during the first week of life is 30–50 µg/day, suggesting that the iodine requirement in term newborns is 8–10 µg/kg/day [64].

A 3-day metabolic balance study of 29 preterm infants and 20 full-term controls in Belgium showed that 40% of the preterm infants had a negative iodine balance even when iodine intake was 17–25 µg/100 kcal [65].

Rogahn et al. [62] randomized 121 preterm infants with an average birth weight of 1.4 kg to receive preterm formula with standard (68 µg/l) or increased (272 µg/l) iodine concentrations, resulting in iodine intakes of 10–13 vs. 32–52 µg/kg/day. No significant difference was observed in TSH, T_3, free T_4 or total T_4 up to term age, suggesting that the lower intake may be sufficient. Long-term effects on neurodevelopment were not assessed in this study, which was performed in the UK where iodine deficiency is rare in the general population [33]. It is unclear whether iodine-containing topical antiseptics were used on the infants in this study.

A Cochrane analysis has found that there is still insufficient data to determine whether iodine supplements improve health outcomes in preterm infants [66]. There is an ongoing randomized, controlled trial in the UK (ClinicalTrials.gov identifier NCT00638092) investigating the effect of iodine supplementation (30 µg/kg/day) on neurodevelopment at 2 years.

Previous recommendations for enteral intakes in preterms are 10–42 µg/kg/day according to Tsang et al. [32] and 11–55 µg/kg/day according to ESPGHAN [33].

There have been reports of clinical cases of iodine deficiency in patients receiving long-term parenteral nutrition. A preterm infant with short bowel syndrome was diagnosed with hypothyroidism due to iodine deficiency at 11 months of age. The infant was being fed almost exclusively parenteral nutrition and was receiving only chlorhexidine-based skin antisepsis after 3 months of age [67].

Current recommendations for parenteral iodine intake in preterms is 1 µg/kg/day [32, 57], even though this is far below the estimated requirement. The reason is that it is assumed that iodine-containing antiseptics will provide sufficient iodine. However, partly due to the risk of excessive iodine intakes, many hospitals have now discontinued the use of iodine-containing antiseptics.

Recommendations
We recommend an enteral intake of 10–55 µg/kg/day and a parenteral intake of about 10 µg/kg/day, reduced to about 1 µg/kg/day if iodine containing topical disinfectants are used (table 2).

Chromium

Chromium is considered to be an essential nutrient, even though this recently has been challenged [68]. Its proposed main role is to potentiate the action of insulin and thereby improve glucose tolerance through a mechanism which has not yet been elucidated.

There have been no clinical reports of chromium deficiency in infants or preterms. Also, there have been no reports of adverse effects of excessive chromium intakes from enteral or parenteral nutrition. There are a few case reports of adult patients with long-term parenteral nutrition who have developed chromium deficiency but there are also some reports of high serum chromium concentrations in this patient group since parenteral nutrition solutions can be contaminated with chromium [57].

There is a large variation between different studies with regard to reported chromium concentrations in breast milk, with mean concentrations ranging between 180 and 1,000 ng/l. Even higher concentrations have been reported, but these may be caused by contamination of samples. In previous reviews, a chromium concentration or 250–500 ng/l in breast milk has been assumed [28, 32].

Chromium concentrations in preterm formulas are generally much higher than in breast milk and have been reported to range between 7.5 and 22 µg/l [28].

Chromium is poorly bioavailable with intestinal absorption in adults being <2% [70]. Urinary excretion is proportional to dietary intake [69].

Recommendations

There is insufficient scientific data upon which to base recommendations for chromium intake in preterms. However, we see no reason to change previous recommendations for enteral chromium intake in preterms of 0.1–2.25 µg/kg/day [32] or 0.03–1.23 µg/kg/day [33], which were based on the concentrations of chromium in breast milk and preterm formulas (table 2), and consider a chromium supply in the range of 0.03–2.25 µg/kg/day as prudent. Similarly, we see no reason to change previous recommendations for parenteral chromium which are 0.05–0.3 µg/kg/day according to Tsang et al. [32] and 0.2 µg/kg/day according to ESPEN/ESPGHAN [57]. It is not needed to add chromium for short-term parenteral nutrition and supplementary chromium may not be needed even for long-term parenteral nutrition since chromium is a common contaminant in these solutions.

Molybdenum

Molybdenum is an essential cofactor for several enzymes involved in oxidation and reduction, including xanthine oxidase, sulfite oxidase and aldehyde oxidase.

There is only a single report of molybdenum deficiency in humans, this was an adult patient receiving long-term parenteral nutrition without molybdenum who developed neurological symptoms and biochemical findings suggesting impaired metabolism of sulfur-containing amino acids, purines and pyrimidines. The biochemical abnormalities in this case were normalized after administration of molybdenum. There are no reports of molybdenum deficiency in children, including preterms.

Molybdenum has a very high bioavailability and >90% of dietary molybdenum is absorbed in infants [70]. Molybdenum homeostasis is regulated primarily by urinary excretion and a large proportion of absorbed molybdenum is excreted in the urine.

Balance studies in adults have suggested a minimum requirement of 25 µg/day, corresponding to 0.4 µg/kg/day [71].

Molybdenum concentrations in breast milk vary between mothers but the mean concentration is regarded to be approximately 2 µg/l [72], corresponding to an intake of 0.3 µg/kg/day, assuming an intake of 150 ml/kg/day. Molybdenum concentrations in preterm formulas are generally much higher than in breast milk, often between 20 and 30 µg/l [28], corresponding to an intake of 3–4.5 µg/kg/day.

There have been no randomized trials of different molybdenum intakes in preterms. Based on an observational balance study in 16 VLBW infants, Friel et al. [73] suggested that an enteral intake of 4–6 μg/kg/day or a parenteral intake of 1 μg/kg/day would be adequate. A stable isotope metabolic balance study in preterms by Sievers et al. [74] suggested that an intake of 3 μg/kg/day or lower may be sufficient.

Recommendations
There is no convincing evidence to change the previous recommendations for enteral (0.3–5 μg/kg/day) and parenteral (approx. 0.25 μg/kg/day) intakes (table 2). Since molybdenum deficiency has not been reported in children, supplemental parenteral molybdenum is only recommended for long-term parenteral nutrition.

Practical Considerations Regarding Microminerals

Parenteral Nutrition
The microminerals zinc, copper, selenium and iodine should be added to parenteral nutrition to VLBW infants within a few days after birth. Parenteral supplementation of iron, manganese, chromium and molybdenum is rarely needed in VLBW infants but should be considered in cases with intestinal failure who require prolonged total or near-total parenteral nutrition.

In Europe, the only available parenteral micromineral supplement is Peditrace® (Fresenius, Germany). As shown in table 1, supplementation with 1–2 ml/kg/day of Peditrace® will give intakes which are reasonably close to the recommended supply with the exception of iodine, which will depend on enteral intake. Development of optimized parenteral micromineral supplements would benefit VLBW infants with intestinal failure who need long-term parenteral nutrition.

Enteral Nutrition
It is important that VLBW infants receive adequate amounts of iron, zinc, copper, selenium and iodine from foods such as human milk with added fortifier, or preterm formula, or from supplements (iron drops). Human milk fortifiers and preterm formulas are normally fortified with zinc, copper, selenium and iodine. Some human milk fortifiers contain adequate amounts of iron but some do not contain iron and should be used in combination with iron drops. The need of food fortification is less clear with regard to manganese, chromium and molybdenum. In conclusion, the evidence base for defining advisable intakes of trace elements other than iron is limited. The intake ranges defined here appear prudent based on current knowledge and clinical experience with such intakes. However, future scientific results may justify deviations from these suggested ranges.

References

1 Domellof M, Braegger C, Campoy C, et al: Iron requirements of infants and toddlers: a position paper by the ESPGHAN Committee on Nutrition. J Pediatr Gastroenterol Nutr 2014;58:119–129.

2 Sachdev H, Gera T, Nestel P: Effect of iron supplementation on mental and motor development in children: systematic review of randomised controlled trials. Public Health Nutr 2005;8:117–132.

3 Szajewska H, Ruszczynski M, Chmielewska A: Effects of iron supplementation in nonanemic pregnant women, infants, and young children on the mental performance and psychomotor development of children: a systematic review of randomized controlled trials. Am J Clin Nutr 2010;91:1684–1690.

4 Domellof M: Iron requirements in infancy. Ann Nutr Metab 2011;59:59–63.

5 Ohlsson A, Aher SM: Early erythropoietin for preventing red blood cell transfusion in preterm and/or low birth weight infants. Cochrane Database Syst Rev 2006;3:CD004863.

6 Zlotkin SH, Lay DM, Kjarsgaard J, Longley T: Determination of iron absorption using erythrocyte iron incorporation of two stable isotopes of iron (^{57}Fe and ^{58}Fe) in very low birth weight premature infants. J Pediatr Gastroenterol Nutr 1995;21:190–199.

7 Ehrenkranz RA, Gettner PA, Nelli CM, et al: Iron absorption and incorporation into red blood cells by very low birth weight infants: studies with the stable isotope ^{58}Fe. J Pediatr Gastroenterol Nutr 1992;15: 270–278.

8 McDonald MC, Abrams SA, Schanler RJ: Iron absorption and red blood cell incorporation in premature infants fed an iron-fortified infant formula. Pediatr Res 1998;44:507–511.

9 Griffin I, Cooke RJ: Iron retention in preterm infants fed low iron intakes: a metabolic balance study. Early Hum Dev 2010;86(suppl 1):49–53.

10 Fomon SJ, Nelson SE, Ziegler EE: Retention of iron by infants. Annu Rev Nutr 2000;20:273–290.

11 Domellöf M, Lönnerdal B, Dewey KG, Cohen RJ, Hernell O: Iron, zinc, and copper concentrations in breast milk are independent of maternal mineral status. Am J Clin Nutr 2004;79:111–115.

12 Ng PC, Lam CW, Lee CH, et al: Hepatic iron storage in very low birth weight infants after multiple blood transfusions. Arch Dis Child Fetal Neonatal Ed 2001; 84:F101–F105.

13 Rabe H, Diaz-Rossello JL, Duley L, Dowswell T: Effect of timing of umbilical cord clamping and other strategies to influence placental transfusion at preterm birth on maternal and infant outcomes. Cochrane Database Syst Rev 2012;8:CD003248.

14 Lundström U, Siimes MA, Dallman PR: At what age does iron supplementation become necessary in low-birth-weight infants? J Pediatr 1977;91:878–883.

15 Doyle JJ, Zipursky A: Neonatal blood disorders; in Sinclair JC, Bracken MB (eds): Effective Care of the Newborn Infant. Oxford, Oxford University Press, 1992, pp 425–453.

16 Berglund SK, Westrup B, Hägglöf B, Hernell O, Domellöf M: Effects of iron supplementation of LBW infants on cognition and behavior at 3 years. Pediatrics 2013;131:47–55.

17 Friel JK, Andrews WL, Aziz K, Kwa PG, Lepage G, L'Abbe MR: A randomized trial of two levels of iron supplementation and developmental outcome in low birth weight infants. J Pediatr 2001;139:254–260.

18 Barclay SM, Aggett PJ, Lloyd DJ, Duffty P: Reduced erythrocyte superoxide dismutase activity in low birth weight infants given iron supplements. Pediatr Res 1991;29:297–301.

19 Taylor TA, Kennedy KA: Randomized trial of iron supplementation versus routine iron intake in VLBW infants. Pediatrics 2013;131:e433–e438.

20 Franz AR, Mihatsch WA, Sander S, Kron M, Pohlandt F: Prospective randomized trial of early versus late enteral iron supplementation in infants with a birth weight of less than 1,301 grams. Pediatrics 2000;106:700–706.

21 Berseth CL, Van Aerde JE, Gross S, Stolz SI, Harris CL, Hansen JW: Growth, efficacy, and safety of feeding an iron-fortified human milk fortifier. Pediatrics 2004;114:e699–e706.

22 Berger HM, Mumby S, Gutteridge JM: Ferrous ions detected in iron-overloaded cord blood plasma from preterm and term babies: implications for oxidative stress. Free Radic Res 1995;22:555–559.

23 Ridley FC, Harris J, Gottstein R, Emmerson AJ: Is supplementary iron useful when preterm infants are treated with erythropoietin? Arch Dis Child 2006;91: 1036–1038.

24 Friel JK, Andrews WL, Hall MS, et al: Intravenous iron administration to very-low-birth-weight newborns receiving total and partial parenteral nutrition. JPEN J Parenter Enteral Nutr 1995;19:114–118.

25 Hambidge M: Human zinc deficiency. J Nutr 2000; 130(suppl):1344S–1349S.

26 Sugiura T, Goto K, Ito K, Ueta A, Fujimoto S, Togari H: Chronic zinc toxicity in an infant who received zinc therapy for atopic dermatitis. Acta Paediatr 2005;94:1333–1335.

27 King JC, Shames DM, Woodhouse LR: Zinc homeostasis in humans. J Nutr 2000;130(suppl):1360S–1366S.

28 Klein CJ: Nutrient requirements for preterm infant formulas. J Nutr 2002;132(suppl 1):1395S–1577S.

29 Bhatia J, Griffin I, Anderson D, Kler N, Domellof M: Selected macro/micronutrient needs of the routine preterm infant. J Pediatr 2013;162(suppl):S48–S55.

30 Díaz-Gómez NM, Doménech E, Barroso F, Castells S, Cortabarria C, Jiménez A: The effect of zinc supplementation on linear growth, body composition, and growth factors in preterm infants Pediatrics 2003;111:1002–1009.

31 Friel JK, Andrews WL, Matthew JD, et al: Zinc supplementation in very-low-birth-weight infants. J Pediatr Gastroenterol Nutr 1993;17:97–104.

32 Tsang RC, Uauy R, Koletzko B, Zlotkin S: Nutritional Needs of the Preterm Infant. Scientific Basis and Practical Guidelines, ed 2. Baltimore, Williams & Wilkins, 2005.

33 Agostoni C, Buonocore G, Carnielli VP, et al: Enteral nutrient supply for preterm infants: commentary from the European Society of Paediatric Gastroenterology, Hepatology and Nutrition Committee on Nutrition. J Pediatr Gastroenterol Nutr 2010;50: 85–91.

34 Kleinman RE: Pediatric Nutrition Handbook, ed 6. Elk Grove Village, American Academy of Pediatrics, 2009.

35 Cordano A: Clinical manifestations of nutritional copper deficiency in infants and children. Am J Clin Nutr 1998;67(suppl):1012S–1016S.

36 Sutton AM, Harvie A, Cockburn F, Farquharson J, Logan RW: Copper deficiency in the preterm infant of very low birth weight. Four cases and a reference range for plasma copper. Arch Dis Child 1985;60: 644–651.

37 Widdowson EM: Trace elements in foetal and early postnatal development. Proc Nutr Soc 1974;33:275–284.

38 Casey CE, Neville MC, Hambidge KM: Studies in human lactation: secretion of zinc, copper, and manganese in human milk. Am J Clin Nutr 1989;49:773–785.

39 Cai L, Li XK, Song Y, Cherian MG: Essentiality, toxicology and chelation therapy of zinc and copper. Curr Med Chem 2005;12:2753–2763.

40 Araya M, Kelleher SL, Arredondo MA, et al: Effects of chronic copper exposure during early life in rhesus monkeys. Am J Clin Nutr 2005;81:1065–1071.

41 Manser JI, Crawford CS, Tyrala EE, Brodsky NL, Grover WD: Serum copper concentrations in sick and well preterm infants. J Pediatr 1980;97:795–799.

42 Tyrala EE: Zinc and copper balances in preterm infants. Pediatrics 1986;77:513–517.

43 Vinton NE, Dahlstrom KA, Strobel CT, Ament ME: Macrocytosis and pseudoalbinism: manifestations of selenium deficiency. J Pediatr 1987;111:711–717.

44 Loui A, Raab A, Braetter P, Obladen M, de Braetter VN: Selenium status in term and preterm infants during the first months of life. Eur J Clin Nutr 2008; 62:349–355.

45 Mostafa-Gharehbaghi M, Mostafa-Gharabaghi P, Ghanbari F, Abdolmohammad-Zadeh H, Sadeghi GH, Jouyban A: Determination of selenium in serum samples of preterm newborn infants with bronchopulmonary dysplasia using a validated hydride generation system. Biol Trace Elem Res 2012;147:1–7.

46 Daniels L, Gibson R, Simmer K: Randomised clinical trial of parenteral selenium supplementation in preterm infants. Arch Dis Child Fetal Neonatal Ed 1996; 74:F158–F164.

47 Tyrala EE, Borschel MW, Jacobs JR: Selenate fortification of infant formulas improves the selenium status of preterm infants. Am J Clin Nutr 1996;64:860–865.

48 Darlow BA, Winterbourn CC, Inder TE, et al: The effect of selenium supplementation on outcome in very low birth weight infants: a randomized controlled trial. The New Zealand Neonatal Study Group. J Pediatr 2000;136:473–480.

49 Ehrenkranz RA, Gettner PA, Nelli CM, et al: Selenium absorption and retention by very-low-birth-weight infants: studies with the extrinsic stable isotope tag ^{74}Se. J Pediatr Gastroenterol Nutr 1991;13: 125–133.

50 Friedman BJ, Freeland-Graves JH, Bales CW, et al: Manganese balance and clinical observations in young men fed a manganese-deficient diet. J Nutr 1987;117:133–143.

51 Freeland-Graves JH, Turnlund JR: Deliberations and evaluations of the approaches, endpoints and paradigms for manganese and molybdenum dietary recommendations. J Nutr 1996;126(suppl):2435S–2440S.

52 Roels HA, Bowler RM, Kim Y, et al: Manganese exposure and cognitive deficits: a growing concern for manganese neurotoxicity. Neurotoxicology 2012;33: 872–880.

53 Abdalian R, Saqui O, Fernandes G, Allard JP: Effects of Manganese from a commercial multi-trace element supplement in a population sample of Canadian patients on long-term parenteral nutrition. JPEN J Parenter Enteral Nutr 2012;37:538–543.

54 Davidsson L, Cederblad A, Lonnerdal B, Sandstrom B: Manganese absorption from human milk, cow's milk, and infant formulas in humans. Am J Dis Child 1989;143:823–827.

55 Knudsen E, Sandstrom B, Andersen O: Zinc and manganese bioavailability from human milk and infant formula used for very low birth weight infants, evaluated in a rat pup model. Biol Trace Elem Res 1995;49:53–65.

56 Casey CE, Robinson MF: Copper, manganese, zinc, nickel, cadmium and lead in human foetal tissues. Br J Nutr 1978;39:639–646.

57 Iron, Minerals and Trace Elements (ESPEN/ESPGHAN recommendations). J Pediatr Gastroenterol Nutr 2005;41:S39–S46.

58 Vermiglio F, Lo Presti VP, Moleti M, et al: Attention deficit and hyperactivity disorders in the offspring of mothers exposed to mild-moderate iodine deficiency: a possible novel iodine deficiency disorder in developed countries. J Clin Endocrinol Metab 2004;89:6054–6060.

59 Zimmermann MB, Andersson M: Prevalence of iodine deficiency in Europe in 2010. Ann Endocrinol (Paris) 2011;72:164–166.

60 Khashu M, Chessex P, Chanoine JP: Iodine overload and severe hypothyroidism in a premature neonate. J Pediatr Surg 2005;40:E1–E4.

61 Smith VC, Svoren BM, Wolfsdorf JI: Hypothyroidism in a breast-fed preterm infant resulting from maternal topical iodine exposure. J Pediatr 2006;149:566–567.

62 Rogahn J, Ryan S, Wells J, et al: Randomised trial of iodine intake and thyroid status in preterm infants. Arch Dis Child Fetal Neonatal Ed 2000;83:F86–F90.

63 Belfort MB, Pearce EN, Braverman LE, He X, Brown RS: Low iodine content in the diets of hospitalized preterm infants. J Clin Endocrinol Metab 2012;97:E632–E636.

64 Dorey CM, Zimmermann MB: Reference values for spot urinary iodine concentrations in iodine-sufficient newborns using a new pad collection method. Thyroid 2008;18:347–352.

65 Delange F, Bourdoux P, Chanoine JP, Ermans AM: Physiopathology of iodine nutrition during pregnancy, lactation and early postnatal life; in Berg H (ed): Vitamins and Minerals in Pregnancy and Lactation. New York, Raven Press, 1988, vol 16, pp 205–214.

66 Ibrahim M, Sinn J, McGuire W: Iodine supplementation for the prevention of mortality and adverse neurodevelopmental outcomes in preterm infants. Cochrane Database Syst Rev 2006;2:CD005253.

67 Crill C, Norman J, Hak E, Christensen M, Helms R: Iodine deficiency and hypothyroidism in an infant receiving parenteral nutrition. Nutr Clin Pract 2009;24:137–138.

68 Di Bona KR, Love S, Rhodes NR, et al: Chromium is not an essential trace element for mammals: effects of a 'low-chromium' diet. J Biol Inorg Chem 2011;16:381–390.

69 Anderson RA, Kozlovsky AS: Chromium intake, absorption and excretion of subjects consuming self-selected diets. Am J Clin Nutr 1985;41:1177–1183.

70 Sievers E, Dorner K, Garbe-Schonberg D, Schaub J: Molybdenum metabolism: stable isotope studies in infancy. J Trace Elem Med Biol 2001;15:185–191.

71 Turnlund JR, Keyes WR, Peiffer GL: Molybdenum absorption, excretion, and retention studied with stable isotopes in young men at five intakes of dietary molybdenum. Am J Clin Nutr 1995;62:790–796.

72 Institute of Medicine: Dietary Reference Intakes for Vitamin A, Vitamin K, Arsenic, Boron, Chromium, Copper, Iodine, Iron, Manganese, Molybdenum, Nickel, Silicon, Vanadium, and Zinc. Washington, National Academy Press, 2001.

73 Friel JK, MacDonald AC, Mercer CN, et al: Molybdenum requirements in low-birth-weight infants receiving parenteral and enteral nutrition. JPEN J Parenter Enteral Nutr 1999;23:155–159.

74 Sievers E, Oldigs HD, Dorner K, Kollmann M, Schaub J: Molybdenum balance studies in premature male infants. Eur J Pediatr 2001;160:109–113.

Magnus Domellöf, MD, PhD
Division of Pediatrics, Department of Clinical Sciences
Umea University
SE–90185 Umea (Sweden)
E-Mail magnus.domellof@pediatri.umu.se

Koletzko B, Poindexter B, Uauy R (eds): Nutritional Care of Preterm Infants: Scientific Basis and Practical Guidelines.
World Rev Nutr Diet. Basel, Karger, 2014, vol 110, pp 140–151 (DOI: 10.1159/000358463)

Calcium, Phosphorus, Magnesium and Vitamin D Requirements of the Preterm Infant

Francis B. Mimouni[a, b, d] · Dror Mandel[a, c, d] · Ronit Lubetzky[b, d] · Thibault Senterre[e]

Departments of [a]Neonatology, Shaare Zedek Medical Center, Jerusalem, [b]Pediatrics and [c]Neonatology, Dana Dwek Children's Hospital and Lis Maternity Hospital, Tel Aviv Medical Center, and [d]Sackler School of Medicine, Tel Aviv University, Tel Aviv, Israel; [e]University of Liège, Department of Neonatology, CHU de Liège, CHR de la Citadelle, Liège, Belgium

Reviewed by Magnus Domellöf, Department of Pediatrics, Umea University, Umea, Sweden; Alison Leaf, National Institute for Health Research, University of Southampton, Southhampton, UK

Abstract

Proper mineral and vitamin D nutrition in preterm infants is essential for adequate bone health because preterm infants are at a risk of prematurely developing osteopenia. This chapter focuses on nutritional aspects of the requirements after a brief description of the perinatal physiology of minerals and vitamin D. The rationale for estimation of nutritional mineral requirements of the preterm infant (based upon estimates of the intrauterine skeletal accretion rate of minerals, and upon estimates of the coefficient of intestinal absorption) is first described. Previous expert recommendations are reviewed and compared to the present recommendations. Finally, vitamin D requirements are thoroughly reviewed based upon what is known of the physiology of vitamin D in preterm infants. A suggestion that each extremely preterm infant should be monitored for adequate vitamin D status is made.   © 2014 S. Karger AG, Basel

Proper mineral and vitamin D nutrition in preterm infants is essential for adequate bone health. Indeed, preterm infants are at risk of developing osteopenia of prematurity for multiple reasons. Among them: (1) low mineral stores at birth due to reduced gestation (80% of minerals are accreted in bone during the third trimester) [1]; (2) difficulties to rapidly establish adequate enteral nutrient supply [1]; (3) inability to provide an amount of minerals similar to that provided by placental transport during a normal pregnancy using parenteral nutrition [1]; (4) use of medications deleterious to the skeleton such as loop diuretics and corticosteroids [1]; (5) contamination of parenteral nutrition solutions with toxins such as aluminum [1]; (6) immobilization in critically ill infants [1], and (7) possibly vitamin D deficiency in some subgroups of preterm infants [2–4]. In this chapter, we will only focus on nutritional aspects of the requirements, after a brief description of the perinatal physiology of minerals and vitamin D.

Perinatal Mineral Homeostasis

During the third trimester, the human fetus is exposed to a hormonal milieu particularly prone for ideal bone mineralization [5]. Abundant substrate is provided through active transport of calcium (Ca) against a concentration gradient with relative hypercalcemia leading to decreased bone resorption (due to relatively low parathyroid hormone and low 1,25-dihydroxyvitamin D ($1,25(OH)_2D$)), and increased bone mineralization (due to high calcitonin and possibly also to high $24,25(OH)_2D$) [5]. During the third trimester, the average accretion rates are 100–120 mg/kg/day for Ca and 50–65 mg/kg/day for phosphorus (P) (up to 150 mg/kg/day for Ca and 75 mg/kg/day for P). Similarly, the term fetus accretes about 760 mg of magnesium (Mg) until birth (on average 3–5 mg/day), just over half of it in bone, and a third in muscles and soft tissues [6]. The intracellular concentration of Mg is about ten times that of the extracellular fluid.

Intrauterine accretion rates are extremely difficult to match in an extrauterine environment. Given issues of mineral solubility, there is a limit to how much Ca and P can be introduced in parenteral solution [7]. Human milk, the ideal 'food' for human term babies, is probably also the ideal nutrition for preterm babies, if it were only for the improved survival and decreased morbidity such as a reduced incidence of necrotizing enterocolitis [8, 9]. However, reduced growth, and inadequate Ca and in particular P intake are inherent to exclusive human milk feeding, and may lead to a particular form of rickets of prematurity, with severe hypophosphatemia and hypercalcemia [10]. Thus the need to 'fortify' human milk with minerals, which efficiently increases linear growth during the in-hospital period [11], with less convincing effects when fortifiers are used after discharge [12]. An alternative to fortified human milk is the administration of formulas designed to meet or approximate the mineral (and the other nutritional) needs of the preterm infant. Nevertheless, one must not assume that all minerals added to formulas or to human milk fortifiers are necessarily absorbed. Indeed, multiple factors regulate mineral intestinal absorption. These include the vitamin D status of the infant, the concentration of Ca and P and their ratio, the concentration and physical properties of major macronutrients such as protein or lactose, the amount and source of fat, and the production process (heat treatment of liquid formulae may promote a Maillard reaction that may decrease Ca absorption [13]). In addition, other elements may theoretically compete with intestinal Ca absorption, such as sodium, zinc, or iron. Thus, 'more' mineral intake is not necessarily translated in more mineral accreted, and a high mineral supply has the potential for more soap formation with dietary fat, more fecal Ca, more fat and energy losses, and more con-

Table 1. Recommendations on the daily intake of Ca, P, Mg and vitamin D for preterm VLBW infants issued by different bodies and authors

Intake recommendation	ESPGAN 1987	ESPGHAN 2010	LSRO, 2002	Atkinson and Tsang, 2005	Rigo, 2007	AAP, 2013	Current authors' proposal, 2013
Ca, mg/kg/day	70–140	120–140	150–220	120–200	100–160	150–220	120–200
P, mg/kg/day	50–90	60–90	100–130	70–120	60–90	75–140	60–140
Mg, mg/kg/day	4.85–9.7	8–15	6.8–17 mg/100 kcal	7.2–9.6	not provided	not provided	8–15
Vitamin D, IU/day	800–1,600	800–1,000	90–225	200–1,000	800–1,000	200–400	400–1,000

stipation [14, 15]. Under certain circumstances, high Ca intakes can result in the formation of precipitates with casein and long-chain fatty acids that may lead to intestinal obstruction [16].

The intestinal absorption of Mg is poorly understood. Approximately 40% of ingested Mg is absorbed from formula, mostly in the proximal gut [17], and Mg absorbed and retained from human milk averages 41% of intake in preterm infants, with a range of 17–66% [18]. This coefficient of absorption in preterm infants is affected by the luminal concentration of Mg and its solubility. Ca and Mg do not compete with each other for intestinal absorption in preterm infants, but high phosphate content in formula may decrease intestinal Mg through formation of insoluble complexes [17].

Enteral Calcium, Phosphorus and Magnesium Requirements

In term infants, the model followed is usually that of human milk. Human milk is adapted to the needs of the human infant, and formulas are for the most part designed in order to mimic either the composition or the functions of human milk. In contrast, it cannot be assumed that human milk, naturally 'designed' to fit the extrauterine needs of the term infant, can be used as the 'perfect' model for the preterm infant. Indeed, intrauterine and extrauterine growth rates, nutrient accretion, etc., are not identical. Thus, nutritional mineral requirements of the preterm infant have been traditionally estimated upon two major bases: the first one relates to the intrauterine accretion rate of minerals by the skeleton, and the other one relates to the coefficient of absorption of minerals by the preterm intestine. Subsequently, several sets of recommendations have been published by various experts. There are the 1987 ESPGAN recommendations [19], commented upon and revised in 2010 [20], the Life Science Research Office recommendations (LSRO) [21], the Atkinson and Tsang recommendations [22], and the recommendations by Rigo et al. [23, 24] together with recent AAP recommendations [25] (table 1). These recommendations apply to very low birth weight infants until they reach a postmenstrual age of approximately 40 weeks and a birth weight close to normal term birth weight.

Mimouni · Mandel · Lubetzky · Senterre

Mineral accretion estimates during pregnancy are essentially all based upon the cornerstones studies of Widdowson et al. [6], who carefully analyzed the body composition of a large number of aborted fetuses at various gestational ages, including the exact mineral composition of their ashes. According to Widdowson's work, during the last 3 months of gestation the fetal accretion of Ca, P and Mg is about 20 g, 10 g and 700 mg, respectively, which represents accretion rates of approximately 100–120 mg/kg/day for Ca, 50–65 mg/kg/day for P, and 3–5 mg/kg/day for Mg [6].

The assumptions used for intestinal absorption estimates in the above-mentioned recommendations are based upon either older balance studies, or upon studies using stable isotopes of Ca and Mg [26]. Although these studies have allowed improving massively our knowledge on mineral metabolism and balance, they have shown that there is a significant variability of mineral absorption among preterm infants. The coefficient of absorption of Ca ranges grossly between 40 and 70%, that of P between 60 and 95%, and that of Mg approximates 40% [27, 28]. These variations explain most of the differences among the various experts' recommendations. The lowest estimate of Ca requirements in mg/kg/day is that of ESPGHAN [19] and the highest is by the LSRO [21] and the AAP [25]. Similarly, the lowest estimate of P requirement is by the ESPGHAN [19] and the highest is by AAP [25] (table 1). In view of the fact that most recent data using stable isotopes of Ca are consistent with relatively lower coefficients of absorption of Ca than older data showed, we favor the higher estimates as proposed by Atkinson and Tsang [22]. We suggest that the daily requirements for Ca should be 120–200 mg/kg. The ESPGHAN [20] used an estimate of 90% of coefficient of absorption for P, an optimistic estimate when considering for instance the data of Lapillonne et al. [29] who found coefficients of absorption of 76% in fortified human milk fed preterm infants and 65.3% in those fed a preterm formula. We suggest that the daily requirements of P should cover a wider range than that recommended by ESPGHAN, and be similar to the Atkinson and Tsang proposals (60–140 mg/kg).

In human milk, the Ca:P ratio is 2:1 in mass, close to the actual composition of skeletal minerals (2.2:1) [20]. Thus, it would seem logical that the Ca:P ratio (by weight) be maintained approximately at the level present in human milk, i.e. approximately 2:1. However, it might be more appropriate taking into account P accretion with lean body mass, especially when optimizing preterm infant macronutrient intakes, and a ratio of 1.6:1–1.8:1 has been suggested by Mize et al. [30], based upon careful balance studies. As far as Mg is concerned, it has been calculated that preterm infants fed human milk are provided with an intake of 5.5–7.5 mg/kg/day [22]. ESPGHAN assumed an absorption coefficient of 40%, and calculated a net accretion of 2.2–3 mg/kg/day, i.e. less than the 3–5 mg/kg/day of intrauterine accretion (for a 1-kg baby) [19, 20]. ESPGHAN recommended that infants fed formula be provided with Mg intakes of 8–12 mg/kg/day, because they had a retention rate within the range of intrauterine accretion [31]. Lapillonne et al. [29] found a 37.5% coefficient of absorption for Mg in their balance studies both in fortified human milk-fed preterm infants and in those fed a preterm formula. In contrast, Koo and Tsang [32] assumed that the coefficient of absorption of Mg is 50%, and thus estimated the requirements to be 8 mg/kg/day (0.33 mmol). We consider coefficient of absorption of approximately 40% a more realistic [18, 29] and recommend a daily Mg intake of 8–15 mg/kg, as suggested by ESPGHAN.

Vitamin D Requirements

The issue of vitamin D requirements in preterm infants is complex. Requirements may be theoretically affected by the availability of substrates such as Ca, P, Mg and vitamin D itself. In addition, it is unclear whether all the elements of adequate vitamin D metabolism (including production, absorption, action and degradation) are mature in preterm infants. Thus, circulating values of vitamin D and its metabolites at concentrations that appear to be adequate in term infants may not be adequate in preterm infants.

Vitamin D Stores at Birth
In humans, 25-hydroxyvitamin D (25(OH)D), the major circulating metabolite of vitamin D after its 25-hydroxylation in the liver, is also the vitamin D metabolite involved in transplacental passage [33]. Theoretically vitamin D stores of preterm infants at birth may be lower than those of term infants, because of shortened gestation. However, Pittard et al. [34] found that serum 25(OH)D concentrations are not influenced by gestational age, while Chan et al. [35] found them to increase with gestational age. In a more recent study of infants born between 25 and 35 weeks, serum 25(OH)D at 1 week of age were unaffected by gestational age [36]. Moreover, vitamin D stores at birth (as evaluated by cord blood 25(OH)D concentrations) correlate with maternal serum concentrations, and are mostly influenced by maternal race, sun exposure and dietary intake rather than gestational age at birth [33]. Specific populations, such as subcontinental Indians [2], or Middle-Eastern Arabs [3], and in the USA to a certain extent, African-American preterm infants [4] are at a greater risk of vitamin D deficiency at birth, presumably due to poorer maternal vitamin D status. A recent study in the USA showed that at the latitude of Cincinnati, 64% of very preterm infants (<32 weeks at birth) were vitamin D deficient at birth [37].

Vitamin D Production in Skin
To our knowledge, no studies have been published evaluating vitamin D production in the skin production in preterm infants exposed to UVB. Preterm infants are generally not exposed to UVB during their stay in the NICU. They also are not likely to not be routinely exposed to UVB after discharge. Indeed, the American Academy of Pediatrics (AAP) recommends to use sunblock in infants >6 months of age (in order to protect them from skin cancer), and to avoid exposure to direct sunlight in infants <6 months [38]. Thus, we assume that vitamin D skin production should be negligible in preterm infants who become essentially dependent on preformed vitamin D supply.

Mimouni · Mandel · Lubetzky · Senterre

Intestinal Vitamin D Absorption

Studies on preterm infants given doses as low as 108 IU/day [39] and as high as 1,000 IU/day [40] show that preterm infants have increases in serum 25(OH)D concentrations similar to those of term infants, which supports the concept of similar vitamin D absorption (and 25-hydroxylation). With daily intakes of 400 IU, 87% of preterm infants <1,500 g at birth achieve 25(OH)D concentrations >50 nmol/l (20 ng/ml), level covering requirements in terms of skeletal health, and 8% achieve concentrations >125 nmol/l, a level associated with potential risk of harm [41]. In contrast, a recent study in the USA showed that 35% of very preterm infants were vitamin D deficient at discharge despite 200–400 IU/day vitamin D intakes [37]. In another study, intakes of 1,000 IU/day allowed to correct vitamin D deficiency at birth by day 10 on average [42]. In one study from Japan, where preterm infant formulae have very high vitamin D content, as high as 2,700 IU/l, 75% of serum samples obtained from preterm infants had 25(OH)D values >100 nmol/l [43]. Importantly, in these infants, urinary Ca/creatinine ratios were not reliable indicators of excessive vitamin D intake [43].

Liver 25-Hydroxylation

Although the 25-hydroxylation process has not been directly investigated, many studies have shown adequate 25(OH)D increases after administration of vitamin D in preterm infants [34, 39, 40, 44, 45] which support the concept that both absorption and 25-hydroxylation of vitamin D are adequate.

1-Hydroxylation in the Kidney

Most studies have reported higher values of $1,25(OH_2)D$ in preterm infants than in term infants [46]. Those infants with rickets of prematurity and or fractures have actually the highest values [46, 47]. Thus, it appears that the regulation of renal 1-hydroxylation is effective and in place in small preterm infants.

Action of $1,25(OH_2)D$

Ravid et al. [48] have suggested that in vitro $1,25(OH_2)D$ effect on lymphocytes is blunted as compared to adults. However, in their study there were no differences between lymphocytes obtained from term and those obtained from preterm infants. In an in vivo study, 90 preterm infants <32 weeks' gestation received in a non-randomized fashion doses of $1,25(OH_2)D$ varying from 0.1 to 3 µg/kg [49]. In all infants, serum Ca decreased at 24 h and increased again by 72 h. The authors thus concluded that preterm infants were somewhat refractory to $1,25(OH_2)D$, although there was no control group [49]. Indeed, a dose of 0.68 µg/day in adults with renal failure is capable of eliciting a calcemic response [49]. In a further study from the same group, Koo et al. [50] administered $1,25(OH_2)D$ (4 µg/kg) or no medication. The difference between treated infants and controls was striking. Thus, preterm infants responded well to supraphysiologic doses of $1,25(OH_2)D$. Whether or not they respond to physiologic doses has not been determined.

As reviewed in the preceding paragraphs, there is no strong evidence that metabolism of vitamin D in preterm infants is different from that of term infants. Moreover, mean serum 25(OH)D concentrations in small preterm infants with rickets or fractures are not different from those of preterm infants without rickets or fractures. In 1989, Evans et al. [51] randomized 81 small preterm infants (<1,500 g at birth) to daily 400 versus 200 IU of vitamin D and 2 months later did not find any differences in bone outcome. Koo et al. [52] randomized VLBW infants fed high Ca and high P preterm formula to a vitamin D daily intake of 200, 400 or 800 IU. They found no biochemical or radiological differences between groups. Backström et al. [53] randomized preterm infants to 500 versus 1,000 IU daily and reported no difference in bone mass between groups at either 3 months or at age 11 years [54]. In a recent study, 48 preterm infants were randomized to three groups of vitamin D intake (200, 400, or 800 IU daily) [55]. Serum Ca and P were not different among groups after 2 weeks of treatment, and serum osteocalcin (an index of bone formation and turnover) increased similarly in all three groups. The highest intake group had a significant increase in urine deoxypyridinoline, an index of bone resorption [55]. This study was small and did not attempt to directly study bone density. Finally, a comparative study of 32 preterm infants with enamel defects and 64 controls failed to demonstrate that a daily vitamin D dose of 500 or 100 IU reduced the prevalence of such defects [56].

We conclude that the advisable vitamin D intake for preterm infants ranges from 400 to 1,000 IU/day according to their vitamin D status. A dose of 400 IU/day is probably sufficient to maintain adequate (>50 nmol/l) serum concentrations of 25(OH)D in most preterm infants and to prevent vitamin D deficiency rickets, without exposing them to significant risks of vitamin D intoxication. In vitamin D deficient newborns, a daily intake of 1,000 IU vitamin is probably required to normalize neonatal stores. Whether or not it is also sufficient to provide infants with extraskeletal benefits of vitamin D is not known at this moment [39, 57]. Nevertheless, as methods for the measurement of 25(OH)D concentrations are more standardized and readily available than in the past [58], we suggest that each extremely preterm infant should be monitored for adequate vitamin D status.

Parenteral Requirements

During the first week of life, VLBW infants usually receive the majority of their nutritional intakes by the intravenous route. Therefore, parenteral nutrition represents a major therapeutic issue in VLBW infants that at times requires several weeks of treatment until they can be completely fed by the enteral route [59, 60]. Although the minerals provided in parenteral nutrition are directly available for metabolism, a significant limiting factor is the relatively poor mineral salt solubility that restricts one's ability to provide infants with a supply that would match intrauterine needs. In addition, preterm infants at birth are at high risk for perturbations of mineral homeostasis, particularly hypocalcemia and hypophosphatemia [24]. Thus, adequate provision of Ca immediately after birth is necessary to reduce the risk of early-onset hypocalcemia [24]. A similar concept is emerging for early P intakes [61–63]. Indeed, beside its important role in bone metabolism, P plays a critical role in energy metabolism and represents a major intracellular anion that is essential for cell membrane function, and adenosine triphosphate and nucleic acids formation. Early hypophosphatemia is particularly frequent in intrauterine growth-restricted preterm infants and might be underestimated due to the fact that laboratories frequently report adult references with lower thresholds. Hypophosphatemia is generally characterized by reduced urinary phosphate excretion and a higher rate of bone resorption that may induce hypercalcemia and/or hypercalciuria [64]. Hypophosphatemia is generally considered when plasma phosphate levels decrease below 5 mg/dl (1.6 mmol/l) [24]. Recent studies have demonstrated an association between optimization of macronutrient intakes and hypophosphatemia during the first weeks of life in VLBW infants [61–63]. P retention is linked to both bone and lean body mass accretion with a Ca:P ratio of ~2.15 (mg) in the bone and nitrogen:P ratio of ~16 (mg) in lean body mass [24, 64]. This is important to consider when optimizing nutritional intakes during parenteral nutrition, particularly during the first week of life. Indeed, improving early postnatal growth with positive nitrogen retention implies that P requirements in preterm infants are probably higher than previously estimated for parenteral nutrition [59, 64]. Thus, the 'ideal' Ca:P ratio on parenteral nutrition is different than for enteral nutrition and is probably between 1 and 1.5 (mg) [24].

Mg intakes are rarely indispensable during the first days of life except when hypomagnesemia is associated with refractory hypocalcemia [24]. Moreover, neonatal hypermagnesemia might be observed in case of maternal treatment with Mg sulfate or high P intakes [24]. Therefore, recent recommendations [59, 60, 65] are that, on the first day of life, mineral requirements on parenteral nutrition be 25–40 mg/kg/day for Ca (1 mmol/kg/day), 18–30 mg/kg/day for P (1 mmol/kg/day), and 0–3 mg/kg/day for Mg (0–0.12 mmol/kg/day). Afterwards, Ca intake might be increased up to 65–100 mg/kg/day (1.6–2.5 mmol/kg/day), P intake up to 50–80 mg/kg/day (1.6–2.5 mmol/kg/day) and Mg intakes up to 7–10 mg/kg/day (0.3–0.4 mmol/kg/day). In spite of the fact that such intakes are lower than the mean fetal accretion during the third trimester of gestation, they might allow similar or higher accretion than on enteral nutrition with current preterm infant formula [24, 59].

Post-Discharge Requirements

As discussed extensively in a medical position paper by the ESPGHAN Committee on Nutrition in 2006, at the time of discharge, many VLBW and ELBW infants have 'cumulative deficits in the accretion of energy, protein, minerals and other nutrients, resulting in higher nutrient requirements per kilogram body weight than healthy appropriate for gestational age infants' [66]. The 2006 ESPGHAN position statement recommended that if preterm infants are fed formula, they should receive a special post-discharge formula with high content of protein, minerals and trace elements as well as LC-PUFA [66]. However, a 2012 Cochrane review of nutrient-enriched formula versus standard term formula for preterm infants following hospital discharge concluded that current recommendations to prescribe 'post-discharge formula' for preterm infants following hospital discharge are not supported by the available evidence; it also stated that some limited evidence exists that feeding preterm infants following hospital discharge with 'preterm formula' (which is generally only available for in-hospital use) may increase growth rates up to 18 months' corrected age [67]. Furthermore, a 2013 Cochrane review of multinutrient fortification of human breast milk for preterm infants following hospital discharge concluded that the limited available data do not provide convincing evidence that feeding preterm infants with multinutrient-fortified breast milk compared with unfortified breast milk following hospital discharge affects important outcomes including growth rates during infancy [68]. At the current time, we are aware of only one report that systematically studied mineral metabolism, to the inclusion of bone mineral content, in such infants after discharge, and concluded that such fortified formulas are beneficial for bone [69].

References

1 Koo WWK, Mimouni F: Calcium and magnesium metabolism in preterm infants; in Tsang RC (ed): Calcium and Magnesium Metabolism in Early Life. Boca Raton, CRC Press, 1995, pp 55–70.

2 Agarwal R, Virmani D, Jaipal ML, Gupta S, Gupta N, Sankar MJ, Bhatia S, Agarwal A, Devgan V, Deorari A, Paul VK; Investigators of LBW Micronutrient Study Group, Departments of Pediatrics and Endocrinology: Vitamin D status of low birth weight infants in Delhi: a comparative study. J Trop Pediatr 2012;58:446–450.

3 Dawodu A, Nath R: High prevalence of moderately severe vitamin D deficiency in preterm infants. Pediatr Int 2011;53:207–210.

4 Taylor SN, Wagner CL, Fanning D, Quinones L, Hollis BW: Vitamin D status as related to race and feeding type in preterm infants. Breastfeed Med 2006;1:156–163.

5 Mimouni F, Koo WKK: Neonatal mineral metabolism; in Tsang RC (ed): Calcium and Magnesium Metabolism in Early Life. Boca Raton, CRC Press, 1995, pp 71–89.

6 Widdowson EM, McCance RA, Spray CM: The chemical composition of the human body. Clin Sci 1951;10:113–115.

7 Ribeiro Dde O, Lobo BW, Volpato NM, da Veiga VF, Cabral LM, de Sousa VP: Influence of the calcium concentration in the presence of organic phosphorus on the physicochemical compatibility and stability of all-in-one admixtures for neonatal use. Nutr J 2009; 8:51–64.

8 Boyd CA, Quigley MA, Brocklehurst P: Donor breast milk versus infant formula for preterm infants: systematic review and meta-analysis. Arch Dis Child Fetal Neonatal Ed 2007;92:F169–F175.

9 Rønnestad A, Abrahamsen TG, Medbø S, Reigstad H, Lossius K, Kaaresen PI, Egeland T, Engelund IE, Irgens LM, Markestad T: Late-onset septicemia in a Norwegian national cohort of extremely premature infants receiving very early full human milk feeding. Pediatrics 2005;115:e269–e276.

10 Lyon AJ, McIntosh N, Wheeler K, Brooke OG: Hypercalcaemia in extremely low birth weight infants. Arch Dis Child 1984;59:1141–1144.

11 Kuschel CA, Harding JE: Multicomponent fortified human milk for promoting growth in preterm infants. Cochrane Database Syst Rev 2004;1: CD000343.

12 Young L, Embleton ND, McCormick FM, McGuire W: Multinutrient fortification of human breast milk for preterm infants following hospital discharge. Cochrane Database Syst Rev 2013;2:CD004866.

13 Langhendries JP, Hurrell RF, Furniss DE, Hischenhuber C, Finot PA, Bernard A, Battisti O, Bertrand JM, Senterre J: Maillard reaction products and lysinoalanine: urinary excretion and the effects on kidney function of preterm infants fed heat-processed milk formula. J Pediatr Gastroenterol Nutr 1992;14: 62–70.

14 Carnielli VP, Luijendijk IH, Van Goudoever JB, Sulkers EJ, Boerlage AA, Degenhart HJ, Sauer PJ: Structural position and amount of palmitic acid in infant formulas: effects on fat, fatty acid, and mineral balance. J Pediatr Gastroenterol Nutr 1996;23: 553–560.

15 Quinlan PT, Lockton S, Irwin J, Lucas AL: The relationship between stool hardness and stool composition in breast- and formula-fed infants. J Pediatr Gastroenterol Nutr 1995;20:81–90.

16 Koletzko B, Tangermann R, von Kries R, Stannigel H, Willberg B, Radde I, Schmidt E: Intestinal milk-bolus obstruction in formula-fed premature infants given high doses of calcium. J Pediatr Gastroenterol Nutr 1988;7:548–553.

17 Mimouni F, Tsang RC: Perinatal magnesium metabolism: personal data and challenges for the 1990s. Magnes Res 1991;4:109–117.

18 Dauncey MJ, Shaw JC, Urman J: The absorption and retention of magnesium, zinc, and copper by low birth weight infants fed pasteurized human breast milk. Pediatr Res 1977;11:1033–1039.

19 Committee on Nutrition of the Preterm Infant, European Society of Paediatric Gastroenterology and Nutrition: Nutrition and feeding of preterm infants. Acta Paediatr Scand Suppl 1987;336:1–14.

20 Agostoni C, Buonocore G, Carnielli VP, De Curtis M, Darmaun D, Decsi T, Domellöf M, Embleton ND, Fusch C, Genzel-Boroviczeny O, Goulet O, Kalhan SC, Kolacek S, Koletzko B, Lapillonne A, Mihatsch W, Moreno L, Neu J, Poindexter B, Puntis J, Putet G, Rigo J, Riskin A, Salle B, Sauer P, Shamir R, Szajewska H, Thureen P, Turck D, van Goudoever JB, Ziegler EE; ESPGHAN Committee on Nutrition: Enteral nutrient supply for preterm infants: commentary from the European Society of Paediatric Gastroenterology, Hepatology and Nutrition Committee on Nutrition. J Pediatr Gastroenterol Nutr 2010;50:85–91.

21 Klein CJ: Nutrient requirements for preterm infant formulas. J Nutr 2002;132:1395S–1577S.

22 Atkinson S, Tsang RC: Calcium and phosphorus; in Tsang RC, Uay R, Koletzko B, Zlotkin SH (eds): Nutrition of the Preterm Infant: Scientific Basis and Practice, ed 2. Cincinnati, Digital Educational Publishing, Inc, 2005, pp 245–275.

23 Rigo J, Pieltain C, Salle B, Senterre J: Enteral calcium, phosphate and vitamin D requirements and bone mineralization in preterm infants. Acta Paediatr 2007;96:969–974.

24 Rigo J, Mohamed MW, de Curtis M: Disorders of calcium, phosphorus, and magnesium metabolism; in Martin RJ, Fanaroff AA, Walsh MC (eds): Fanaroff and Martin Neonatal-Perinatal Medicine, ed 9. St Louis, Elsevier Mosby, 2011, pp 1523–1555.

25 Abrams SA: Calcium and vitamin D requirements of enterally fed preterm infants. Pediatrics 2013;131: e1676–e1683.

26 Abrams SA: Calcium absorption in infants and small children: methods of determination and recent findings. Nutrients 2010;2:474–480.

27 Hicks PD, Rogers SP, Hawthorne KM, Chen Z, Abrams SA: Calcium absorption in very low birth weight infants with and without bronchopulmonary dysplasia. J Pediatr 2011;158:885–890.

28 Rigo J, Senterre J: Nutritional needs of premature infants: current issues. J Pediatr 2006;149:s80–s88.

29 Lapillonne AA, Glorieux FH, Salle BL, Braillon PM, Chambon M, Rigo J, Putet G, Senterre J: Mineral balance and whole-body bone mineral content in very low-birth-weight infants. Acta Paediatr Suppl 1994; 405:117–122.

30 Mize CE, Uauy R, Waidelich D, Neylan MJ, Jacobs J: Effect of phosphorus supply on mineral balance at high calcium intakes in very low birth weight infants. Am J Clin Nutr 1995;62:385–391.

31 Rigo J, De Curtis M: Disorders of calcium, phosphorus and magnesium metabolism; in Martin RJ, Fanaroff AA (eds): Neonatal-Perinatal Medicine: Diseases of the Fetus and the Infant, ed 8. Philadelphia, Elsevier, 2006, pp 1491–1522.

32 Koo WW, Tsang RC: Mineral requirements of low-birth-weight infants. J Am Coll Nutr 1991;10:474–486.

33 Gray TK, Lowe W, Lester GE: Vitamin D and pregnancy: the maternal-fetal metabolism of vitamin D. Endocr Rev 1981;2:264–274.

34 Pittard WB 3rd, Geddes KM, Hulsey TC, Hollis BW: How much vitamin D for neonates? Am J Dis Child 1991;145:1147–1149.

35 Chan GM, Tsang RC, Chen IW, DeLuca HF, Steichen JJ: The effect of $1,25(OH)_2$ vitamin D_3 supplementation in premature infants. J Pediatr 1978;93: 91–96.

36 Henriksen C, Helland IB, Rønnestad A, Grønn M, Iversen PO, Drevon CA: Fat-soluble vitamins in breast-fed preterm and term infants. Eur J Clin Nutr 2006;60:756–762.

37 Monangi N, Slaughter JL, Dawodu A, Smith C, Akinbi HT: Vitamin D status of early preterm infants and the effects of vitamin D intake during hospital stay. Arch Dis Child Fetal Neonatal Ed 2014;99:F166–F168.

38 Council on Environmental Health, Section on Dermatology, Balk SJ: Policy statement – ultraviolet radiation: a hazard to children and adolescents. Pediatrics 2011;127:588–597.

39 Hillman LS, Haddad JG: Perinatal vitamin D metabolism. II. Serial 25-hydroxyvitamin D concentrations in sera of term and premature infants. J Pediatr 1975;86:928–935.

40 Delmas PD, Glorieux FH, Delvin EE, Salle BL, Melki I: Perinatal serum bone Gla-protein and vitamin D metabolites in preterm and full-term neonates. J Clin Endocrinol Metab 1987;65:588–591.

41 McCarthy RA, McKenna MJ, Oyefeso O, Uduma O, Murray BF, Brady JJ, Kilbane MT, Murphy JF, Twomey A, Donnell CP, Murphy NP, Molloy EJ: Vitamin D nutritional status in preterm infants and response to supplementation. Br J Nutr 2012;27:1–8.

42 Salle BL, Delvin EE, Lapillonne A, Bishop NJ, Glorieux FH: Perinatal metabolism of vitamin D. Am J Clin Nutr 2000;71(suppl):1317S–1324S.

43 Nako Y, Tomomasa T, Morikawa A: Risk of hypervitaminosis D from prolonged feeding of high vitamin D premature infant formula. Pediatr Int 2004; 46:439–443.

44 Markestad T, Aksnes L, Finne PH, Aarskog D: Vitamin D nutritional status of premature infants supplemented with 500 IU vitamin D_2 per day. Acta Paediatr Scand 1983;72:517–520.

45 Hillman LS, Hollis B, Salmons S, Martin L, Slatopolsky E, McAlister W, Haddad J: Absorption, dosage, and effect on mineral homeostasis of 25-hydroxycholecalciferol in premature infants: comparison with 400 and 800 IU vitamin D_2 supplementation. J Pediatr 1985;106:981–989.

46 Steichen JJ, Tsang RC, Greer FR, Ho M, Hug G: Elevated serum 1,25-dihydroxyvitamin D concentrations in rickets of very low-birth-weight infants. J Pediatr 1981;99:293–298.

47 Koo WW, Sherman R, Succop P, Ho M, Buckley D, Tsang RC: Serum vitamin D metabolites in very low birth weight infants with and without rickets and fractures. J Pediatr 1989;114:1017–1022.

48 Ravid A, Koren R, Rotem C, Amir Y, Reisner S, Novogrodsky A, Liberman UA: Mononuclear cells from human neonates are partially resistant to the action of 1,25-dihydroxyvitamin D. J Clin Endocrinol Metab 1988;67:755–759.

49 Venkataraman PS, Tsang RC, Steichen JJ, Grey I, Neylan M, Fleischman AR: Early neonatal hypocalcemia in extremely preterm infants. High incidence, early onset, and refractoriness to supraphysiologic doses of calcitriol. Am J Dis Child 1986;140:1004–1008.

50 Koo WW, Tsang RC, Poser JW, Laskarzewski P, Buckley D, Johnson R, Steichen JJ: Elevated serum calcium and osteocalcin levels from calcitriol in preterm infants. A prospective randomized study. Am J Dis Child 1986;140:1152–1158.

51 Evans JR, Allen AC, Stinson DA, Hamilton DC, St John Brown B, Vincer MJ, Raad MA, Gundberg CM, Cole DE: Effect of high-dose vitamin D supplementation on radiographically detectable bone disease of very low birth weight infants. J Pediatr 1989;115: 779–786.

52 Koo WW, Krug-Wispe S, Neylan M, Succop P, Oestreich AE, Tsang RC: Effect of three levels of vitamin D intake in preterm infants receiving high mineral-containing milk. J Pediatr Gastroenterol Nutr 1995; 21:182–189.

53 Backström MC, Mäki R, Kuusela AL, Sievänen H, Koivisto AM, Ikonen RS, Kouri T, Mäki M: Randomised controlled trial of vitamin D supplementation on bone density and biochemical indices in preterm infants. Arch Dis Child Fetal Neonatal Ed 1999; 80:F161–F166.

54 Backström MC, Mäki R, Kuusela AL, Sievänen H, Koivisto AM, Koskinen M, Ikonen RS, Mäki M: The long-term effect of early mineral, vitamin D, and breast milk intake on bone mineral status in 9- to 11-year-old children born prematurely. J Pediatr Gastroenterol Nutr 1999;29:575–582.

55 Kislal FM, Dilmen U: Effect of different doses of vitamin D on osteocalcin and deoxypyridinoline in preterm infants. Pediatr Int 2008;50:204–207.

56 Aine L, Backström MC, Mäki R, Kuusela AL, Koivisto AM, Ikonen RS, Mäki M: Enamel defects in primary and permanent teeth of children born prematurely. J Oral Pathol Med 2000;29:403–409.

57 Wagner CL, Greer FR; American Academy of Pediatrics Section on Breastfeeding; American Academy of Pediatrics Committee on Nutrition: Prevention of rickets and vitamin D deficiency in infants, children, and adolescents. Pediatrics 2008;122:1142–1152.

58 Mimouni FB: Vitamin D status in growing children: should we routinely screen for vitamin D adequacy? J Pediatr Gastroenterol Nutr 2010;51(suppl 3):S121–S122.

59 Senterre T, Rigo J: Parenteral nutrition in premature infants: practical aspects to optimize postnatal growth and development (in French). Arch Pediatr 2013;20:986–993.

60 Koletzko B, Goulet O, Hunt J, Krohn K, Shamir R: 1. Guidelines on Paediatric Parenteral Nutrition of the European Society of Paediatric Gastroenterology, Hepatology and Nutrition (ESPGHAN) and the European Society for Clinical Nutrition and Metabolism (ESPEN), Supported by the European Society of Paediatric Research (ESPR). J Pediatr Gastroenterol Nutr 2005;41(suppl 2):S1–S87.

61 Mizumoto H, Mikami M, Oda H, Hata D: Refeeding syndrome in a small-for-dates micro-preemie receiving early parenteral nutrition. Pediatr Int 2012; 54:715–717.

62 Ichikawa G, Watabe Y, Suzumura H, Sairenchi T, Muto T, Arisaka O: Hypophosphatemia in small for gestational age extremely low birth weight infants receiving parenteral nutrition in the first week after birth. J Pediatr Endocrinol Metab 2012;25:317–321.

63 Moltu SJ, Strommen K, Blakstad EW, Almaas AN, Westerberg AC, Braekke K, et al: Enhanced feeding in very-low-birth-weight infants may cause electrolyte disturbances and septicemia – a randomized, controlled trial. Clin Nutr 2012;32:207–212.

64 Pieltain C, de Halleux V, Senterre T, Rigo J: Prematurity and bone health. World Rev Nutr Diet 2013; 106:181–188.

65 Fusch C, Bauer K, Böhles HJ, Jochum F, Koletzko B, Krawinkel M, Krohn K, et al; Working Group for Developing the Guidelines for Parenteral Nutrition of the German Society for Nutritional Medicine: Neonatology/paediatrics – guidelines on parenteral nutrition, chapt 13. Ger Med Sci 2009;7:Doc15.

66 ESPGHAN Committee on Nutrition, Aggett PJ, Agostoni C, Axelsson I, De Curtis M, Goulet O, Hernell O, Koletzko B, Lafeber HN, Michaelsen KF, Puntis JW, Rigo J, Shamir R, Szajewska H, Turck D, Weaver LT: Feeding preterm infants after hospital discharge: a commentary by the ESPGHAN Committee on Nutrition. J Pediatr Gastroenterol Nutr 2006;42:596–603.

67 Young L, Morgan J, McCormick FM, McGuire W: Nutrient-enriched formula versus standard term formula for preterm infants following hospital discharge. Cochrane Database Syst Rev 2012;3: CD004696.

68 Young L, Embleton ND, McCormick FM, McGuire W: Multinutrient fortification of human breast milk for preterm infants following hospital discharge. Cochrane Database Syst Rev 2013;2:CD004866.

69 Lapillonne A, Salle BL, Glorieux FH, Claris O: Bone mineralization and growth are enhanced in preterm infants fed an isocaloric, nutrient-enriched preterm formula through term. Am J Clin Nutr 2004;80: 1595–1603.

Francis B. Mimouni, MD
Department of Pediatrics, Tel Aviv Medical Center
6 Weizman Street
Tel Aviv 64239 (Israel)
E-Mail fbmimouni@gmail.com

Koletzko B, Poindexter B, Uauy R (eds): Nutritional Care of Preterm Infants: Scientific Basis and Practical Guidelines.
World Rev Nutr Diet. Basel, Karger, 2014, vol 110, pp 152–166 (DOI: 10.1159/000358464)

Vitamins – Conventional Uses and New Insights

Alison Leaf · Zoe Lansdowne

Southampton Biomedical Research Centre, University of Southampton, Southampton, UK

Reviewed by Ricardo Uauy, National Institute of Nutrition and Food Technology, University of Chile, Santiago de
Chile, Chile; Brenda Poindexter, Riley Hospital for Children at Indiana University Health, Indianapolis, Ind., USA

Abstract

There are 13 nutrients classified as vitamins: 4 'fat-soluble' and 9 'water-soluble'. All are essential to
maintain healthy homeostasis and metabolic function. Preterm infants are born with low levels and
reduced stores of fat-soluble vitamins. Active placental transfer of water-soluble vitamins ensures
high levels at birth, but as they are not stored, levels fall rapidly. All VLBW and ELBW infants require
vitamins to be provided soon after birth. Quantifying exact requirements of each vitamin which will
meet the needs for all infants is difficult due to a limited evidence base. However, timely prescription
of vitamin supplements and awareness of situations where delivery or uptake might be compromised will help to ensure that these vulnerable patients do not suffer from vitamin deficiencies. Multivitamin preparations are available for parenteral and enteral use. Vitamins A, C and E have important functions as antioxidants. Further research is required to understand optimal doses and routes
of administration for initial and ongoing nutritional support.   © 2014 S. Karger AG, Basel

Vitamins are essential nutrients required in small amounts, predominantly to support
enzyme reactions and maintain intermediary metabolism. There are 4 fat-soluble vitamins (A, D, E and K) and 9 water-soluble vitamins (vitamin C and 8 vitamins as-
cribed to the 'B' group). Vitamins A, E and C have important roles as antioxidants.

During pregnancy the placenta is the conduit for all nutrient delivery from the
mother to fetus. Following birth, breast milk is the natural source of nutrition for a
healthy infant born at term. However, for preterm infants the vitamin content of human milk may be insufficient. In addition, preterm infants may be too sick or unstable
to commence enteral feeding immediately, thus parenteral nutrition may be the initial
mode of vitamin delivery. Infant formula and breast-milk fortifiers generally have a
significantly higher vitamin content than breast milk.

Assessing adequacy of vitamin intakes is difficult. Individual requirement depends
on existing levels and stores, which for preterm infants will depend on maternal status,
gestation, and also on an individual baby's unique metabolic capacity and demands. The

Table 1. Effect of heat, light and freezing on vitamin activity

Vitamin	Heat (pasteurization) – inactivates	Light – inactivates	Freezing – inactivates
A	yes [8, 9]; no [41]	no [35]; yes [42]	preserved levels [43, 44]
D	no [41]	*	*
E	no [41]	no [35]; some [42]	yes, but still within reference ranges [43]
K	already low	no [35]	already low
C	yes [41]	yes [45]	yes [44, 46]
Thiamine	yes [27]	*	*
Riboflavin	no [41]	yes [27, 45, 47]	*
Niacin	no [27]	*	no [48]
Pyridoxine	yes [41]	yes [27]	reduced [49]
Biotin	*	*	no [48]
Pantothenic acid	*	*	*
Folate	yes [41]	yes	no [48]
Cobalamin	no [41]	*	*

* No information available.

location of critical importance might be at intracellular or membrane level, yet measurements are usually only possible in blood or urine, or by indirect functional methods.

In this chapter we will summarize for each vitamin their actions and effects, what is known about placental transfer and status at preterm birth and the effect of maternal diet and stores. We will consider the immediate physiological needs following preterm birth and review the basis for current recommendations for ongoing daily intakes as well as measures of adequacy. We will consider dietary sources of vitamins for preterm infants and situations in which extra supplementation may be beneficial. We will discuss the role of vitamins as antioxidants and also consider potential damaging effects of heat, freezing and photodegradation (table 1), with particular reference to pasteurization of breast milk and light exposure of parenteral nutrition solutions.

Fat-Soluble Vitamins

Vitamins A, D, E and K are the fat-soluble vitamins; vitamin D is discussed in another chapter [see chapter by Mimouni, pp. 140–151]. Vitamins A and E act as antioxidants by scavenging free radicals and may offer therapeutic potential for diseases of

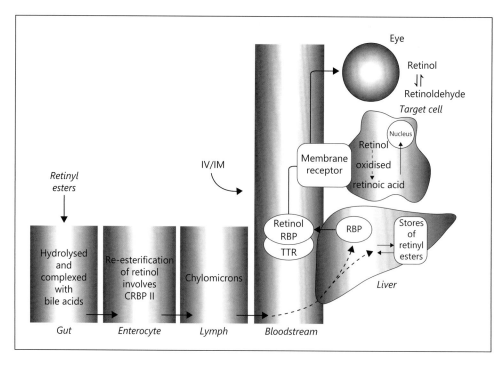

Fig. 1. Uptake and metabolism of vitamin A. CRBP II = Cellular retinol-binding protein type 2; IV = intravenous; IM = intramuscular; RBP = retinol-binding protein; TTR = transthyretin. Reproduced from [5] with permission from BMJ Publishing Group Ltd.

prematurity including bronchopulmonary dysplasia, retinopathy, intraventricular haemorrhage, and necrotizing enterocolitis [1]. Vitamin K is a co-factor in carboxylation reactions and it plays an important role in blood clotting by contributing in the vitamin K-dependent conversion of preprothombin to the active carboxylated prothombin [2]. Beyond its role in blood coagulation, vitamin K is also important for cell cycle regulation and cell-cell adhesion [3].

Vitamin A (fig. 1)

Vitamin A is the collective term for a group of compounds chemically defined as retinoids since they share a common structure with the carotenoids found in the retina; it is found in green and yellow vegetables, egg yolk and fish liver oil. Vitamin A includes retinol (preformed vitamin A), β-carotene and the carotenoids. Vitamin A has an essential role in vision, growth, healing, reproduction, cell differentiation and immune function [4]. Vitamin A is required in the fetal lung for cellular differentiation and surfactant synthesis [5] and the individual surfactant proteins are selectively regulated by retinoic acid which interacts with retinoic acid nuclear receptor in regulating gene expression [6]. Vitamin A deficiency in premature infants may contribute to the development of bronchopulmonary dysplasia and respiratory tract infections.

Cord blood concentrations of vitamin A are lower in premature than term infants [7] and also in multiple gestations [8]. As the fetus accumulates vitamin A in the third trimester, premature infants have reduced hepatic stores at birth [9]. In the human body, retinol is the predominant form with 90% stored in the liver [8]. In the plasma, it is bound to retinol-binding protein synthesized in the liver [5]. Premature infants also have reduced levels of retinol-binding protein, which is necessary to transport retinol to target organs [5]. Vitamin A concentrations in breast milk vary according to maternal dietary intake. Colostrum contains relatively high levels (400–600 IU/dl), but this rapidly decreases to that of mature milk after the first few weeks (60–200 IU/dl) [8]. 90% is in the form of retinyl esters contained in the milk fat globules, with the rest as free retinol [8]. Pancreatic hydrolases convert dietary carotene and retinyl esters to free retinol, and bile salts are then needed to solubilize it into micelles [8]. Decreased levels of enzymes and intraluminal bile acid can negatively affect this process reducing absorption of vitamin A from the intestine [8].

Plasma concentrations <200 µg/l (0.70 µmol/l) are considered deficient in premature infants, and concentrations <100 µg/l (0.35 µmol/l) indicate severe deficiency and depleted liver stores [8]. Plasma concentrations of retinol are maintained at the expense of hepatic stores and reflect body stores only in states of critical depletion or excess, making it difficult to measure vitamin A status [6]. The relative dose response can be measured, but this requires blood tests 5 h apart [5] which may be impractical in ELBW or VLBW infants. In a large randomized controlled trial (RCT) published by Tyson et al. [10], ELBW infants received 5,000 IU vitamin A by intramuscular injections 3 times a week, or 'sham' treatment. The primary outcome of death or chronic lung disease, defined as need for oxygen at 36 weeks, was significantly lower in the intervention group (RR 0.89; 95% CI 0.8–0.99). A considerable number of treated infants still had borderline plasma retinol concentrations and biochemical evidence of a low hepatic store [10]. Giving the same dose orally on a daily basis showed no significant differences in either plasma levels or BPD [9]. As vitamin A is fat-soluble it is possible for accumulation to occur, although this has not been observed in premature infants given the doses used in these studies. Signs of toxicity can include vomiting, changes in skin and mucous membranes and a raised intracranial pressure [9]. Intramuscular injections may be painful and carry the risk of muscle damage. No published study to date has directly compared intramuscular with intravenous administration of vitamin A in VLBW infants in terms of morbidity, mortality, or vitamin A status.

A recent Cochrane review concluded that vitamin A supplementation was beneficial in reducing death or oxygen requirement at 1 month, and reduced oxygen requirement at 36 weeks' post-menstrual age, with a number needed to treat of 13 [11]. There was no evidence of benefit or harm on long-term neurodevelopmental outcomes [11].

Pooled data of vitamin-A-supplemented premature infants has also shown a nonsignificant reduction in retinopathy of prematurity, no effect on the spontaneous closure rate of patent ductus arteriosus, a non-significant reduction in culture-positive nosocomial sepsis and no significant difference in the incidence of intraventricular haemorrhage [11].

Vitamin E

Vitamin E refers to eight naturally occurring compounds with characteristic and similar biological activities [8]. The most abundant and active isomer is α-tocopherol [8]. Vitamin E is an antioxidant that prevents the propagation of free radicals in membranes and plasma lipoproteins [12], thus protecting cell membranes from oxidative stress [12]. By maintaining the structural and functional integrity of polyunsaturated fatty acids, structural components of membranes, vitamin E is critical for the developing nervous system, skeletal muscle and retina [13]. The retina is particularly vulnerable to oxidative damage since photoreceptors (retinal rod outer segments) are composed of highly unsaturated n–3 and n–6 lipids that can be easily oxidized [6].

The combination of limited placental transfer of vitamin E and lower proportion of total body fat relative to body weight results in low total body content of vitamin E in premature infants [8].

Colostrum has high concentrations of vitamin E, approximately 600 mg/l, but this can fall to about one third in mature milk [6]. The amount of tocopherol in milk increases during the course of a breastfeed; hind milk has approximately 4 times the amount compared to foremilk [6].

Vitamin E is transported by lipoproteins [6] and is dependent on lipid and lipoprotein metabolism for tissue delivery [12]. Plasma α-tocopherol concentrations are regulated by the liver, specifically by the α-tocopherol transfer protein, as well as by metabolism and excretion [12]. The absorption of tocopherols depends on total lipid absorption and the actions of pancreatic enzymes and bile salts, as with vitamin A. Vitamin E is stored in the liver, adipose tissue and skeletal muscle.

Measuring vitamin E levels in a premature infant is challenging as serum tocopherol levels may not reflect tissue levels and depend on serum lipid levels [4]. A plasma tocopherol/total lipid ratio >0.8 mg/g indicates vitamin E sufficiency [4].

In preterm infants, lack of vitamin E intake or fat malabsorption results in oedema, thrombocytosis and haemolytic anaemia, and could eventually result in spinocerebellar degeneration [14]. Deficiency typically presents in infants of about 6–8 weeks of age. Reports of vitamin E toxicity in infants are rare, but levels >35 mg/l (81 μmol/l) have been associated with an increased incidence of sepsis and necrotizing enterocolitis [14], explained in part by decreased killing capacity of polymorphonuclear cells which is dependent on free radical formation. Pharmacological doses of parenteral vitamin E (between 50 and 200 mg/kg in divided doses) given in the first few days after birth have been considered as a potential treatment to reduce free radical-mediated diseases in preterm infants. A Cochrane review published in 2003 summarized 26 RCTs involving over 2,000 infants and identified that while vitamin E supplementation reduced the risk of severe retinopathy and blindness [14], it significantly increased the risk of sepsis. The conclusion was that the evidence did not support the routine use of high-dose vitamin E supplementation by the intravenous route, and that serum tocopherol levels >35 mg/l should be avoided [14]. In a recent RCT, 93 ELBW infants were randomized to receive an oral dose of 50 IU/kg vitamin E or placebo within 4 h of birth [15]. α-Tocopherol levels were significantly higher at 24 h and 7 days in infants receiving the vitamin E, with fewer infants showing deficiency; in 4% levels were >35 mg/l.

Vitamin K

Vitamin K exists in two forms: vitamin K_1, phylloquinone, which is the plant form, and vitamin K_2, menaquinones, which are a series of compounds synthesized by bacteria [2] and referred to as MK1–14 depending on specific molecular structure. The vitamin functions post-ribosomally as a co-factor in the metabolic conversion of intracellular precursors of vitamin K-dependent proteins to their active forms [2]. This includes factors II (prothrombin), VII, IX, X, and proteins C, S and Z. Vitamin K-dependent proteins can be found in nearly all tissues in the human body [2]. As well as its role in blood coagulation, vitamin K is important for cell cycle regulation and cell-cell adhesion [3] and in bone metabolism through synthesis of the protein osteocalcin in osteoblasts, which is vitamin K-dependent.

Low, sometimes undetectable, quantities of vitamin K are found in cord blood suggesting that only a very small amount crosses the placenta [8]. The concentration in human milk is also low, at <10 μg/l, making newborn infants prone to deficiency [8]. Neonates are born with a mostly sterile colon which becomes colonized soon after birth and under normal conditions vitamin K is produced by the colonic flora. However, as many VLBW and LBW infants are at risk for infection and given broad-spectrum antibiotics, these infants are particularly dependent on prophylactic administration of vitamin K. Moreover, it is not known to which extent colonic vitamin K may enter the systemic circulation. Unless vitamin K is given at birth, most preterm infants will develop at least subclinical deficiency within 7–10 days after birth [16]. Infants fed exclusively breast milk comprise a group at high risk of vitamin K deficit and should receive vitamin K prophylaxis [1]. Low circulating vitamin K and reduced concentrations of coagulation factors II, VII, IX and X at birth result in increased risk of haemorrhage (haemorrhagic disease of the newborn) [17]. A parenteral or enteral supply is required to prevent vitamin K deficiency bleeding which may kill or cause permanent, serious handicap in newborn infants [2]. The best markers for assessment of neonatal vitamin K status are concentrations of vitamin K_1 and PIVKA-II ('protein induced by vitamin K absence', which is undercarboxylated prothrombin) [2]. Assessment of undercarboxylated osteocalcin concentration may also be used to assess potential deficiency. Circulating vitamin K levels directly reflect storage, intake and transport [2]. Vitamin K absorption is similar to that of other fat-soluble vitamins; from the intestine into the lymphatic system via chylomicrons, requiring both bile salts and pancreatic secretions [8]. A recent RCT showed that intramuscular prophylaxis at birth with a reduced dose of 0.2 mg of vitamin K_1 maintained satisfactory vitamin K status in preterm infants born <32 weeks' gestation without producing evidence of hepatic overload [18]. Infants >1 kg were not included in the trial so they should continue to receive 1 mg intramuscularly [19]. Vitamin K can also be provided intravenously to preterm infants which circumvents the risks of pain, inflammation and hematoma associated with intramuscular or subcutaneous injection [20, 21]. Plasma concentrations of vitamin K rapidly increase after intravenous application and may temporarily reduce albumin-binding capacity for unconjugated bilirubin. Therefore, it is recommended not to exceed a dosage of 0.4 mg/kg body weight with intravenous infusion, which achieves plasma concentrations similar to those observed after oral supply of 3 mg or intramuscular supply of 1.5 mg [22]. Lipid-soluble vitamin preparations for use in parenteral nutrition appear to contain sufficient amounts of vitamin K [23]. No toxicity has been reported so far [8], but it is prudent to be cautious of high plasma vitamin K concentrations, as vitamin K-dependent proteins are also ligands for tyrosine kinase that may affect cell growth [3].

In 2010, the Cochrane Collaboration published a review protocol to determine the effectiveness of vitamin K prophylaxis in the prevention of vitamin K deficiency bleeding in preterm infants, so we should await the results of this systematic review [24].

Water-Soluble Vitamins

The water-soluble vitamins include vitamin C (ascorbic acid) and eight nutrients included in the B group: thiamine (B_1), riboflavin (B_2), niacin (B_3), pyridoxine (B_6), biotin, pantothenic acid, folic acid and cyanocobalamin (B_{12}). Vitamin B was initially thought to be one compound, however subsequent investigations gradually revealed eight separate components, often found in similar foods, and all involved in intermediary metabolism. Some were given numerical labels, while others discovered independently were given names [25]. For simplicity, each vitamin will be referred to by name, with number in parenthesis.

Functions, Acquisition and Metabolism of Individual Water-Soluble Vitamins
The information provided here is extracted and summarized from Truswell [25], Skeaff [26] and Schanler [27] unless individually referenced.

Thiamine (B_1) in the form of the diphosphate or pyrophosphate is an important co-enzyme for major decarboxylation reactions in carbohydrate metabolism and also may have a role in neurophysiology and nerve conduction [27]. It is absorbed by active transport in the small intestine, and by passive transport at high concentration. There is a high turnover and no significant storage. Deficiency is rarely diagnosed in VLBW infants, but it should be considered if an increased carbohydrate load results in accumulation of pyruvate and lactate [28]. Tests of sufficiency include measuring levels in plasma, or indirectly by the 'transketolase test': adequate thiamine status <15% activity, mild deficiency 15–25%, and severe deficiency >25%.

Riboflavin is an important component of two co-enzymes: flavin mononucleotide and flavin adenine dinucleotide which are important oxidizing agents and participate in the oxidation chain in mitochondria. They are also co-factors for other enzymes such as NADH dehydrogenase (see below) and xanthine oxidase [25]. Absorption involves a special carrier system in proximal small intestine, and a little is stored in muscle. Riboflavin is highly conserved and deficiency is rare. Functional adequacy can be determined by red blood cell glutathione reductase activity and measures of urinary excretion. While plasma and urine levels will fall rapidly on a riboflavin-free diet [29], most preterm infants receiving parenteral nutrition or preterm formula have elevated levels, suggesting current standard regimens may be excessive [29] in the context of immature renal function.

Niacin is a generic name for a group of compounds including nicotinic acid and nicotinamide which form part of the co-enzymes nicotinamide adenine dinucleotide (NAD) and nicotinamide adenine dinucleotide phosphate (NADP). It is important in oxidative phosphorylation and fatty acid oxidation within mitochondria. Absorption is from the stomach and small intestine and little is stored. Niacin is also synthesized in the liver from tryptophan – 60 mg of tryptophan is considered equivalent to 1 mg niacin and is referred to as one 'niacin equivalent' (NE). Clinical deficiency is rare in infants, however data on optimal intakes are lacking. Toxicity in infants has not been described. Tests of adequacy include urinary N-methylnicotinamide, red cell NAD concentration and fasting plasma tryptophan.

Pyridoxine (B$_6$) is found in three interconvertible forms: pyridoxine, pyridoxal and pyridoxamine. Each has a phosphorylated derivative of which pyridoxal 5′-phosphate is most abundant in the human body. It has a function in almost all reactions of amino acid metabolism and is also important in release of glucose from glycogen and in synthesis of sphingomyelin and phosphatidylcholine. It is involved in the synthesis of taurine in bile and the conversion of tryptophan to niacin. It is passively absorbed in the small intestine and some is stored tightly bound in tissues. Deficiency results in dermatitis and neurological dysfunction (including seizures) and poor growth. Toxicity is rare: sensory neuropathy has been described in adults on prolonged high intakes. Tests of adequacy include measurement of plasma pyridoxal 5′-phosphate as well as urinary metabolites.

Biotin is a co-enzyme for carboxylase reactions in carbohydrate, amino acid and fatty acid metabolism. It is widespread in the diet and also synthesized by bacteria in the lower intestine; it is present in lower concentration in breast milk than in cow's milk. Deficiency results in increased cholesterol and 3-hydroxyisovaleric acid and may rarely manifest as skin rashes, alopecia and depression. Urinary biotin gives a measure of adequacy.

Pantothenic acid is an essential part of the structure of CoA and acyl carrier protein. It is important in the tricarboxylic acid cycle and in lipid synthesis. It is widespread in food sources and deficiency is very rare. Urinary levels can be measured.

Folate is the name given to a group of related compounds which have an essential role in 1-carbon transfers (methyl transfer) in purine and pyrimidine synthesis and are therefore essential in cell division. Folic acid is the synthetic form of the vitamin, whereas folate acts in the body as tetrahydrofolate. Folates including folic acid are absorbed in the small intestine and are present in high concentrations in erythrocytes. Small stores are present in the liver and folates are re-cycled via the enterohepatic circulation. Deficiency results in reduced ability of cells to double their DNA and divide. Serum folate measurements indicate recent intake while red cell folate reflects 'cellular status'. Hypersegmentation of neutrophils may also be seen in deficiency. The importance of folic acid in pregnancy is well recognized in the prevention of neural tube defects and it is increasingly recognized that metabolic interactions between folic acid and other nutrients including choline and methionine may be important in modulating epigenetic phenomena [30].

Cobalamin (B_{12}) consists of two co-enzymes involved in metabolism of propionate and synthesis of methionine. Vitamin B_{12} is synthesized by bacteria and is found in meat, fish, eggs and dairy products. It is absorbed in the small intestine but requires 'intrinsic factor' produced by parietal cells in the stomach. There is a high retention and deficiency is rare except in those lacking intrinsic factor, or consuming a vegan diet. Megaloblastic anaemia and neuropathy resulting from impaired myelination due to methionine deficiency are clinical features. B_{12} is also important in maintaining the action of folate in nuclear division. Adequacy can be assessed by serum B_{12} levels; elevated methylmalonate may also be observed in deficiency states.

Ascorbic acid (vitamin C) is required for hydroxylation of proline and lysine in collagen synthesis. It is involved in many other metabolic pathways including synthesis of noradrenaline from dopamine, synthesis of carnitine, activation of neuropeptides, and catabolism of tyrosine, and is an important antioxidant. A high concentration is found in fetal and neonatal brain. Ascorbic acid is produced from glucose and galactose by many animals but not by primates or guinea pigs. Food sources include fruit, liver, kidney but there is little in cow's milk. It is actively absorbed in the small intestine and is not stored for long. Vitamin C enhances the absorption of non-heme iron. Classical features of 'scurvy' are only now seen in situations of famine and extreme diets, and include fatigue and muscle weakness. Measurements can be made of serum and white blood cell vitamin C levels [26].

Placental Transfer and Status at Preterm Birth
Active transport of water-soluble vitamins across the placenta ensures relatively high concentrations in the fetus and newborn [27] even following preterm birth [7]. For pyridoxine (B_6), maternal intake in the third trimester determines the infant's status [27]. However as there is little or no storage, circulating levels fall relatively rapidly after

birth if intake is not assured. As preterm infants have a relatively high metabolic rate and a need for rapid tissue turnover for growth, even those without significant complications will require a steady intake of water-soluble vitamins from soon after birth.

Defining Recommended Intakes for VLBW and ELBW Infants

Adequate intakes for term infants have mainly been derived from measurement of the quantities in breast milk of healthy term infants of healthy mothers who are well and gaining weight appropriately [31]. Estimating intakes for VLBW and ELBW infants is more difficult: their need for growth and laying down of body tissues is greater than for more mature infants, however their absorptive and metabolic capacity may be less and their dietary intakes are more variable. They frequently experience periods on parenteral nutrition, periods of intestinal dysfunction, periods of low nutrient intake on donor breast milk and then periods of enhanced intakes on fortified breast milk or preterm formula. The relative intakes of carbohydrate and protein will vary considerably on these different diets and with it the requirements for and indeed intakes of different water-soluble vitamins. The thorough reviews by Greer [8] and Schanler [27] remain the most comprehensive assessments of vitamin requirements in VLBW and ELBW infants during the transitional first few days after birth and while on parenteral or enteral nutrition (table 2) [8].

Recommendations for enteral intakes were further refined by ESPGHAN in 2010 [32] with expanded reference material available at http://links.lww.com/A1480. Two studies of intakes and circulating levels of water-soluble vitamins in VLBW preterm infants (mean gestation 29–30 weeks) showed that daily intakes of thiamine, riboflavin, pyridoxine, folic acid, vitamin B_{12} and vitamin C were often higher than those recommended, particularly while on parenteral nutrition, and plasma levels were generally maintained within the normal range [33, 34]. Care should be taken to avoid excessive intakes of riboflavin (>670 µg/100 kcal). Niacin requirement reflects protein intake and as this is increased, a higher intake of niacin is recommended. Vitamin C levels were significantly higher when on enteral feeds than on parenteral nutrition with similar documented daily intake, suggesting enteral delivery is more effective.

Provision of Vitamins following Preterm Birth

Early/Transition Period

As very preterm infants are born with low or minimal stores of both fat- and water-soluble vitamins, 'dietary' provision should be ensured from an early age – ideally within the first 24 h. Oxygen-induced injuries to the lung and retina may occur very early in post-natal life, thus provision of antioxidant vitamins is particularly important. Intravenous preparations are available to provide the full range of vitamins. However, care must be taken to ensure that infusions are not stopped or reduced and that products are protected from light (see table 1). Vitamins for parenteral use

Table 2. Acceptable range of vitamin intakes for VLBW and ELBW infants

Vitamin	ESPGHAN 2010	Reasonable nutrient intakes, units/kg/day	
		VLBW (ELBW if different)	highest evidence
A	400–1,000 µg/kg	400–3,330 IU/kg/day (5,000 IU 3× weekly i.m. to reduce BPD)	large RCT; systematic review; review articles; plasma levels
E	2.2–11 mg	2.2–11 mg/kg (= 3.3–16.4 IU/kg)	small clinical trials
K	4.4–28	4.4–28 µg/kg/day	small trials of preterm infants on fortified breast milk and formula
Thiamine (B_1)	140–300	140–300 µg/kg	small clinical studies
Riboflavin (B_2)	200–400	200–400 µg/kg	small clinical studies; avoid high intakes in renal impairment
Niacin (B_3)	0.38–5.5 mg/kg	1–5.5 mg/kg	no recent research evidence; requirement depends on tryptophan in diet
Pyridoxine (B_6)	45–300 µg	50–300 µg/kg	small clinical studies; levels in breast milk and breast-fed infants
Biotin	1.7–16.5 µg	1.7–16.5 µg/kg	very little data; RNI estimated from content in breast milk and need for rapid growth
Pantothenic acid	0.33–2.1 mg	0.5–2.1 mg	very little data; lower RNI based on amount that would be obtained in approximately 150 ml/kg/day of breast milk
Folic acid	35–100 µg	35–100 µg	small RCT in VLBW infants
Cobalamin (B_{12})	0.1–0.77	0.1–0.8 µg/kg/day	based on content of breast milk and plasma levels; higher dose of 3 µg/kg/day may be appropriate on erythropoietin (RCT) [37]
C (L-ascorbic acid)	11–46	20–55 mg/kg/day	small clinical trials; well-absorbed enterally; important antioxidant – avoid excessive doses (pro-oxidant) but accommodate deterioration over product shelf life

may be added separately: water-soluble in aqueous solution and fat-soluble in lipid solution, or together in the lipid solution. Administering fat-soluble vitamins in aqueous parenteral nutrition results in poor delivery and should be avoided if possible [35]. On prolonged parenteral nutrition, plasma vitamin levels should be measured.

Enteral Feeding
Maternal breast milk will not provide adequate intakes of vitamins A and D for VLBW and ELBW infants and supplements should be given. For water-soluble vitamins, breast milk content generally reflects maternal intakes. Content tends to be

lower in colostrum and gradually increases in mature milk. In mothers who are vitamin-deficient, concentration can be increased by dietary supplementation [27]; for riboflavin and niacin, breast milk concentration will increase even in adequately nourished mothers. The concentration of thiamine, riboflavin and niacin in breast milk is generally too low to meet preterm infant requirements [27]. Pyridoxine content is lower in preterm than term breast milk [36] and also may be insufficient. Folate content increases throughout lactation but is probably inadequate for preterm without fortification; supplementation should be considered with erythropoietin treatment [37]. The B_{12} level declines from first week to 6 months, is low in women on vegan diet and under these conditions can be increased to normal level by maternal B_{12} supplementation. There are, however, no reports of B_{12} deficiency in preterm infants fed on breast milk from mothers on a normal omnivorous diet. Pantothenic acid content is higher in preterm than term breast milk [38], at approximately 3.5 µg/ml of milk, but would be unlikely to provide the recommended daily intake for VLBW and ELBW infants and recent evidence suggests that biotin deficiency may be common in preterm infants fed breast milk or standard formula [39]. Breast milk does contain reasonable amounts of vitamin C which can be increased by maternal supplementation, however this may still be insufficient for growing preterm infants. Excessive intakes may reduce absorption of B_{12} and act as pro-oxidant.

It would thus appear that even from a well-nourished mother, unfortified breast milk will be unlikely to provide adequate water-soluble vitamins. Donor breast milk may be nutritionally inferior to mother's expressed milk, and vitamin content may be further affected by pasteurization and freezing (table 1). Preterm infants for whom donor milk is a significant part of the diet should be high priority for early vitamin supplementation, including both fat- and water-soluble vitamins (table 1).

Preterm formula and breast milk fortifiers are usually supplemented with all vitamins, however absolute content varies between different products. Local products should be checked against recommended intakes: breast milk fortifiers frequently do not contain sufficient fat-soluble vitamins to meet recommendations. Infants receiving part or all of their diet as unfortified breast milk should receive a multivitamin supplement containing at minimum vitamins A, D, C, thiamine and riboflavin.

Effects of Heat and Light on Vitamin Function
Some vitamins are destroyed or inactivated by heat or light, and lipid emulsions may undergo oxidation when exposed to both ambient light and phototherapy lights [40]. It is important to be aware of these potential hazards, particularly for delivery of parenteral nutrition and when using pasteurized (heat-treated) breast milk [41]. Delivery of vitamins A and E in lipid emulsion rather than in aqueous solution significantly improves both overall bioavailability and risk of degradation due to light exposure [35]. Consideration of light exposure should also be given during storage of vitamin

preparations – for example avoiding use of glass-fronted refrigerators. What is known about the effects of heat, light and freezing on fat and water-soluble vitamins is summarized in table 1.

Summary and Conclusions

- Fat-soluble vitamins have critical roles in haemostasis and antioxidant protection and can prevent serious morbidity and mortality.
- Water-soluble vitamins are vital for all aspects of metabolism: they are not stored, and levels decline rapidly.
- Optimizing early vitamin intake for VLBW and ELBW infants is thus important.
- Breast milk will not meet all requirements, and content is further depleted by pasteurization or freezing.
- Breast milk fortifier and preterm formula provide all vitamins, however, as products vary, further supplements may be required.
- Multivitamin preparations are selective and rarely contain all vitamins.
- Evidence base for optimal intake of vitamins for ELBW infants is weak.

Topics for Research and Development

- Development of more comprehensive enteral multivitamin supplements for premature infants.
- Balance studies of water-soluble vitamins in ELBW infants – thiamine, riboflavin and niacin.
- Effects of heat, light and freezing on vitamin content of human milk and other nutritional products, where this information is lacking.

References

1 Leaf A, Subramanian S, Cherian S: Vitamins for preterm infants. Curr Paediatr 2004;14:298–305.
2 Greer FR: Vitamin K the basics – what's new? Early Hum Dev 2010;86(suppl 1):43–47.
3 Costakos DT, Greer FR, Love LA, Dahlen LR, Suttie JW: Vitamin K prophylaxis for premature infants: 1 mg versus 0.5 mg. Am J Perinatol 2003;20:485–490.
4 Greer FR: Vitamin metabolism and requirements in the micropremie. Clin Perinatol 2000;27:95–118, vi.
5 Mactier H, Weaver LT: Vitamin A and preterm infants: what we know, what we don't know, and what we need to know. Arch Dis Child Fetal Neonatal Ed 2005;90:F103–F108.
6 Bohles H: Antioxidative vitamins in prematurely and maturely born infants. Int J Vitam Nutr Res 1997;67:321–328.
7 Baydas G, Karatas F, Gursu MF, Bozkurt HA, Ilhan N, Yasar A, et al: Antioxidant vitamin levels in term and preterm infants and their relation to maternal vitamin status. Arch Med Res 2002;33:276–280.
8 Greer FR: Vitamins A, E and K; in Tsang RC, Uauy R, Koletzko BV, Zlotkin SH (eds): Nutrition of the Preterm Infant, ed 2. Cincinnati, Digital Educational Publishing, 2005, pp 141–172.

9 Wardle SP, Hughes A, Chen S, Shaw NJ: Randomised controlled trial of oral vitamin A supplementation in preterm infants to prevent chronic lung disease. Arch Dis Child Fetal Neonatal Ed 2001;84:F9–F13.

10 Tyson JE, Wright LL, Oh W, Kennedy KA, Mele L, Ehrenkranz RA, et al: Vitamin A supplementation for extremely-low-birth-weight infants. National Institute of Child Health and Human Development Neonatal Research Network. N Engl J Med 1999;340: 1962–1968.

11 Darlow BA, Graham PJ: Vitamin A supplementation to prevent mortality and short- and long-term morbidity in very low birth weight infants. Cochrane Database Syst Rev 2011;10:CD000501.

12 Traber MG, Stevens JF: Vitamins C and E: beneficial effects from a mechanistic perspective. Free Radic Biol Med 2011;51:1000–1013.

13 Thakur ML, Srivastava US: Vitamin E metabolism and its application. Nutr Res 1996;16:1767–1809.

14 Brion LP, Bell EF, Raghuveer TS: Vitamin E supplementation for prevention of morbidity and mortality in preterm infants. Cochrane Database Syst Rev 2003;4:CD003665.

15 Bell EF, Hansen NI, Brion LP, et al: Tocopherol levels in very preterm infants after a single enteral dose of vitamin E given soon after birth. Boston, Pediatric Academic Societies, 2012.

16 Clarke P: Vitamin K prophylaxis for preterm infants. Early Hum Dev 2010;86(suppl):17–20.

17 Puckett RM, Offringa M: Prophylactic vitamin K for vitamin K deficiency bleeding in neonates. Cochrane Database Syst Rev 2000;4:CD002776.

18 Clarke P, Mitchell SJ, Wynn R, Sundaram S, Speed V, Gardener E, et al: Vitamin K prophylaxis for preterm infants: a randomized, controlled trial of three regimens. Pediatrics 2006;118:e1657–e1666.

19 BNF for Children: London, BMJ Publishing Group, 2005.

20 Bührer C, Genzel-Boroviczény O, Kauth T, Kersting M, Koletzko B, et al; Ernährungskommission-der-Deutschen-Gesellschaft-für-Kinder-und-Jugend-medizin: Vitamin-K-Prophylaxe bei Neugeborenen. Ergänzung zu den Empfehlungen der Ernährungskommission der Deutschen Gesellschaft für Kinder- und Jugendmedizin (DGKJ). Monatsschr Kinderheilkd, in press.

21 Shearer MJ: Vitamin K in parenteral nutrition. Gastroenterology 2009;137(suppl):S105–S118.

22 Raith W, Fauler G, Pichler G, Muntean W: Plasma concentrations after intravenous administration of phylloquinone (vitamin K_1) in preterm and sick neonates. Thromb Res 2000;99:467–472.

23 Clarke P: Vitamin K prophylaxis for preterm infants. Early Hum Dev 2010;86(suppl 1):17–20.

24 Ardell S, Offringa M, Soll R: Prophylactic vitamin K for the prevention of vitamin K deficiency bleeding in preterm neonates. Cochrane Database Systc Rev 2010;1:CD008342.

25 Truswell AS: The B vitamins; in Mann J, Truswell AS (eds): Essentials of Human Nutrition, ed 3. Oxford, Oxford University Press, 2007, pp 184–200.

26 Skeaff M: Vitamins C and E; in Mann J, Truswell AS (eds): Essentials of Human Nutrition, ed 3. Oxford, Oxford University Press, 2007, pp 201–213.

27 Schanler RJ: Water-soluble vitamins for premature infants; in Tsang RC, Uauy R, Koletzko BV, Zlotkin SH (eds): Nutrition of the Preterm Infant, ed 2. Cincinnati, Digital Educational Publishing, 2005, pp 173–199.

28 Oguz SS, Ergenekon E, Tumer L, Koc E, Turan O, Onal E, et al: A rare case of severe lactic acidosis in a preterm infant: lack of thiamine during total parenteral nutrition. J Pediatr Endocrinol Metab 2011;24: 843–845.

29 Porcelli PJ, Rosser ML, DelPaggio D, Adcock EW, Swift L, Greene H: Plasma and urine riboflavin during riboflavin-free nutrition in very-low-birth-weight infants. J Pediatr Gastroenterol Nutr 2000;31:142–148.

30 Zeisel SH: Choline: critical role during fetal development and dietary requirements in adults. Annu Rev Nutr 2006;26:229–250.

31 Powers HJ: Vitamin requirements for term infants: considerations for infant formulae. Nutr Res Rev 1997;10:1–33.

32 Agostoni C, Buonocore G, Carnielli VP, De Curtis M, Darmaun D, Decsi T, et al: Enteral nutrient supply for preterm infants: commentary from the European Society of Paediatric Gastroenterology, Hepatology and Nutrition Committee on Nutrition. J Pediatr Gastroenterol Nutr 2010;50:85–91.

33 Friel JK, Bessie JC, Belkhode SL, Edgecombe C, Steele-Rodway M, Downton G, et al: Thiamine, riboflavin, pyridoxine, and vitamin C status in premature infants receiving parenteral and enteral nutrition. J Pediatr Gastroenterol Nutr 2001;33:64–69.

34 Levy R, Herzberg GR, Andrews WL, Sutradhar B, Friel JK: Thiamine, riboflavin, folate, and vitamin B_{12} status of low birth weight infants receiving parenteral and enteral nutrition. JPEN J Parenter Enteral Nutr 1992;16:241–247.

35 Haas C, Genzel-Boroviczeny O, Koletzko B: Losses of vitamin A and E in parenteral nutrition suitable for premature infants. Eur J Clin Nutr 2002;56:906–912.

36 Udipi SA, Kirksey A, West K, Giacoia G: Vitamin B_6, vitamin C and folacin levels in milk from mothers of term and preterm infants during the neonatal period. Am J Clin Nutr 1985;42:522–530.

37 Haiden N, Klebermass K, Cardona F, Schwindt J, Berger A, Kohlhauser-Vollmuth C, et al: A randomized, controlled trial of the effects of adding vitamin B_{12} and folate to erythropoietin for the treatment of anemia of prematurity. Pediatrics 2006;118:180–188.

38 Song WO, Chan GM, Wyse BW, Hansen RG: Effect of pantothenic acid status on the content of the vitamin in human milk. Am J Clin Nutr 1984;40:317–324.

39 Tokuriki S, Hayashi H, Okuno T, Yoshioka K, Okazaki S, Kawakita A, et al: Biotin and carnitine profiles in preterm infants in Japan. Pediatr Int 2013;55:342–345.

40 Neuzil J, Darlow BA, Inder TE, Sluis KB, Winterbourn CC, Stocker R: Oxidation of parenteral lipid emulsion by ambient and phototherapy lights: potential toxicity of routine parenteral feeding. J Pediatr 1995;126:785–790.

41 Van Zoeren-Grobben D, Schrijver J, Van den Berg H, Berger HM: Human milk vitamin content after pasteurisation, storage, or tube feeding. Arch Dis Child 1987;62:161–165.

42 Allwood MC, Martin HJ: The photodegradation of vitamins A and E in parenteral nutrition mixtures during infusion. Clin Nutr 2000;19:339–342.

43 Ezz El Din ZM, Abd El Ghaffar S, El Gabry EK, Fahmi WA, Bedair RF: Is stored expressed breast milk an alternative for working Egyptian mothers? East Mediterr Health J 2004;10:815–821.

44 Rechtman DJ, Lee ML, Berg H: Effect of environmental conditions on unpasteurized donor human milk. Breastfeed Med 2006;1:24–26.

45 Hoff DS, Michaelson AS: Effects of light exposure on total parenteral nutrition and its implications in the neonatal population. J Pediatr Pharmacol Ther 2009;14:132–143.

46 Buss IH, McGill F, Darlow BA, Winterbourn CC: Vitamin C is reduced in human milk after storage. Acta Paediatr 2001;90:813–815.

47 Sisson TR: Photodegradation of riboflavin in neonates. Fed Proc 1987;46:1883–1885.

48 Friend BA, Shahani KM, Long CA, Vaughn LA: The effect of processing and storage on key enzymes, B vitamins, and lipids of mature human milk. I. Evaluation of fresh samples and effects of freezing and frozen storage. Pediatr Res 1983;17:61–64.

49 Lawrence RA: Storage of human milk and the influence of procedures on immunological components of human milk. Acta Paediatr Suppl 1999;88:14–18.

Dr. Alison Leaf, MD, FRCPCH, MBChB, BSc
NIHR, Southampton Biomedical Research Centre, University of Southampton
Mailpoint 803, Child Health, Level F, South Block, Southampton General Hospital
Tremona Road, Southampton SO16 6YD (UK)
E-Mail a.a.leaf@soton.ac.uk

Koletzko B, Poindexter B, Uauy R (eds): Nutritional Care of Preterm Infants: Scientific Basis and Practical Guidelines.
World Rev Nutr Diet. Basel, Karger, 2014, vol 110, pp 167–176 (DOI: 10.1159/000358465)

The Developing Intestinal Microbiome: Probiotics and Prebiotics

Josef Neu

Department of Pediatrics/Neonatology, University of Florida, Gainesville, Fla., USA

Reviewed by Johannes B. van Goudoever, Department of Pediatrics, Emma Children's Hospital Amsterdam,
The Netherlands; Hania Szajewska, Department of Paediatrics, The Medical University of Warsaw, Warsaw, Poland

Abstract

The microbes in the human intestinal tract interact with the host to form a 'superorganism'. The functional aspects of the host microbe interactions are being increasingly scrutinized and it is becoming evident that this interaction in early life is critical for development of the immune system and metabolic function and aberrations may result in life-long health consequences. Evidence is suggesting that such interactions occur even before birth, where the microbes may be either beneficial or harmful, and possibly even triggering preterm birth. Mode of delivery, use of antibiotics, and other perturbations may have life-long consequences in terms of health and disease. Manipulating the microbiota by use of pro- and prebiotics may offer a means for maintenance of 'healthy' host microbe interactions, but over-exuberance in their use also has the potential to cause harm. Considerable controversy exists concerning the routine use of probiotics in the prevention of necrotizing enterocolitis. This chapter will provide a brief overview of the developing intestinal microbiome and discuss the use of pro- and prebiotics in preterm infants.   © 2014 S. Karger AG, Basel

Emerging non-culture-based technologies derived largely from the Human Genome Project are increasingly being applied to evaluate the intestinal microbiota. The Human Microbiome Roadmap has thus been proposed as a stimulus to evaluate the role of the intestinal microbiome in health and disease [1]. It is becoming increasingly evident that the intestinal microbiota comprises a complex ecosystem that has been shaped by millennia of evolution that usually exists in a symbiotic relationship with the host. During early development, the microbiota undergoes changes based on the individual's genetic program, diet, and other environmental factors. The resident gastrointestinal microbes play major roles in nutrition and the developing immune system [2, 3]. Previous studies have demonstrated that germ-free animals have extensive defects in the development of gut-associated lymphoid tissue [4], arrested capillary network development in the gut and reduced antibody production. Its role in the de-

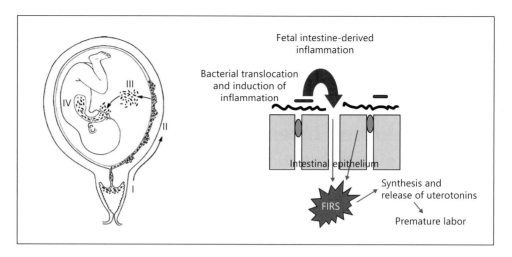

Fig. 1. Model showing how ascending vaginal bacteria translocate through the maternofetal membranes and the fetus swallows the colonized amniotic fluid (left) and how this leads to fetal inflammatory response syndrome (FIRS) that is of fetal intestinal origin (right).

veloping human immune system is well known and much of this interaction occurs in the first years after birth.

The microbial composition of the intestine during early development may provide the milieu that prevents or enhances certain diseases such as neonatal sepsis, necrotizing enterocolitis (NEC), type 1 diabetes, asthma, allergies, celiac disease, inflammatory bowel disease and obesity [5–8]. In this chapter, several aspects of the developing intestinal microbiome based on new technologies are discussed in relation to health. We further discuss the role of antibiotics, probiotics and prebiotics, especially as they pertain to the newborn infant and his/her subsequent development.

Development of the Intestinal Microbiota

Fetal Microbial Ecology
Although a commonly held belief is that the intestinal tract of the fetus is sterile, recent studies using a combination of culture and non-culture-based techniques suggest that many preterm infants are exposed to microbes found in the amniotic fluid, even without a history of rupture of membranes or culture-positive chorioamnionitis [9]. This has led to speculation that the microbial ecology of the swallowed amniotic fluid may play a role not only in the fetal intestinal physiology and inflammation but perhaps in premature labor (fig. 1) [10].

It needs to be noted that the fetus swallows large quantities of amniotic fluid in the last trimester of pregnancy and the highly immunoreactive intestine is exposed to large quantities of these microbes and microbial components. One study from our group used high-throughput 16S-based techniques to analyze intestinal microbial ecology in premature neonates in 23 neonates born at 23–32 weeks' gestational age [11]. Surprisingly, microbial DNA was detected in meconium, suggesting an intrauterine origin. This suggests the possibility that meconium might be a reasonable source for evaluation of the intrauterine microbial milieu.

Microbiota Development in Term Infants

One of the first comprehensive non-culture-based studies of intestinal microbes in 14 healthy term infants, using a ribosomal DNA microarray-based approach, suggested that the composition of microbes within each baby evolved over time but showed similarity during the first year, but 'temporal patterns of the microbial communities varied widely from baby to baby, suggesting a broader definition of 'healthy colonization' than previously recognized [12]. By 1 year of age, the profile of microbial communities begins to converge toward a profile characteristic of the adult gastrointestinal tract' [12]. Another study from Norway (the 'NoMic' study) evaluated 85 healthy term breastfed infants at 4 and 120 days [13]. These were vaginally delivered, healthy, term infants, who were not exposed to antibiotics, exclusively breastfed during their first month of life and at least partially breastfed up to 4 months. Selected microbial groups were identified by targeting small subunit microbial ribosomal RNA genes. In contrast to more recent studies [12], but in agreement with older culture-based studies, almost all the infants in this study harbored Gammaproteobacteria and *Bifidobacterium*. The authors found that non-cultivable species belonging to *Bacteroides*, as well as microbes identified as Lachnospiraceae 2, were highly represented. This study also showed a relative abundance of *Staphylococcus* genera that decreased over the evaluated time period. Furthermore, the bifidobacteria were represented in relatively high abundance. Whether the differences in bifidobacteria in this study and in the previous study [12] were due to choice of primer (resulting in primer bias), infant health status, use of antibiotics, diet or geographic region remain speculative.

Preterm Infant Microbiota

As in the neonate born at term, the preterm infants' gastrointestinal tracts may already have been exposed to an intrauterine microbial milieu that has influenced development prior to birth. Studies on 29 consecutive extremely preterm infants fecal microbiota was collected between 3 and 56 days of life and analyzed using 'fingerprinting' (gel separation, elution of bands from gels and subsequent analysis of band sequences) correlated clinical factors such as growth, digestive tolerance, nutrition and antibiotic use to the major taxa present in the feces [14]. The diversity score (related to number of operational taxonomic units) increased 0.45 units/week. *Staphylococcus* species were by far the as the major group with *Bifidobacterium* being poorly represented. Gestational age (≥28 weeks) and cesarean delivery independently correlated with better diversity scores during follow-up. The 6-week diversity score inversely correlated with the duration of antibiotic use and parenteral feeding. A predominance

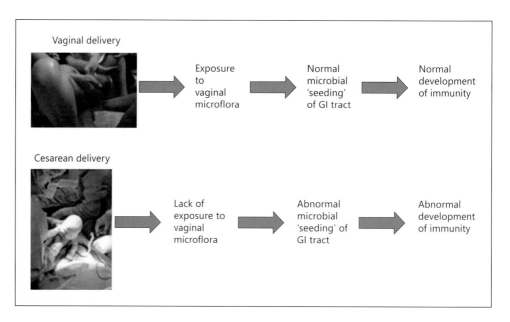

Fig. 2. Colonization after vaginal versus cesarean delivery.

of *Staphylococcus* seen during this time is of interest since these are the most commonly represented genera with late-onset sepsis in the neonate. It is of interest but speculative that these are organisms that may translocate through the intestinal barrier and cause bacteremia and subsequent sepsis.

Mode of Delivery
During birth and rapidly thereafter, bacteria from the mother and the surrounding environment colonize the infant's gut. Microbial colonization after vaginal delivery may be very different than after cesarean delivery (fig. 2) [15]. During vaginal delivery, the contact with the mother's vaginal and intestinal flora is an important source for the start of the infant's colonization with predominance of *Lactobacillus*, *Prevotella* and other *Bifidobacterium* [16–27]. During cesarean delivery, direct contact of the mouth of the newborn with the vaginal and intestinal microbiota is absent, and non-maternally derived environmental bacteria play an important role for infants' intestinal colonization which has a less diverse flora and a bacterial community similar to those found on the skin surface dominated by *Staphylococcus* and with a delayed intestinal colonization by *Lactobacillus*, *Bifidobacterium* and *Bacteroides* [8, 17].

With increasing concern over rising rates of cesarean delivery and insufficient exclusive breastfeeding of infants in developed countries, a Canadian group characterized the gut microbiota of healthy Canadian infants and described the influence of cesarean delivery and formula feeding [18]. Fecal samples were collected at 4 months of age, and microbiota composition was characterized using high-throughput DNA sequencing. 'Compared with breastfed infants, formula-fed infants had increased richness of species, with overrepresentation of *Clostridium difficile. Escherichia-Shigella* and *Bacteroides* species were underrepresented in infants born by cesarean delivery. Infants born by elective cesarean delivery had particularly low bacterial richness and diversity.' These findings support the accumulating evidence that delivery mode and interaction with infant diet serve as important antecedents to the development of the microbial community.

Some authors have suggested that the composition of the very first human microbiota could have lasting effects on the intestine [8]. Of major importance is the evidence that intestinal microbiota's interaction with the intestinal mucosa plays a critical role in development of the immune system [19]. Thus, depending on the mode of delivery, differences in microbial colonization patterns in the infant's gastrointestinal tract may lead to differences in the development of immunity. Available epidemiological data show that atopic diseases, asthma, type 1 diabetes and food allergies appear more often in infants after cesarean delivery than after vaginal delivery [20–23]. Studies in adults using non-culture-based analysis of the intestinal microbiota show that antibiotics may perturb the gastrointestinal tract for years [24, 25]. Nevertheless, the increase in cesarean deliveries in many countries could have significant consequences in public health with higher allergies, asthma, celiac and other diseases [15].

Necrotizing Enterocolitis and Intestinal Microbiota

In another study, designed to determine differences in microbial patterns that may be critical to the development of NEC, microbial analysis from fecal samples from NEC patients distinctly clustered separately from controls [26]. As described by the authors, 'Patients with NEC had less diversity, an increase in abundance of Gammaproteobacteria, a decrease in other bacteria species, and had received a higher mean number of previous days of antibiotics'. These results suggested 'that NEC is associated with severe lack of microbiota diversity that may accentuate the impact of single dominant microorganisms favored by empiric and widespread use of antibiotics' [27].

Manipulations of the Intestinal Microbiota and Their Consequences

Antibiotics
In the USA, a large number of mothers giving birth prematurely are treated with antibiotics. Additionally, most (nearly 90%) of VLBW infants are treated with a course of broad-spectrum antibiotics [28]. Two studies so far have suggested an increased incidence of NEC related to this practice [26, 27]. In studies of adults, the abundance of specific resistance genes to antibiotics was greater in those patients treated with antibiotics [24, 25].

Probiotics

Probiotics are defined as live microorganism which when administered confer a health benefit to the host [29]. It is common belief that probiotic microbes confer benefits similar to the commensal and symbiotic microbes that reside within the gastrointestinal tract. These provide a number of benefits for the host. They compete for nutrient-binding sites to provide a protective barrier against incoming bacteria and have, in some cases, antimicrobial action. Probiotics may also interfere with the adherence of pathogenic bacteria, increase the physical and immunological barrier function of the intestine, increase mucus production, decrease ischemic injury through nitric oxide production, and modulate the inflammatory response. In addition, there is some evidence linking probiotic use with improved intestinal motility [30]. Despite the numerous beneficial actions that are being attributed to probiotics, there are also several risks that also need to be considered [31].

There is evidence that probiotics have immunomodulatory actions, which may be beneficial for diseases with high pro-inflammatory activity in the bowel such as inflammatory bowel disease and NEC. The immunomodulatory effect may be mediated by strengthening the interepithelial intestinal barrier, whereby bacterial translocation across the epithelium and activation of the secondary inflammatory cascade are reduced. In addition, there is a specific immune stimulation by probiotics through processes involving dendritic cells that present antigens to undifferentiated T cells, directing their differentiation to effector versus regulatory phenotypes. Dendritic cells also sample commensal organisms, incorporate them, and transport them to mesenteric lymph nodes where they induce a local immune response by activating specific B cells to produce specific secretory IgA [32].

Probiotics and NEC

Prospective randomized trials have evaluated the effects of different probiotics on the prevention of NEC [33–43]. A multicenter trial of probiotic suggested a beneficial preventive effect against NEC. However, there was a trend for a higher incidence of sepsis in infants receiving probiotics [34], especially in those with a birth weight <750 g, thus warranting caution, despite recent recommendations for the routine use of probiotics based on a meta-analysis of the current data [35]. There is currently considerable controversy over the routine use of probiotics for the prevention of NEC in preterm infants. The meta-analyses [35, 36] have been questioned on the basis of several considerations, one of the major concerns being that different probiotics were used in the different studies, and the quality level of several of the studies included in the meta-analysis [37], hence rendering the meta-analyses flawed [38]. Of note, recently, in preterm pigs an increased NEC incidence has been reported following a specific probiotic administration [39].

Therefore, in conclusion, the observed effects of individual probiotic preparations on the incidence of NEC have to be reconfirmed in large independent adequately powered high-quality RCT. One of the largest studies reported thus far did not show a significant decrease in sepsis, death or NEC [40]. Since probiotics may influence host gene expression and ongoing bacterial colonization, long-term outcome data are desirable. Furthermore, probiotic products in the USA and Europe have not been subjected to rigorous manufacturing quality control or FDA approval. Despite encouraging data of beneficial effects of some probiotics, more studies are needed to determine which probiotic is appropriate for a given disease or neonatal population [41]. We also need to attain a better understand of their mechanism of action, determine the appropriate dose and safety (both short and long term) in the neonate. Neither the American Academy of Pediatrics nor the European Society for Pediatric Gastroenterology, Hepatology and Nutrition has endorsed the use of probiotics for this purpose. Nevertheless, these agents are already being used and guidelines for their use have been published [42].

Monitoring of Probiotics

If probiotics are to be used in newborns, the incidence of sepsis secondary to probiotic translocation and antibiotic resistance, changes in growth, development, immune function, and allergic diseases, and long-term changes must be monitored. Further, to document possible associations between the supplemented probiotic and sepsis, it will be important to use molecular probes to identify infectious agents because they are more sensitive and strain-specific than culture-based methods and may be less prone to bias.

Prebiotics

Prebiotics are selectively fermented ingredients that allow changes in the composition in the gastrointestinal microflora, that confer benefits upon host well-being. Prebiotics are not fully digested in the small intestine and, thus, can act in the lower intestinal tract to preferentially promote the growth of non-pathogenic organisms such as bifidobacteria and lactobacilli.

Some prebiotic agents include the oligosaccharides inulin, galactose oligosaccharide, fructose oligosaccharide, acidic oligosaccharides and/or lactulose [43]. Although these compounds increase fecal bifidobacteria counts, reduce stool pH, reduce stool viscosity, accelerate gastrointestinal transport, and improve gastric motility [44–46], their efficacy in prevention of NEC is unclear. The theoretical benefit of such preparations has been reviewed [43]. So far, no convincing benefit in the prevention of NEC has been found in the first controlled randomized trials [45, 47–49]. One study in an animal model suggested increased intestinal bacterial translocation after the administration of prebiotics [50].

Human milk contains considerable amounts of a variety of different oligosaccharides, which, in part, undergo fermentation in the colon. The concentration of oligosaccharides changes with the duration of lactation. Levels are highest in colostrum at 20–23 g/l then decline to about 20 g/l on day 4 of lactation and to 9 g/l on day 120 of lactation [51]. These oligosaccharides are thought to maintain normal gut flora. They inhibit growth of pathogenic bacteria. Short-chain fatty acids, some of their fermentation products, are important energy fuels for colonocytes and for the body following absorption. Human milk oligosaccharides are also thought to have important roles as anti-infective agents.

Key Points

- With the development of high-throughput sequencing technologies, a much better understanding of the composition, function and effects of medical interventions in the intestinal microbiota and its relationship with the host is being developed. Analysis of entire microbial population sequences also allows for evaluation of the functional characteristics of the microbial population via functional metagenomics.
- While it is being debated, there is no conclusive evidence to recommend the routine use of probiotics or prebiotics all preterm infants. The available trials do not indicate that an optimal probiotic strain or prebiotic, dosing regimen, or protocol has been identified. Safety and efficacy of each probiotic strain must be tested separately. Data generated with one probiotic strain do not necessarily apply to another strain.
- Despite the progress made in the care of sick preterm babies, more studies are needed to understand the effects of therapeutic interventions on the intestinal microbiota. Precautions to minimize negative alterations in the intestinal microbiota with current medical practices (e.g. antibiotics) and the use of bioactive agents such as pro- and prebiotics are warranted in the neonate.

References

1 Turnbaugh PJ, et al: The human microbiome project. Nature 2007;449:804–810.
2 Penders J, et al: Factors influencing the composition of the intestinal microbiota in early infancy. Pediatrics 2006;118:511–512.
3 Lee YK, Mazmanian SK: Has the microbiota played a critical role in the evolution of the adaptive immune system? Science 2010;330:1768–1773.
4 Bauer H, Horowitz RE, Levenson SM, Popper H: The response of the lymphatic tissue to the microbial flora. Studies on germ-free mice. Am J Pathol 1963;42: 741–783.
5 Strachan DP: Hay fever, hygiene, and household size. BMJ 1989;299:1259–1260.
6 Larsen N, et al: Gut microbiota in human adults with type 2 diabetes differs from non-diabetic adults. PLoS One 2010;5:e9085.
7 De Palma G, et al: Intestinal dysbiosis and reduced immunoglobulin-coated bacteria associated with coeliac disease in children. BMC Microbiol 2010;10:63.
8 Turnbaugh PJ, et al: A core gut microbiome in obese and lean twins. Nature 2009;457:480–484.
9 DiGiulio DB, et al: Microbial prevalence, diversity and abundance in amniotic fluid during preterm labor: a molecular and culture-based investigation. PLoS One 2008;3:33056.
10 Mshvildadze M, Neu J, Mai V: Intestinal microbiota development in the premature neonate: establishment of a lasting commensal relationship? Nutr Rev 2008;66:658–663.
11 Mshvildadze M, et al: Intestinal microbial ecology in premature infants assessed with non-culture-based techniques. J Pediatr 2010;156:20–25.

12 Palmer C, Bik EM, Digiulio DB, Relman DA, Brown PO: Development of the human infant intestinal microbiota. PLoS Biol 2007;5:e177.

13 Eggesbø M, et al: Development of gut microbiota in infants not exposed to medical interventions. APMIS 2011;119:17–35.

14 Jacquot A, et al: Dynamics and clinical evolution of bacterial gut microflora in extremely premature patients. J Pediatr 2011;158:390–396.

15 Rushing J, Neu J: Cesarean versus vaginal delivery: long-term infant outcomes and the hygiene hypothesis. Clin Perinatol 2011;38:321–331.

16 Dominguez-Bello MG, et al: Delivery mode shapes the acquisition and structure of the initial microbiota across multiple body habitats in newborns. Proc Natl Acad Sci USA 2010;107:11971–11975.

17 Biasucci G, Benenati B, Morelli L, Bessi E, Boehm G: Cesarean delivery may affect the early biodiversity of intestinal bacteria. J Nutr 2008;138:1796S–1800S.

18 Azad MB, et al: Gut microbiota of healthy Canadian infants: profiles by mode of delivery and infant diet at 4 months. CMAJ 2013;185:385–394.

19 Björkstén B: Effects of intestinal microflora and the environment on the development of asthma and allergy. Springer Semin Immunopathol 2004;25:257–270.

20 Negele K, et al: Mode of delivery and development of atopic disease during the first 2 years of life. Pediatr Allergy Immunol 2004;15:48–54.

21 Debley JS, Smith JM, Redding GJ, Critchlow CW: Childhood asthma hospitalization risk after cesarean delivery in former term and premature infants. Ann Allergy Asthma Immunol 2005;94:228–233.

22 Laubereau B, et al: Caesarean section and gastrointestinal symptoms, atopic dermatitis, and sensitisation during the first year of life. Arch Dis Child 2004; 89:993–997.

23 Eggesbø M, Botten G, Stigum H, Nafstad P, Magnus P: Is delivery by cesarean section a risk factor for food allergy? J Allergy Clin Immunol 2003;112:420–426.

24 Jernberg C, Löfmark S, Edlund C, Jansson JK: Long-term ecological impacts of antibiotic administration on the human intestinal microbiota. ISME J 2007;1: 56–66.

25 Jakobsson HE, et al: Short-term antibiotic treatment has differing long-term impacts on the human throat and gut microbiome. PLoS One 2010;5:e9836.

26 Wang Y, et al: 16S rRNA gene-based analysis of fecal microbiota from preterm infants with and without necrotizing enterocolitis. ISME J 2009;3:944–954.

27 Cotten CM, et al: Prolonged duration of initial empirical antibiotic treatment is associated with increased rates of necrotizing enterocolitis and death for extremely low birth weight infants. Pediatrics 2009;123:58–66.

28 Clark RH, Bloom BT, Spitzer AR, Gerstmann DR: Reported medication use in the neonatal intensive care unit: data from a large national data set. Pediatrics 2006;117:1979–1987.

29 Guarner F, Requena T, Marcos A: Consensus statements from the Workshop 'Probiotics and Health: Scientific Evidence'. Nutr Hosp 2010;25:700–704.

30 Indrio F, et al: The effects of probiotics on feeding tolerance, bowel habits, and gastrointestinal motility in preterm newborns. J Pediatr 2008;152:801–806.

31 Boyle RJ, Robins-Browne RM, Tang ML: Probiotic use in clinical practice: what are the risks? Am J Clin Nutr 2006;83:1256–1264.

32 Macpherson AJ, Uhr T: Induction of protective IgA by intestinal dendritic cells carrying commensal bacteria. Science 2004;303:1662–1665.

33 Bin-Nun A, et al: Oral probiotics prevent necrotizing enterocolitis in very low birth weight neonates. J Pediatr 2005;147:192–196.

34 Lin HC, et al: Oral probiotics prevent necrotizing enterocolitis in very low birth weight preterm infants: a multicenter, randomized, controlled trial. Pediatrics 2008;122:693–700.

35 Deshpande G, Rao S, Patole S, Bulsara M: Updated meta-analysis of probiotics for preventing necrotizing enterocolitis in preterm neonates. Pediatrics 2010;125:921–930.

36 Alfaleh K, Bassler D: Probiotics for prevention of necrotizing enterocolitis in preterm infants. Cochrane Database Syst Rev 2008;23:CD005496.

37 Mihatsch WA, et al: Critical systematic review of the level of evidence for routine use of probiotics for reduction of mortality and prevention of necrotizing enterocolitis and sepsis in preterm infants. Clin Nutr 2012;31:6–15.

38 Soll RF: Probiotics: are we ready for routine use? Pediatrics 2010;125:1071–1072.

39 Cilieborg MS, Boye M, Molbak L, Thymann T, Sangild PT: Preterm birth and necrotizing enterocolitis alter gut colonization in pigs. Pediatr Res 2011;69: 10–16.

40 Rojas MA, et al: Prophylactic probiotics to prevent death and nosocomial infection in preterm infants. Pediatrics 2012;130:e1113–e1120.

41 Sanders ME, et al: An update on the use and investigation of probiotics in health and disease. Gut 2013; 62:787–796.

42 Deshpande GC, Rao SC, Keil AD, Patole SK: Evidence-based guidelines for use of probiotics in preterm neonates. BMC Med 2011;9:92.

43 Sherman PM, et al: Potential roles and clinical utility of prebiotics in newborns, infants, and children: proceedings from a global prebiotic summit meeting, New York City, June 27–28, 2008. J Pediatr 2009;155: S61–S70.

44 Boehm G, et al: Supplementation of a bovine milk formula with an oligosaccharide mixture increases counts of faecal bifidobacteria in preterm infants. Arch Dis Child Fetal Neonatal Ed 2002;86:F178–F181.

45 Mihatsch WA, Hoegel J, Pohlandt F: Prebiotic oligosaccharides reduce stool viscosity and accelerate gastrointestinal transport in preterm infants. Acta Paediatr 2006;95:843–848.

46 Indrio F, et al: Prebiotics improve gastric motility and gastric electrical activity in preterm newborns. J Pediatr Gastroenterol Nutr 2009;49:258–261.

47 Modi N, Uthaya S, Fell J, Kulinskaya E: A randomized, double-blind, controlled trial of the effect of prebiotic oligosaccharides on enteral tolerance in preterm infants (ISRCTN77444690). Pediatr Res 2010;68:440–445.

48 Westerbeek EA, et al: Neutral and acidic oligosaccharides in preterm infants: a randomized, double-blind, placebo-controlled trial. Am J Clin Nutr 2010; 91:679–686.

49 Riskin A, et al: The effects of lactulose supplementation to enteral feedings in premature infants: a pilot study. J Pediatr 2010;156:209–214.

50 Barrat E, et al: Supplementation with galactooligosaccharides and inulin increases bacterial translocation in artificially reared newborn rats. Pediatr Res 2008;64:34–39.

51 Coppa GV, et al: Changes in carbohydrate composition in human milk over 4 months of lactation. Pediatrics 1993;91:637–641.

Prof. Josef Neu, MD
Pediatrics/Neonatology, University of Florida
1600 SW Archer Road
Gainesville, FL 32610 (USA)
E-Mail neuj@peds.ufl.edu

Koletzko B, Poindexter B, Uauy R (eds): Nutritional Care of Preterm Infants: Scientific Basis and Practical Guidelines.
World Rev Nutr Diet. Basel, Karger, 2014, vol 110, pp 177–189 (DOI: 10.1159/000358466)

Practice of Parenteral Nutrition in VLBW and ELBW Infants

Nicholas D. Embleton[a] · Karen Simmer[b]

[a]Newcastle Neonatal Service, Newcastle Hospitals NHS Foundation Trust, Institute of Health and Society, Newcastle University, Newcastle upon Tyne, UK; [b]Centre for Neonatal Research and Education, School of Paediatrics and Child Health, University of Western, Crawley, W.A., Australia

Reviewed by Berthold Koletzko, Dr. von Hauner Children's Hospital, University of Munich Medical Centre, Munich, Germany; Brenda Poindexter, Riley Hospital for Children at Indiana University Health, Indianapolis, Ind., USA

Abstract

Preterm infants have limited nutrient stores at birth, take time to establish enteral feeding, are at risk of accumulating significant nutrient deficits, and frequently suffer poor growth – all risks which are associated with poorer neurodevelopmental outcome. Parenteral nutrition (PN) provides a relatively safe means of meeting nutrient intakes, and is widely used in preterm infants in the initial period after birth. PN is also important for infants who may not tolerate enteral feeds such as those with congenital or acquired gut disorders such as necrotizing enterocolitis (NEC). PN is associated with several short-term benefits, but clear evidence of long-term benefit from controlled trials in neonates is lacking. There are many compositional, practical and risk aspects involved in neonatal PN. In most preterm infants, authorities recommend amino acid intakes approximating to 3.5–4 g/kg/day of protein, lipid intakes of 3–4 g/kg/day and sufficient carbohydrate to meet a total energy intake of 90–110 kcal/kg/day. Where PN is the sole source of nutrition, careful attention to micronutrient requirements is necessary. PN may be administered via peripheral venous access if the osmolality allows, but in many cases requires central venous access. Standardized PN bags may meet the nutrient needs of many preterm infants over the first few days, although restricted fluid intakes mean that many receive inadequate amounts especially of amino acids. PN can be associated with increased rates of bacterial and fungal sepsis, mechanical complications related to venous line placement and miscalculations and errors in manufacture, supply and administration. PN is also associated with metabolic derangements, hepatic dysfunction, and risks contamination with toxins such as aluminum, which enter the solutions during manufacturing. PN must only be administered in units with good quality control, strict asepsis in manufacture and administration and multidisciplinary teams focused on nutrient needs and intakes. © 2014 S. Karger AG, Basel

Preterm infants are born with limited nutrient stores. Their nutritional status is further compromised by gastrointestinal immaturity meaning that enteral milk feeds take time to establish. Infants born at around 24 completed weeks' gestation are composed of approximately 90% water, with the remainder being protein with virtually no lipid (except in neural structures) and tiny amounts of minerals [1, 2]. Protein in organs and muscle represent the largest potential energy 'store' but if catabolized for energy will no longer be functionally available. Heird and others [3, 4] have estimated that ELBW infants only have sufficient energy for the first 2–3 days of life without exogenous administration. A typical 500 g baby at 24 weeks is only composed of approximately 50 g of dry tissue. Even if one third of that protein could be utilized for energy that still only represents potential energy stores of around 50 kcal, barely enough to meet basal metabolic energy requirements for the first 24 h [5]. Delivery of an extremely preterm infant (e.g. <28 weeks' gestation) deserves to be viewed as a nutritional emergency.

Administration of parenteral nutrition (PN) is now considered standard of care for most (extremely) preterm infants over the first few postnatal days, and is essential for those with gastrointestinal malfunction secondary to diseases such as necrotizing enterocolitis (NEC) [6]. Neonatal PN (aqueous solutions of glucose, electrolytes and amino acids ± intravenous lipids and other nutrients) initially evolved in the late 1960s with the first case report of an infant 'receiving all nutrients by vein' [7]. Recent reviews have highlighted the major obstacles that needed to be overcome for that to occur including: formulation of a suitable solution, challenges of concentrating nutrients into a hyperosmolar solution without precipitation, securing of venous access (typically via the central vein), maintenance of asepsis in production and supply, and anticipating, monitoring and correcting of metabolic balances that might arise [8, 9]. The practice of neonatal PN has developed dramatically over the last two to three decades, but uncertainties persist around indications, compositional aspects, practical aspects of supply and delivery, need for central venous access, and monitoring strategies. Systematic reviews have examined the role of supplementation with nutrients such as carnitine [10], cysteine [11], glutamine [12] and taurine [13], the timing of introduction of lipid [14, 15] and practical aspects of delivery such as use of heparin [16], and percutaneous lines for delivery [17], but few studies have examined the optimal macronutrient intakes with which PN is initiated, or how quickly those amounts can be increased over the first few postnatal days.

Indications and Benefits

PN is associated with important risks and benefits, and clinical judgment is required to balance these competing outcomes. There is general agreement that infants born extremely preterm or very low birth weight (<1,500 g) will benefit from PN, but it is less clear whether the nutritional benefits outweigh the risks in larger, more stable infants e.g. those >32 weeks' gestation. No study has defined the optimal population cut-off indications for PN but most units in developed countries use PN routinely

<30 weeks and/or <1,250 g birth weight. Many would recommend PN use in infants <32 weeks or <1,500 g, and some would use in more mature infants whilst enteral feeds are established. The average duration of 'bridging' PN until full enteral feeding is achieved is typically 1–2 weeks, and closely linked to degree of prematurity [18, 19].

In addition to PN used as a 'bridge' to establishing nutrient intakes via the enteral route, PN is also indicated for infants who have gastrointestinal malfunction or failure, typified by infants who develop NEC, in both the pre- and postoperative period. In these infants, PN is generally the sole source of nutrients for several days or weeks and much closer attention must be paid to ensuring that nutrient deficits do not accumulate, specifically for micronutrients (e.g. zinc, manganese, and iodine [20, 21]) and vitamins (especially fat-soluble vitamins). PN is associated with an oxidant load, and combined with other factors is associated with hepatic dysfunction [22, 23], further compounded by a lack of enteral feeds. Hepatic dysfunction is a major issue for infants on long-term PN but usually of only minor importance for well stable infants receiving 'bridging' PN.

Whilst PN is designed to meet nutrient requirements, achieving the intakes with enteral nutrition (especially breast milk) will always be preferable where this is possible. PN may allow more gradual increases in milk feeds: although rapid feed advancements have been associated with increased rates of NEC in some non-controlled studies there are no adequately powered studies comparing rates of feed increase although such studies are in progress (see www.npeu.ox.ac.uk/sift). PN avoids negative nitrogen balance (Evidence base: high quality) [24–27], promotes weight gain (Evidence base: high quality) [28] and is associated with neurocognitive benefit (Evidence base: low quality) [29, 30]. Although there are few controlled trials with long-term neurodevelopmental status as an outcome, most clinicians would now lack equipoise to compare the effects of PN versus placebo (dextrose) on long-term outcomes such as cognition, although uncertainties persist [31].

Risks of Parenteral Nutrition

There are significant risks associated with use of PN, and issues around composition, supply, formulation, hepatic dysfunction and oxidant load are discussed later in the chapter. Most units administer PN via a central venous catheter, typically inserted in the umbilical vein or percutaneously (PICC, peripherally inserted central catheter). Umbilical venous catheters are rarely associated with hepatic thrombosis, whilst PICCs are also associated with localized skin infections, thrombophlebitis and invasive bacterial and fungal sepsis. PICCs have been associated with fatal pericardial tamponade (due to erosion of the catheter tip through the atrial wall) and misplacement into organs (e.g. liver) or body cavity (e.g. thorax, abdomen, etc.). PN can be administered via the peripheral vein [17], thereby avoiding or reducing many of those risks, but is associated with increased local complications such as extravasations that may result in permanent harm. Aqueous PN solutions are always hypertonic and hyperosmolar but there is little agreement on the upper limit for peripheral administration. Institutional guidelines often quote an upper limit of between 800 and 1,200 mosm/l to enable 'safe' peripheral administration, but these limits are based on scant evidence (Evidence base: low quality). The co-administration of intravenous lipid appears to reduce the associated phlebitis.

PN use frequently involves the inadvertent administration of potential toxins, particularly aluminum, that may contaminate solutions. Controlled studies have shown that aluminum intake in PN is associated with worse neurodevelopmental outcome [32] and worse measures of bone mineralization in the lumbar spine and hip bone in adolescents [33]. These long-term adverse effects are of major concern and efforts are being undertaken to reduce or completely avoid aluminum in the raw material supply chain. There are also concerns regarding the adverse effects of intravenous lipid administration, which in the short term is associated with higher circulating levels of cholesterol and triglycerides. However, in a recent study, cholesterol levels were not increased upon early lipid administration, although triglyceride concentrations were increased during the first days of lipid administration [27]. In one small long-term follow-up study, neonatal lipid administration was associated with measures of adverse vascular health in young adults as determined by increased aortic stiffness, a relationship that was strongly associated with serum cholesterol levels during the infusion [34].

Reports of hyperammonemia as a consequence of PN are largely historical, but there remain uncertainties about the optimal amino acid combination [31, 35]. Amino acid solutions consist of essential amino acids and a variable quantity and quality of non-essential amino acids to meet nitrogen requirements, but there is limited research in this area in preterm infants. Measurement of plasma amino acid profiles is expensive and not useful in clinical practice. Most commercial formulations have been designed to result in plasma profiles similar to cord blood or that of a breast milk-fed infant, but the 'gold standard' profile for a preterm infant on PN has not been determined. Whilst excess levels of individual amino acids may be harmful, inadequate levels may prevent appropriate growth.

Physiologically the supply of amino acids via the parenteral compared to the enteral route is not ideal as it provides amino acids that initially pass into the arterial circulation as opposed to enteral substrate that is initially absorbed into the portal vasculature after splanchnic uptake and metabolism. Very high rates of energy expenditure and protein synthesis have been documented in portally-drained tissues, where catabolism of amino acids for energy is a normal process. Stable isotope studies show that there are large differences in utilization between the amino acids, and emphasize that our current knowledge of optimal intakes as determined by, for example, plasma amino acid levels, are extremely limited [36].

Practical Aspects of Supply and Composition

A PN strategy that is often referred to as 'aggressive PN' has become a priority in the NICU and refers to the clinical practice of commencing relatively high dose amino acids (2–3 g/kg/day) as PN within hours of birth with the aim of reducing the incidence and severity of ex-utero growth retardation [37]. Many would argue that the term 'aggressive' is a misnomer and that early administration of amino acids at a level capable of meeting nutrient requirements might be better termed 'appropriate'.

Thureen et al. [38] demonstrated using isotope infusions and indirect calorimetry measurements, that very preterm infants tolerate infusions of 3 g/kg/day early in life with plasma amino acid levels similar to the fetus and with improved protein accretion and nitrogen balance (185.6 vs. –41.6 mg N kg^{-1} day^{-1}). A systematic review of randomized clinical trials comparing a high versus a low dose of parenteral amino acids concluded that 3.5 g/kg/day in the first week was safe but further trials are needed to determine if even more is beneficial [26]. Protein:energy ratios are crucial but the optimal ratio (and optimal carbohydrate/lipid energy source) has not been determined. Most authorities suggest approximately 20–25 kcal of non-protein energy are required per gram of (protein equivalent) amino acids to promote lean mass accretion (Evidence base: moderate quality) [39]. Inadequate energy availability may have been a limiting factor in trials examining higher nitrogen intakes [40].

Preventing nutrient deficiencies, ex-utero growth retardation and associated morbidities have become a priority in contemporary neonatal intensive care. In a prospective non-randomized consecutive observational study of 102 infants with birth weight <1,250 g, Senterre and Rigo [41] demonstrated that if nutritional protocols were optimized to meet recent recommendations, that is using 'aggressive' PN, the incidence of postnatal growth restriction can be dramatically reduced. They used standardized PN solution prepared by their hospital pharmacy (2.7 g amino acids and 12 g dextrose/100 ml with electrolytes and minerals) to achieve a mean intake in week 1 of 3.2 g/kg/day amino acids and 80 kcal/kg/day.

Lipid is a good source of energy and is safe to start early [15] at 2 g/kg/day on day 1 (Evidence base: moderate quality) [27, 42, 43]. The optimal lipid emulsion needs to provide essential fatty acids, maintain long-chain polyunsaturated fatty acids (PUFA) levels and immune function, and reduce lipid peroxidation. Until recently, the only emulsion widely available for neonates was a soybean oil (SO) emulsion. SO is rich in the omega–6 PUFA linoleic acid, and its metabolites include peroxides that may induce toxic effects as well as pro-inflammatory cytokines. Novel preparations are now available and have been recently reviewed [14, 44]. In these, some of the SO is replaced with other oils including coconut oil (rich in medium-chain triglyceride), olive oil thereby reducing the content of linoleic acid. Also, emulsions containing fish oil which is rich in long-chain omega–3 fatty acids (EPA, DHA) have become available. Long-chain omega–3 fatty acids are precursors of anti-inflammatory mediators. Short-term benefits include a reduction in lipid peroxidation [45] and fatty acid pro-

Table 1. Suggested monitoring strategy for PN

Parameter	Timing and frequency of measurement
Sodium, potassium, chloride, bicarbonate and glucose	Daily over at least first 3–4 days
Calcium and phosphate (± magnesium)	Twice weekly until stable
Plasma triglycerides	Twice weekly (or if lipemic serum)
Liver function tests	Weekly
Weight	Daily or alternate days
Length and head circumference	Weekly

files [46]. Intestinal failure-associated liver disease has been reported to improve with modification of PN, including reducing or stopping SO emulsion, using mixed emulsions with some fish oil, or using low dosages of emulsions based on fish oil only. However these have not been approved for use in pediatric patients [47, 48], and there are few trials in preterm infants that help determine the optimal intravenous lipid source (Evidence base: low quality).

Carbohydrate intake may be limited in preterm and sick neonates because hyperglycemia is common. The upper rate of glucose administration (7–12 mg/kg/min) is determined by glucose oxidative capacity for energy production and glycogen deposition and is influenced by gestational age and clinical condition. The level at which a raised plasma glucose results in adverse outcome has never been well defined, but hyperglycemia (>10 mmol/l) is common after preterm birth, and may be related to surges in catecholamines, decrease in insulin production and insulin resistance. Hyperglycemia is associated with increased mortality, intraventricular hemorrhage, sepsis and chronic lung disease. Hyperglycemia is most easily treated by reducing glucose intake down to a minimum intake of 4 mg/kg/min, although the use of insulin is common in many units. Provision of protein (as amino acids) in PN results in lower glucose levels [49] possibly through stimulation of the insulin/IGF-1 axis, a mechanism likely, in particular, to involve amino acids such as arginine and branched chain amino acids. Routine basal insulin infusion is not helpful, and is associated with hypoglycemia and associated morbidity (Evidence base: moderate quality) [50].

The optimal way to assess the safety and efficacy of PN has not been determined and monitoring PN in preterm infants varies from unit to unit. A typical strategy is suggested in table 1 (Evidence base: low quality). Some units screen for catheter-related sepsis by monitoring CRP twice a week.

Manufacture and Supply

Compositional/technical issues with PN are comprehensively covered in the Lawrence and Trissel Handbook of Injectable Drugs (2013) [51]. PN conventionally consists of solutions of amino acids/glucose/electrolytes, and fat emulsion that are infused separately. Amino acid, glucose and electrolyte solutions that are hypertonic and solutions with high glucose concentrations (>12.5–15%) generally need be infused centrally.

PN solutions, whether prepared in-house or manufactured commercially, need to be prepared under stringent 'clean room' conditions including a laminar flow hood, using appropriate ingredients. The process should be validated and the prepared solutions monitored regularly for sterility and quality, and staff trained in the preparation process. Electrolytes added to solutions must be compatible when mixed together. Calcium and phosphate salts have a potential to form an insoluble precipitate limiting the quantity that can be added to solutions. All solutions must be visually checked for clarity, particles and leaks. Computer-generated worksheets and labels help eliminate calculation errors, as will the use of standardized formulae.

Solutions are filtered in the pharmacy during preparation on PN. Some groups recommend the additional use of in-line filters on PN lines to protect patients from precipitates such as calcium phosphate, particles that may be present in containers, or inadvertent microbial contamination [52]. However, the incidence of sepsis does not appear to be reduced in neonatal patients by adding in-line filters [53] and the additional cost may be significant.

Potentially toxic peroxides may be formed in PN solutions by an oxygenation reaction in the presence of light [54–56]. Protecting the PN container from light will reduce this problem and many also advise the use of amber tubing to reduce the contamination further. Lipid emulsions are also sources of peroxides and may undergo further peroxidation on exposure to light. The degree of peroxidation varies with the source of fat used. Lipid containers should be protected from light and amber tubing used.

Solutions may be supplied in either single-use containers such as bags, bottles, or syringes. The containers should not be punctured more than once to reduce microbial contamination. Medications should not be added to PN solutions at ward level as this may cause incompatibilities or contaminate the solution, and care should be taken if running PN in conjunction with other solutions (e.g. through a Y connection) for similar reasons.

Adding both fat- and water-soluble vitamins to lipid solutions is used as a strategy in some units as the lipid emulsion may provide an additional degree of light protection. Vitamins added to the lipid emulsion rather than to amino acid/dextrose may enable more predictable amounts to be delivered to the infant, but vitamins may still adsorb onto the containers or lines used. Adding vitamins in this way allows the preparation to be purchased commercially, or made in-house in batches. Stability of PN solutions is dependent on composition. Commercially available preparations of amino acids/dextrose/electrolytes have shelf lives of up to several months. Concerns about microbiological contamination, both during in-house manufacture or on the ward, limit expiry time to 48 h once connected.

Standardized Parenteral Nutrition

Individual prescriptions for PN (IPN) are written and prepared every 24–48 h and therefore are unavailable for much of the first day of life. Devlieger et al. [57] and others proposed that most patients in the NICU can tolerate some variation in intake and hence may be managed with few combinations of standard PN (SPN) without significant electrolyte disturbances. SPN can be readily available in the NICU enabling initiation of the PN within an hour of birth. SPN has other advantages over IPN including better provision of nutrients, less prescription and administration errors, decreased risk of infection, and cost savings (Evidence base: moderate quality) [58–60].

Some units provide SPN in fixed low volume to ensure complete nutritional requirements are met when fluid is restricted or while enteral feeds are introduced. One such unit is in Auckland, New Zealand, where starter solutions provide 2 g/kg/day amino acids in 30 ml for patients born <1,000 g in the first 3 days and, thereafter and for bigger patients, 3.5–4 g/kg/day provided in 90–100 ml. Recently, a large UK trial has examined the use of standardized concentrated PN (SCAMP) where the amino acid requirements can be met in a similarly small volume, meaning that nutrition is not compromised when fluids are restricted. Initial results are promising, but complete trial data reporting is awaited [61]. Whether standardized PN bags are prepared in-house or ordered commercially depends on the quantity required and collaboration between units.

A recent study examined a commercially designed multichamber ready-to-use solution in preterm infants enrolled in a multicenter prospective non-comparative study [62]. The pack contained three chambers (the third lipid chamber being optional to activate) and provided 3.1 g amino acids, 13.3 g dextrose and 2.5 g lipid/100 ml. The benefits are thought to be sterility, longer shelf life (18 months) and increased ability to deliver early nutrition. To improve stability and reduce peroxidation, vitamins and trace elements were added by the hospital pharmacy, but frequent electrolyte supplementation was still requested by physicians (43%). This enabled reasonable nutritional intakes (>2.5 g/kg/day amino acids and >75 kcal/kg/day) in the first week and promoted acceptable weight gain (22 g/kg/day after the first week).

Quality Assurance, Control and Good Practice in Neonates

A recent confidential enquiry into the practice of providing PN in the UK reviewed 264 cases of neonatal PN administration and determined that a 'good' standard of care overall was only achieved in 24% of cases. There were delays in recognizing the need for PN in 28% cases, and delays in administration once a decision to administer had been made (17% cases). The PN requirements were often not documented in the infants' case record, in 37% the initial PN prescription was deemed to be inadequate for

Table 2. Suggested target intakes of nutrients from PN in first week

Nutrient	Day 0[a]	Days 1–2	Day 3[b]
Amino acids[c], g/kg/day	≥2	≥3.5	3.5–4
Lipid, g/kg/day	≥2	3–4	3–4
Total energy intake, kcal/kg/day	60–80	80–100	≥100

[a] First 24 h of life. [b] Assuming minimal contribution from enteral nutrition. [c] In g of protein equivalent.

needs, and in 19% monitoring was considered to be inadequate. At an organizational level, very few hospitals had multidisciplinary nutritional teams. This high variability in aspects of composition, supply and administration, healthcare organization and quality assurance reflect many concerns. They suggest that (1) PN practice does not receive sufficient emphasis as an integral component of modern neonatal care, and (2) the evidence base for optimal practice remains to be determined. The reports note that recommendations from professional bodies are available, but recognize the lack of a strong evidence base for practice [63]. Many cite the ESPEN/ESPGHAN guidelines published in 2005 as a basis for practice [1], but like other recommendations they are based on limited evidence and depend to a large extent on expert judgement. Only very few large randomized controlled trials have been conducted since that report.

Initiating Parenteral Nutrition and Introducing Enteral Nutrition: Suggestions for a Practical Approach

Individual units need to develop an approach that is sensitive to local circumstances, and that maximizes quality outcomes whilst minimizing harm. There are few adequately powered trials and meta-analyses are limited, but suggested intakes are summarized in table 2 (Evidence base: low quality) along with the following guide:

(1) Develop unit-specific, evidence-based guidelines and facilitate access to professionals with expertise in nutrition, ideally including neonatal dieticians as part of a multidisciplinary team.

(2) Standardized PN and lipid solutions available 24 h/day either from the pharmacy or via the use of 'emergency' bags kept in a fridge on the NICU that are capable of providing at least 3.5 g/kg/day of amino acids.

(3) Start PN and lipid on admission to the NICU aiming to achieve intakes as listed in table 1 over the first few days.

(4) Commercially available bags that contain approximately 2.4–2.7 g/100 ml amino acids will meet suggested intakes if administered at 80–100 ml/day on day 1. If this is formulated with approximately 10% dextrose and co-administered with 2 g/kg/day of lipid then caloric intakes can also be met.

(5) Promote the use of breast milk and aim to provide all infants (except those who are very unstable) with breast milk colostrum in the first 24 h.

(6) Increase the volume of PN to approximately 150 ml/kg/day by day 3 along with 3–4 g/kg/day of lipid. At this volume a typical standardized PN bag will provide 3.6 g/kg/day of amino acids, and when combined with lipid will provide a total caloric intake of approximately 100 kcal/kg/day.

(7) Individualize PN administration (composition, volume and/or concentration) in the presence of significant electrolyte disturbances, hyperglycemia, or fluid restrictions and when enteral nutrition is not tolerated.

(8) Decrease PN as breast milk volume intakes increase so that total fluid intakes do not exceed 150–175 ml/kg/day in the first few days. Consider stopping PN when enteral volumes of 125–150 ml/kg/day are tolerated.

(9) Audit outcomes on a regular basis.

Conclusion

Administration of PN to VLBW infants is now an essential component of care, and with careful formulation can meet all nutrient needs over the first few days. However, there are several risks associated with formulation, supply and administration that mean it must only be undertaken in specialist centers with adequate resource and expertise. Despite the clear benefits, data on long-term outcome are lacking and further research is needed.

Research Questions

(1) What is the optimal protein:energy ratio to maximize protein accretion, whilst minimizing metabolic harm?

(2) What composition of individual amino acid optimizes protein accretion but minimizes the risks of toxicity from high individual levels, and the risks of amino acid insufficiency?

(3) What PN regimens maximize infant and childhood neurocognitive outcomes and minimize long-term metabolic risk?

(4) How is PN supply and delivery best optimized in busy NICU environments?

Acknowledgment

The authors thank Ms. Judith Kristensen, Pharmacist, King Edward Memorial Hospital for Women, Subiaco, W.A., Australia.

References

1 Koletzko B, Goulet O, Hunt J, Krohn K, Shamir R: Guidelines on Paediatric Parenteral Nutrition of the European Society of Paediatric Gastroenterology, Hepatology and Nutrition (ESPGHAN) and the European Society for Clinical Nutrition and Metabolism (ESPEN), Supported by the European Society of Paediatric Research (ESPR). J Pediatr Gastroenterol Nutr 2005;41(suppl 2):S1–S87.

2 Ziegler EE, O'Donnell AM, Nelson SE, Fomon SJ: Body composition of the reference fetus. Growth 1976;40:329–341.

3 Heird WC: The importance of early nutritional management of low-birth-weight infants. Pediatr Rev 1999;20:e43–44.

4 Heird WC, Wu C: Nutrition, Growth, and Body Composition. 106th Ross Conference on Pediatric Research, 1996, pp 7–20.

5 Leitch CA, Denne SC: Energy expenditure in the extremely low-birth-weight infant. Clin Perinatol 2000;27:181–195, vii–viii.

6 Koletzko BK, Goulet K, Shamir R: Paediatric Parenteral Nutrition. A Practical Reference Guide. Basel, Karger, 2008.

7 Wilmore DW, Dudrick SJ: Growth and development of an infant receiving all nutrients exclusively by vein. JAMA 1968;203:860–864.

8 Dudrick SJ: History of parenteral nutrition. J Am Coll Nutr 2009;28:243–251.

9 Fusch C, Bauer K, Bohles HJ, et al: Neonatology/Paediatrics – Guidelines on Parenteral Nutrition, Chapt 13. Ger Med Sci 2009;7:Doc15.

10 Cairns PA, Stalker DJ: Carnitine supplementation of parenterally fed neonates. Cochrane Database Syst Rev 2000;4:CD000950.

11 Soghier LM, Brion LP: Cysteine, cystine or N-acetylcysteine supplementation in parenterally fed neonates. Cochrane Database Syst Rev 2006;4: CD004869.

12 Moe-Byrne T, Wagner JVE, McGuire W: Glutamine supplementation to prevent morbidity and mortality in preterm infants. Cochrane Database Syst Rev 2012;3:CD001457.

13 Verner A, Craig S, McGuire W: Effect of taurine supplementation on growth and development in preterm or low birth weight infants. Cochrane Database Syst Rev 2007;4:CD006072.

14 Vlaardingbroek H, Veldhorst MAB, Spronk S, van den Akker CHP, van Goudoever JB: Parenteral lipid administration to very-low-birth-weight infants – early introduction of lipids and use of new lipid emulsions: a systematic review and meta-analysis. Am J Clin Nutr 2012;96:255–268.

15 Simmer K, Rao SC: Early introduction of lipids to parenterally-fed preterm infants. Cochrane Database Syst Rev 2005;2:CD005256.

16 Shah PS, Ng E, Sinha AK: Heparin for prolonging peripheral intravenous catheter use in neonates. Cochrane Database Syst Rev 2002;4:CD002774.

17 Ainsworth SB, Clerihew L, McGuire W: Percutaneous central venous catheters versus peripheral cannulae for delivery of parenteral nutrition in neonates. Cochrane Database Syst Rev 2007;3: CD004219.

18 Tan MJ, Cooke RW: Improving head growth in very preterm infants – a randomised controlled trial I: neonatal outcomes. Arch Dis Child Fetal Neonatal Ed 2008;93:F337–F341.

19 Embleton ND, Pang N, Cooke RJ: Postnatal malnutrition and growth retardation: an inevitable consequence of current recommendations in preterm infants? Pediatrics 2001;107:270–273.

20 Embleton ND: Galvanised by a rash diagnosis. Arch Dis Child Educ Pract Ed 2004;89:ep40–ep45.

21 Shah MD, Shah SR: Nutrient deficiencies in the premature infant. Pediatr Clin North Am 2009;56: 1069–1083.

22 Sherlock R, Chessex P: Shielding parenteral nutrition from light: does the available evidence support a randomized, controlled trial? Pediatrics 2009;123: 1529–1533.

23 Chessex P, Watson C, Kaczala GW, et al: Determinants of oxidant stress in extremely low birth weight premature infants. Free Rad Biol Med 2010;49:1380–1386.

24 Denne SC, Poindexter BB: Evidence supporting early nutritional support with parenteral amino acid infusion. Semin Perinatol 2007;31:56–60.

25 Denne SC: Protein and energy requirements in preterm infants. Semin Neonatol 2001;6:377–382.

26 Embleton ND: Optimal protein and energy intakes in preterm infants. Early Hum Dev 2007;83:831–837.

27 Vlaardingbroek H, Vermeulen MJ, Rook D, et al: Safety and efficacy of early parenteral lipid and high-dose amino acid administration to very low birth weight infants. J Pediatr 2013;163:638–644.e1–e5.

28 Moyses HE, Johnson MJ, Leaf AA, Cornelius VR: Early parenteral nutrition and growth outcomes in preterm infants: a systematic review and meta-analysis. Am J Clin Nutr 2013;97:816–826.

29 Stephens BE, Walden RV, Gargus RA, et al: First-week protein and energy intakes are associated with 18-month developmental outcomes in extremely low birth weight infants. Pediatrics 2009;123:1337–1343.

30 Poindexter BB, Langer JC, Dusick AM, Ehrenkranz RA; National Institute of Child Health and Human Development Neonatal Research Network: Early provision of parenteral amino acids in extremely low birth weight infants: relation to growth and neurodevelopmental outcome. J Pediatr 2006;148:300–305.

31 Blanco CL, Gong AK, Schoolfield J, et al: Impact of early and high amino acid supplementation on ELBW infants at 2 years. J Pediatr Gastroenterol Nutr 2012;54:601–607.

32 Bishop NJ, Morley R, Day JP, Lucas A: Aluminum neurotoxicity in preterm infants receiving intravenous-feeding solutions. N Engl J Med 1997;336:1557–1561.

33 Fewtrell MS, Bishop NJ, Edmonds CJ, Isaacs EB, Lucas A: Aluminum exposure from parenteral nutrition in preterm infants: bone health at 15-year follow-up. Pediatrics 2009;124:1372–1379.

34 Lewandowski AJ, Lazdam M, Davis E, et al: Short-term exposure to exogenous lipids in premature infants and long-term changes in aortic and cardiac function. Arterioscler Thromb Vasc Biol 2011;31:2125–2135.

35 Blanco CL, Gong AK, Green BK, Falck A, Schoolfield J, Liechty EA: Early changes in plasma amino acid concentrations during aggressive nutritional therapy in extremely low birth weight infants. J Pediatr 2011;158:543–548.e1.

36 Vlaardingerbroek H, Van Goudoever JB, Van Den Akker CHP: Safety and efficacy of early and high-dose parenteral amino acid administration to preterm infants. CAB Reviews. Perspect Agric Vet Sci Nutr Nat Res 2009;4:No. 021. DOI:10.1079/PAVSNNR20094021.

37 Wilson DC, Cairns P, Halliday HL, Reid M, McClure G, Dodge JA: Randomised controlled trial of an aggressive nutritional regimen in sick very low birth weight infants. Arch Dis Child Fetal Neonatal Ed 1997;77:F4–F11.

38 Thureen PJ, Melara D, Fennessey PV, Hay WW Jr: Effect of low versus high intravenous amino acid intake on very low birth weight infants in the early neonatal period. Pediatr Res 2003;53:24–32.

39 Te Braake FW, van den Akker CH, Riedijk MA, van Goudoever JB: Parenteral amino acid and energy administration to premature infants in early life. Semin Fetal Neonatal Med 2007;12:11–18.

40 Clark RH, Chace DH, Spitzer AR: Pediatrix Amino Acid Study G. Effects of two different doses of amino acid supplementation on growth and blood amino acid levels in premature neonates admitted to the neonatal intensive care unit: a randomized, controlled trial. Pediatrics 2007;120:1286–1296.

41 Senterre T, Rigo J: Optimizing early nutritional support based on recent recommendations in VLBW infants and postnatal growth restriction. J Pediatr Gastroenterol Nutr 2011;53:536–542.

42 Drenckpohl D, McConnell C, Gaffney S, Niehaus M, Macwan KS: Randomized trial of very low birth weight infants receiving higher rates of infusion of intravenous fat emulsions during the first week of life. Pediatrics 2008;122:743–751.

43 Krohn K, Koletzko B: Parenteral lipid emulsions in paediatrics. Curr Opin Clin Nutr Metab Care 2006;9:319–323.

44 Deshpande G, Simmer K: Lipids for parenteral nutrition in neonates. Curr Opin Clin Nutr Metab Care 2011;14:145–150.

45 Deshpande GC, Simmer K, Mori T, Croft K: Parenteral lipid emulsions based on olive oil compared with soybean oil in preterm (<28 weeks' gestation) neonates: a randomised controlled trial. J Pediatr Gastroenterol Nutr 2009;49:619–625.

46 Rayyan M, Devlieger H, Jochum F, Allegaert K: Short-term use of parenteral nutrition with a lipid emulsion containing a mixture of soybean oil, olive oil, medium-chain triglycerides, and fish oil: a randomized double-blind study in preterm infants. JPEN J Parenter Enteral Nutr 2012;36:81S–94S.

47 Gura KM, Lee S, Valim C, et al: Safety and efficacy of a fish-oil based fat emulsion in the treatment of parenteral nutrition-associated liver disease. Pediatrics 2008;121:e678–e686.

48 Koletzko B, Goulet O: Fish oil containing intravenous lipid emulsions in parenteral nutrition-associated cholestatic liver disease. Curr Opin Clin Nutr Metab Care 2010;13:321–326.

49 Mahaveer A, Grime C, Morgan C: Increasing early protein intake is associated with a reduction in insulin-treated hyperglycemia in very preterm infants. Nutr Clin Pract 2012;27:399–405.

50 Beardsall K, Vanhaesebrouck S, Ogilvy-Stuart AL, et al: Early insulin therapy in very-low-birth-weight infants. N Engl J Med 2008;359:1873–1884.

51 Lawrence A, Trissel F: Handbook on Injectable Drugs, ed 17. Bethesda, American Society of Health-System Pharmacists, 2013.

52 Bethune K, Allwood M, Grainger C, Wormleighton C: Use of filters during the preparation and administration of parenteral nutrition: position paper and guidelines prepared by a British pharmaceutical nutrition group working party. Nutrition 2001;17:403–408.

53 Van Den Hoogen A, Krediet TG, Uiterwaal CSPM, Bolenius JFGA, Gerards LJ, Fleer A: In-line filters in central venous catheters in a neonatal intensive care unit. J Perinat Med 2006;34:71–74.

54 Chessex P, Friel J, Harrison A, Rouleau T, Lavoie JC: The mode of delivery of parenteral multivitamins influences nutrient handling in an animal model of total parenteral nutrition. Clin Nutr 2005;24:281–287.

55 Chessex P, Laborie S, Lavoie JC, Rouleau T: Photoprotection of solutions of parenteral nutrition decreases the infused load as well as the urinary excretion of peroxides in premature infants. Semin Perinatol 2001;25:55–59.

56 Chessex P, Lavoie JC, Rouleau T, et al: Photooxidation of parenteral multivitamins induces hepatic steatosis in a neonatal guinea pig model of intravenous nutrition. Pediatr Res 2002;52:958–963.

57 Devlieger H, De Pourcq L, Casneuf A, et al: Standard two-compartment formulation for total parenteral nutrition in the neonatal intensive care unit: a fluid tolerance-based system. Clin Nutr 1993;12:282–286.

58 Petros WP, Shanke WA Jr: A standardized parenteral nutrition solution: prescribing, use, processing, and material cost implications. Hosp Pharm 1986; 21:648–649, 654–656.

59 Lenclen R, Crauste-Manciet S, Narcy P, et al: Assessment of implementation of a standardized parenteral formulation for early nutritional support of very preterm infants. Eur J Pediatr 2006;165:512–518.

60 Krohn K, Babl J, Reiter K, Koletzko B: Parenteral nutrition with standard solutions in paediatric intensive care patients. Clin Nutr 2005;24:274–280.

61 Morgan C, Herwitker S, Badhawi I, et al: SCAMP: standardised, concentrated, additional macronutrients, parenteral nutrition in very preterm infants: a phase IV randomised, controlled exploratory study of macronutrient intake, growth and other aspects of neonatal care. BMC Pediatr 2011;11:53.

62 Rigo J, Marlowe ML, Bonnot D, et al: Benefits of a new pediatric triple-chamber bag for parenteral nutrition in preterm infants. J Pediatr Gastroenterol Nutr 2012;54:210–217.

63 Mason DG, Puntis JW, McCormick K, Smith N: Parenteral nutrition for neonates and children: a mixed bag. Arch Dis Child 2011;96:209–210.

Nicholas D. Embleton, MBBS, MD, FRCPH
Newcastle Neonatal Service, Newcastle Hospitals NHS Foundation Trust
Institute of Health and Society, Newcastle University
Queen Victoria Road, Newcastle upon Tyne NE1 4LP (UK)
E-Mail Nicholas.embleton@ncl.ac.uk

Koletzko B, Poindexter B, Uauy R (eds): Nutritional Care of Preterm Infants: Scientific Basis and Practical Guidelines.
World Rev Nutr Diet. Basel, Karger, 2014, vol 110, pp 190–200 (DOI: 10.1159/000358467)

Preterm Nutrition and the Brain

Sara E. Ramel · Michael K. Georgieff

Division of Neonatology, University of Minnesota Amplatz Children's Hospital, University of Minnesota
School of Medicine, Minneapolis, Minn., USA

Reviewed by Berthold Koletzko, Dr. von Hauner Children's Hospital, University of Munich Medical Center,
Munich, Germany; Brenda Poindexter, Department of Pediatrics, James W. Riley Hospital for Children, Indiana
University, Indianapolis, Ind., USA; Ricardo Uauy, Institute of Nutrition and Food Technology INTA, Universidad
de Chile, Santiago de Chile, Chile

Abstract

The brain is the most highly metabolic organ in the preterm neonate and consumes the greatest
amount of nutrient resources for its function and growth. As preterm infants survive at greater rates,
neurodevelopment has become the primary morbidity outcome of interest. While many factors influence neurodevelopmental outcomes in preterm infants, nutrition is of particular importance because the healthcare team has a great deal of control over its provision. Studies over the past 30 years
have emphasized the negative neurodevelopmental consequences of poor nutrition and growth in
the preterm infant. While all nutrients are important for brain development, certain ones including
glucose, protein, fats (including long-chain polyunsaturated fatty acids), iron, zinc, copper, iodine,
folate and choline have particularly large roles in the preterm infant. They affect major brain processes such as neurogenesis, neuronal differentiation, myelination and synaptogenesis, all of which
are proceeding at a rapid pace between 22 and 42 weeks' post-conception. At the macronutrient
level, weight gain, linear growth (independent of weight gain) and head circumference growth are
markers of nutritional status. Each has been associated with long-term neurodevelopment. The relationship of micronutrients to neurodevelopment in preterm infants is understudied in spite of the
large effect these nutrients have in other young populations. Nutrients do not function alone to
stimulate brain development, but rather in concert with growth factors, which in turn are dependent
on adequate nutrient status (e.g. protein, zinc) as well as on physiologic status. Non-nutritional factors such as infection, corticosteroids, and inflammation alter how nutrients are accreted and distributed, and also suppress growth factor synthesis. Thus, nutritional strategies to optimize brain growth
and development include assessment of status at birth, aggressive provision of nutrients that are
critical in this time period, control of non-nutritional factors that impede brain growth and repletion
of nutrient deficits.   © 2014 S. Karger AG, Basel

The limit of viability for preterm infants has not really changed in over 30 years,
yet the rate of survival at each gestational age has grown markedly due to improvements in pre- and postnatal care. The main focus of neonatal care has thus

changed from reducing mortality to reducing long-term morbidity. Furthermore, the focus within morbidity has shifted from chronic lung disease to neurodevelopmental outcomes as evidenced by the increasing body of literature devoted to the latter. This shift has occurred for two primary reasons – improved strategies to protect the lungs and a better understanding of how to access and assess the preterm brain. The latter is leading to new strategies to enhance brain growth and development in the preterm infant with the goal of improving long-term outcomes.

A large number of factors have been shown to influence neurodevelopmental outcomes in preterm infants including gestational age, size for dates, intracranial hemorrhage, white matter damage, socioeconomic status, and infections [1]. Strategies have been implemented to try to reduce these risks (e.g. prematurity prevention), but many remain beyond the control of the neonatal care team. In contrast, nutrition is a factor that caregivers can assess and modulate. Nevertheless, achievement of optimal nutritional status to promote brain growth and neurodevelopment in preterm infants remains elusive as evidenced by the high rate of 'extrauterine growth retardation' and its attendant loss of IQ potential [2, 3]. The failure to achieve complete nutritional sufficiency in the NICU is due to a complex set of issues that include (1) lack of complete knowledge of which nutrients to prescribe (and when), (2) failure to prescribe what is known to be beneficial for fear of unintended complications (e.g. necrotizing enterocolitis), (3) failure to deliver what is prescribed (i.e. frequent disruptions of nutrient intake), and, ultimately, (4) whether critically ill infants can accrete nutrients that are provided to them and channel those nutrients toward supporting brain growth and development.

The following sections detail what is known about the effects of specific nutrients on brain development in premature infants. The information for many of the nutrients is based on fetal accretion rates with the assumption that the preterm neonate's requirements are similar to the fetus [4]. Observational studies of neurodevelopmental outcomes as a function of specific nutrient deficits in preterm infants are rare, but becoming more prevalent in the literature [5]. Prospective, randomized trials of specific nutrients with the goal of assessing neurodevelopment are exceedingly rare. Because of the paucity of controlled trials in human preterm infants, developmentally appropriate preclinical models are used to establish which nutrients demonstrate critical periods during late fetal and early neonatal brain development [for review, see 6].

Prior to discussing specific nutrients in detail, several sections will address the rapid growth and development of the preterm brain, the concept of critical periods for nutrients and the mechanisms by which nutrients modulate brain differentiation. After considering the nutrients, a final section will consider the intertwined roles of nutrients and growth factors, and the role of illness in mediating nutrient demand and utilization.

The Plasticity and Vulnerability of the Neonatal Brain

At 25 weeks' post-conceptional age (PCA), the normal human brain resembles a coffee bean; bi-lobed and smooth without sulci or gyri. By 40 weeks' PCA, it resembles a walnut; bi-lobed with extensive sulcation and gyration. Its external appearance is far more similar to an adult brain than the fetal brain after only 15 weeks. This remarkable change in external structure is paralleled by extensive internal growth and differentiation [7]. The role of the neonatologist is to provide the metabolic substrates (i.e. nutrients) that will accomplish this brain development in an extrauterine environment. The nutrients are delivered via different routes and forms than in utero. It is a testament to the brain's remarkably plasticity that brain development can progress so normally in certain NICU patients in spite of the very different circumstances surrounding its growth.

While the rapidly growing preterm brain exhibits far more plasticity than the adult brain, it is also highly vulnerable to insult. Vulnerability generally outweighs plasticity in the developing brain, implying that it is better to continue on a normal developmental trajectory than to fall off and rely on 'catch-up' mechanisms to re-establish trajectory. Prompt nutrient delivery and stabilization of neonatal physiology so that the nutrients can be optimally utilized is of paramount importance if the goal is to achieve the best neurodevelopmental outcome.

Basic Principles of Nutrients and Brain Development

The positive or negative neurodevelopmental effects that nutrients or nutrient deficits have are based on the timing and on the dose/duration of exposure [8]. This occurs because the brain is not a homogeneous organ, instead it is composed of many anatomic regions and processes (e.g. myelination) that have different developmental trajectories and critical periods [7]. Throughout development, the vulnerability of a brain region or process is based on the intersection of two factors: when a nutrient deficit occurs and whether the brain requires that nutrient at that time. Nutrient deficits can affect the anatomy of neurons by reducing proliferation (number of neurons) or differentiation (complexity of neurons). Both are determinants of ultimate neural function. Glial cells, which include oligodendrocytes, astrocytes and microglia are also nutritionally sensitive and their respective functions of myelination, nutrient delivery and neuronal trafficking can be affected by a critically timed nutrient deficiency. Deficits of protein, energy, iron, zinc and long-chain polyunsaturated fatty acids (LC-PUFAs) affect anatomy significantly [for reviews, 6, 9].

Beyond structure, nutrients also regulate neurochemistry through their effects on neurotransmitter concentrations and receptor numbers. Ultimately, neuronal function is driven by synaptic efficacy – the efficiency of the electrical activity of the brain. Nutrients that particularly affect neuroelectrophysiology and neural metabolism include glucose, protein, iron, zinc, LC-PUFAs, and choline [reviewed in 6, 9].

Table 1. Nutrients that particularly affect brain development in preterm infants

Macronutrients
    Protein*
    Specific fats (e.g. LC-PUFAs*)
    Glucose*
Micronutrients
    Iron*
    Zinc*
    Copper*
    Iodine (thyroid)*
Vitamins/co-factors
    Folate*
    Choline*
    Vitamin A
    Vitamin B_6
    Vitamin B_{12}

* Likely exhibits a critical/sensitive period for neurodevelopment between 24 and 44 weeks' post-conception based on human data or preclinical models.

While the goal of nutrition is maintenance of sufficiency or repletion of a deficit, little evidence exists that further supplementation of a nutritionally replete individual results in additional neurodevelopmental benefit. Indeed, many nutrients demonstrate a U-shaped risk curve where over-supplementation may result in damage to a developing system.

Specific Nutrients That Exhibit a Critical Period between 24 and 44 Weeks' PCA

Basically all nutrients are important for brain growth and development. However, some have particularly large effects on the brain between 24 and 44 weeks' PCA (table 1). Several of these exhibit 'critical' or 'sensitive' periods, which are defined as time frames where failure to provide a stimulus results in long-term deficits [10]. Interestingly, similar neurobehavioral sequelae result from each of these particular nutrient deficits when they occur in the neonatal period, suggesting that the common feature underlying the risk is the timing of the insult. This makes sense since many of the nutrients (e.g. glucose, iron, branched chain amino acids, zinc) support basic neuronal metabolism, which in turn regulates differentiation [11]. Brain areas that have the highest metabolic rates (and most tenuous blood supplies) will be at greatest risk from metabolic disruptions. Rapidly developing systems that are therefore at risk at the time of preterm birth include the hippocampus (which underlies learning and memory), myelin (speed of processing), and the cerebellum (balance, motor integration, cognition) [7]. Besides serving their primary purposes, these systems connect with nascent secondary systems (e.g. cortical structures). Abnormal development of the primary systems can result in improper connections being made to the secondary structures with subsequent behavioral manifestations later in life [12, 13].

Macronutrients

Postnatal Growth Failure and Neurodevelopment

Overall growth in the NICU, assessed by anthropometrics such as weight, length and head circumference for age, is a surrogate for macronutrient nutritional status. VLBW premature infants commonly exhibit growth failure, typically defined as inadequate weight for PCA [2]. VLBW preterm infants are largely dependent on parenteral nutritional supplementation in the first few days to weeks of life. During this time they accrue their most significant macronutritional deficits and fall off the greatest amount from the intrauterine growth curve [2]. This growth failure persists beyond hospital discharge, where it has been further characterized as being 'disproportionate' with reduced length/height and increased adiposity [14]. The negative effects specifically of poor weight gain on neurodevelopment are well documented and are reflected in both gray and white matter loss [3, 13] as well as poor neurodevelopmental outcomes [see figure 1 in chapter by Uauy and Koletzko, 'Defining the nutritional needs of preterm infants', pp. 4–10].

The primary determinant of weight gain in the neonate is energy intake, as carbohydrate and fat, that exceeds resting energy expenditure in a protein-sufficient environment. Carbohydrates, particularly glucose, are the main fuel source for the brain. The human has a peculiarly high brain energy demand among mammals, accounting for an estimated 50% of total body oxygen consumption.

Fats clearly play a large role in brain development since they comprise a large percentage of the brain's composition. Fats (including cholesterol) are necessary for myelin synthesis, synaptosome formation and cell membrane fluidity, all of which are crucial for efficient neural processing. A large amount of literature on the role of a specific group of fats, the LC-PUFAs, has evolved over the past 20+ years and are summarized elsewhere in this book. Fundamentally, the preterm neonate has limited capacity to synthesize the LC-PUFAs, including docosohexaenoic acid (DHA; 22:6 omega–3) and arachidonic acid (AA; 20:4 omega–6) from their respective 18 carbon precursors until at least 48 weeks post-conception and potentially beyond. Severe deficiencies of these fatty acids in preclinical models including mice, rats, and non-human primates results in hypomyelination with an altered fatty acid profile in the myelin component accompanied by abnormal behavioral [15, 16]. The literature on LC-PUFA supplementation has focused primarily on formula-fed preterm infants although some studies have assessed supplementation of human milk. Two major outcome domains have been assessed: visual processing and mental development.

Ramel · Georgieff

The most recent Cochrane review on the subject [17] concluded that studies of cognitive and visual outcomes in studies comparing infants consuming cow milk-based preterm formula with LC-PUFAs to those consuming unsupplemented formula have been mixed. In general, there may be short-term positive changes in neural processing that have not been demonstrated to be sustained beyond infancy. The reviews suggest that the studies are underpowered to draw conclusions about long-term efficacy. The findings may be significantly confounded by the highly variable gestational age and health of the infants, and the wide range of sources and doses utilized.

Protein is not only important as structural scaffolding for the brain, but also as a building block for signaling molecules such as growth factors and neurotransmitters which are also influential in cognition. At the cellular level, branched chain amino acids regulate the mTOR-signaling pathway, which in turn determines neuronal complexity by regulating protein translation and actin polymerization rates [11]. Animal models have shown that protein deficit is associated with decreased synapse numbers and myelination [reviewed in 6].

More recent attention has specifically focused on protein accretion/linear growth failure and its potential independent effect on brain development and neonatal outcome. The emphasis stems from the finding that FFM and linear growth index protein accretion and closely reflects brain structural growth. First year linear growth, independent of weight gain, influences later cognitive and language development in preterm and term infants [18, 19]. FFM accretion in the NICU increases speed of processing at 4 months' corrected age in infants born prematurely [20].

Concern for protein toxicity, which in turn limits early administration, stems from studies in the early 1970s showing metabolic acidosis, uremia, growth restriction and worse developmental outcomes in low birth weight infants receiving protein supplementation. However, recent research has shown these concerns to be unfounded as long as high-quality protein at levels much less than reported in these previous studies are utilized [21]. Follow-up studies are now consistently revealing improved head/brain growth and cognitive development in those infants receiving improved amounts of protein supplementation [21–23]. Each 1 g/kg/day increase in protein intake in the first week of life results in an 8.2-point increase in the Mental Development Index at 18 months' corrected age [22]. These improvements are long-lasting. Preterm infants randomized to higher protein and energy intakes during the first few weeks of life have increased brain volume, specifically of the caudate nucleus, as well as improved cognitive scores when imaged and tested as adolescents [23].

Micronutrients and Vitamins

The roles of micronutrients and vitamins in preterm newborn brain development are largely understudied compared to the macronutrients. This is unfortunate because strong epidemiologic data in humans and basic science data in preclinical models emphasize the importance of these factors in normal brain development during the late fetal and early neonatal period [6]. Moreover, deficiencies of iron, copper, iodine and zinc are exceedingly common worldwide, affect mostly women of child-bearing age or young infants, and have an estimated cumulative effect of –10 IQ points [24].

Dosing of these micronutrients to preterm infants in the NICU is based on fetal accretion data, but monitoring of their status is rare. It is unclear how many preterm infants are born with compromised stores of these nutrients or what the effect of nutrient provision in the NICU does to their total body, much less brain micronutrient status.

Iron

Iron is the best studied of the micronutrients in preterm infants. Iron is a critical nutrient for the developing fetal and neonatal brain [25]. Iron-containing enzymes and hemoproteins are involved in important cellular processes in the developing brain including myelination, neuronal and glial energy status, monoamine neurotransmitter homeostasis, and thyroid status. Studies in term infants and preclinical models demonstrate a significant impact of perinatal iron deficiency acutely during the period of deficiency and long-term after iron repletion. These behaviors include learning and memory, speed of processing and socioemotional regulation [25].

The neurodevelopmental roles of iron in preterm infants include effects on general cognition and speed of neural processing. Early iron supplementation of preterm infants results in a higher mental processing composite score at 5.3 years [26]. Preterm infants born with cord ferritin concentrations in the lowest quartile (<76 µg/l) have slower central nerve conduction velocities on auditory brainstem-evoked responses [5].

Zinc

Zinc has a major role in the developing brain by regulating neurotransmission in the hippocampus, rates of DNA, RNA and protein synthesis throughout the brain and IGF-1 gene expression [27, 28]. IGF-1 expression, in turn, regulates metabolic activity of neurons through the mTOR-signaling pathway [11]. Clinical studies and preclinical models suggest that zinc sufficiency between 24 and 40 weeks' PCA is important for the proper development and function of the hippocampus, cerebellum and autonomic nervous systems [reviewed in 6].

To date, no studies of neurodevelopmental outcomes of preterm infants as a function of zinc status at birth or in the NICU have been published.

Copper

The role of copper in perinatal brain biology intersects with that of iron. Copper's primary effects in the brain include regulating dopamine monooxygenase activity and scavenging reactive oxygen species through Cu-Zn superoxide dismutase. Beyond this, it regulates iron transport at the blood-brain barrier through donation of

Ramel · Georgieff

a proton from a multi-copper oxidase to convert ferrous iron to its transportable ferric form. Copper deficiency leads to brain iron deficiency with its attendant sequelae. Thus, copper deficiency alters brain dopamine and cytochrome c status, particularly in highly metabolic areas. In the late fetal and early neonatal period, these areas include the hippocampus and the cerebellum. Developmentally appropriately timed preclinical rodent models confirm behavioral effects on learning/memory and balance [29].

Human populations at risk include young pregnant women (with their own growth needs). Preterm infants and growth-restricted infants are born with low stores relative to the term infant (and have faster growth rates and thus higher requirements) [28]. As with zinc, no studies have isolated the role of copper status on neurodevelopmental function or outcome in preterm infants.

Iodine

The sole requirement of iodine for brain development is in the synthesis of thyroid hormone. Thus, iodine deficiency leads to a state of hypothyroidism, which in turn results in lower brain weight and DNA content, reduced neuronal dendritic arborization and synaptogenesis and hypomyelination. Third-trimester fetal iodine deficiency can result in global cognitive deficits [for review, see 30]. In spite of the known importance of iodine for fetal brain development, no studies of neurodevelopment in preterm infants as a function of their neonatal iodine status have been published.

Folate

Folic acid is a co-factor in numerous enzyme pathways in the brain. Its importance during the periconceptional period to prevent neural tube defects is clear. However, folate remains important throughout the fetal period [31], first enhancing neuronal proliferation and migration from 6–24 weeks' PCA and then regional brain differentiation in the third trimester. The hippocampus appears to be particularly targeted in the latter time frame. Premature infants are at risk for folate deficiency because of immature enzyme systems. Folate deficiency in early infancy results in primarily motor deficits. Some cognitive effects have been suspected, consistent with effects on hippocampal structure and function. In spite of this evidence, no neurodevelopmental outcome studies of preterm infants as a function of folate status have been reported.

Choline

Choline is an intriguing nutrient because it participates in critical brain processes during neurodevelopment including neurotransmitter synthesis (acetylcholine), myelin synthesis (phosphotidylcholine) and epigenetic modification of chromatin (as a methyl donor). Intriguing studies of pre- and postnatal supplementation of normal rodents and models of pathologic conditions (e.g. fetal alcohol syndrome, Rett's syndrome, Downs' syndrome) demonstrate a potent effect on improving hippocampal development and subsequent learning and memory behavior [for review, see 32]. Clinical trials of choline supplementation in humans are now ongoing. If results from the preclinical trials translate into benefits for humans, choline may be an important nutritional adjunct in the NICU, since the developmental equivalent of the last trimester appears to be an important time for brain choline accretion.

Beyond Nutrients: The Role of Growth Factors in Brain Development

The temptation in nutritional therapy is to consider only 'supply side' economics. However, adequate supply of nutrients, essentially providing the 'fuel', is only part of the process of achieving brain growth and differentiation. Growth factors are key in translating nutritional fuel into growth, complex structure and function through a number of signaling pathways including mTOR [11]. Without growth factors, neuronal cells will not differentiate in spite of adequate nutrient supply and conversely, without nutrients, growth factors cannot mediate growth. Growth factors found in the late fetal and newborn brain include general ones such as IGF-1 and more brain-specific ones such as brain-derived neurotrophic factor. Growth factor production can be inhibited by a lack of a specific critical nutrient (e.g. zinc for IGF-1) or by non-nutritional factors. Activation of pro-inflammatory cytokines, a common occurrence during episodes of sepsis and NEC in preterm infants, suppresses synthesis of growth factors, including IGF-1, which is important for brain growth and differentiation [33].

Non-Nutritional Factors That Affect Nutrient Status and Brain Development

As with growth factors, certain nutrients are highly affected by the physiologic state of the infant. Infection, and specifically the activation of hepcidin by IL-6 generated during the infectious state, reduces iron absorption and sequesters already absorbed iron in macrophages, rendering it unavailable for erythropoiesis (i.e. the anemia of inflammation). This lack of iron availability likely also affects delivery to the developing brain. Similarly, during sepsis, surgery or any catabolic state, amino acids are diverted for gluconeogenesis and are not as available for building tissue (including brain). Moreover, the availability of certain (branch chained) amino acids are critical in regulating signaling pathways (e.g. mTOR) that determine rates of actin polymerization and tubulin construction in the neurons. Ultimately, states of chronic inflammation (e.g. infection, BPD) will potentially reduce brain growth and development with consequences for behavioral outcome (see section on linear growth above) [18]. The solution is not likely to reside in supplying more nutrients. Instead, a non-nutrient solution (e.g. controlling infections, reducing severity of BPD), may result in better brain growth and development.

Ramel · Georgieff

Conclusion

Nutritional management represents an important opportunity to improve developmental outcomes in preterm infants because it is a relatively controllable factor in the neonatologist's armamentarium. Certain nutrients have a high impact on brain development between 24 and 44 weeks' PCA. Thus, nutritional support should focus on preventing disruption of the provision of these critical nutrients, assessment of their status and correction of their deficit as soon as possible.

References

1 Allen MC: Outcomes after brain injury in the preterm infant; in Shevell M, Miller S (eds): Acquired Brain Injury in the Fetus and Newborn. London, Mac Keith Press, 2012, pp 99–120.
2 Ehrenkranz RA, Younes N, Lemons JA, Fanaroff AA, Donovan EF, Wright LL, et al: Longitudinal growth of hospitalized very low birth weight infants. Pediatrics 1999;104:280–289.
3 Ehrenkranz RA, Dusick AM, Vohr BR, Wright LL, Wrage LA, Poole WK: Growth in the neonatal intensive care unit influences neurodevelopmental and growth outcomes of extremely low birth weight infants. Pediatrics 2006;117:1253–1261.
4 Ziegler EE, O'Donnell AM, Nelson Se, Fomon SJ: Body composition of the reference fetus. Growth 1976;40:329–341.
5 Amin SB, Orlando M, Eddins A, MacDonald M, Monczynski C, Wang H: In utero iron status and auditory neural maturation in premature infants as evaluated by brainstem response. J Pediatr 2010;156: 377–381.
6 Fuglestad A, Rao R, Georgieff MK: The role of nutrition in cognitive development; in Handbook in Developmental Cognitive Neuroscience, ed 2. Cambridge/MA, MIT Press, 2008, pp 623–641.
7 Thompson RA, Nelson CA: Developmental science and the media. Early brain development. Am Psychol 2001;56:5–15.
8 Kretchmer N, Beard JL, Carlson S: The role of nutrition in the development of normal cognition. Am J Clin Nutr 1996;63:997S–1001S.
9 Georgieff MK: Nutrition and the developing brain: nutrient priorities and management. Am J Clin Nutr 2007;85:614S–620S.
10 Hensch TK: Critical period regulation. Annu Rev Neurosci 2004;27:549–579.
11 Wullschleger S, Loewith R, Hall MN: TOR signaling in growth and metabolism. Cell 2006;124:471–484.

12 Luciana M, Lindeke L, Georgieff MK, Mills MM, Nelson CA: Neurobehavioral evidence for working memory deficits in school-aged children with histories of neonatal intensive care treatment. Dev Med Child Neurol 1999;41:521–533.
13 Huppi PS: Cortical development in the fetus and the newborn: advanced MR techniques. Top Magn Reson Imaging 2011;22:33–38.
14 Johnson MJ, Wootton SA, Leaf AA, Jackson AA: Preterm birth and body composition at term equivalent age: a systematic review and meta-analysis. Pediatrics 2012;130:E640–E649.
15 Neuringer M, Connor WE, Lin DS, Barstad L, Luck S: Biochemical and functional effects of prenatal and postnatal omega–3 fatty acid deficiency on retina and brain in rhesus monkeys. Proc Natl Acad Sci USA 1986;83:4021–4025.
16 Carlson SE: Early determinants of development: a lipid perspective. Am J Clin Nutr 2009;89:1523S–1529S.
17 Schulzke SM, Patole SK, Simmer K: Long-chain polyunsaturated fatty acid supplementation in preterm infants. Cochrane Database Syst Rev 2011;2: CD000375.
18 Ramel SE, Demerath E, Gray H, Younge N, Boys C, Georgieff M: The relationship of poor linear growth velocity with neonatal illness and two-year neurodevelopment in preterm infants. Neonatology 2012; 102:19–24.
19 Pongcharoen T, Ramakrishnan U, DiGirolamo AM, Winichagoon P, Flores R, Singkhornard J, Martorell R: Influence of prenatal and postnatal growth on intellectual functioning in school-aged children. Arch Pediatr Adolesc Med 2012;166:411–416.
20 Pfister KM, Gray HL, Miller NC, Demerath EW, Georgieff MK, Ramel SE: Exploratory study of the relationship of fat-free mass to speed of brain processing in preterm infants. Pediatr Res 2013;74:576–583.

21 Poindexter BB, Langer JC, Dusick AM, Ehrenkranz RA; National Institute of Child Health and Human Development Neonatal Research Network: Early provision of parenteral amino acids in extremely low birth weight infants: relation to growth and neurodevelopmental outcome. J Pediatr 2006;148:300–305.

22 Stephens BE, Walden RV, Gargus RA, Tucker R, McKinley L, Mance M, et al: First-week protein and energy intakes are associated with 18-month developmental outcomes in extremely low birth weight infants. Pediatrics 2009;123:1337–1343.

23 Isaacs EB, Gadian DG, Sabatini S, et al: The effect of early human diet on caudate volumes and IQ. Pediatr Res 2008;63:308–314.

24 Walker SP, Wachs TD, Grantham-McGregor S, Black MM, Nelson CA, Huffman SL, et al: Inequality in early childhood: risk and protective factors for early child development. Lancet 2011;378:1325–1338.

25 Lozoff B, Georgieff MK: Iron deficiency and brain development. Semin Pediatr Neurol 2006;13:158–165.

26 Steinmacher J, Pohlandt F, Bode H, Sander S, Kron M, Franz AR: Randomized trial of early versus late iron supplementation in infants with a birth weight of less than 1,301 grams: neurocognitive development at 5.3 years corrected age. Pediatrics 2007;120:538–546.

27 Gower-Winter SSD, Levenson CW: Zinc in the central nervous system: from molecules to behavior. Biofactors 2012;38:186–193.

28 Sandstead HH: Zinc: essentiality for brain development. Nutr Rev 1985;43:129–137.

29 Prohaska JR: Copper; in Erdman JW, Macdonald IA, Zeisel SH (eds): Present Knowledge in Nutrition, ed 10. Oxford, Wiley, 2012, pp 540–553.

30 Zimmerman MB: The effects of iodine deficiency in pregnancy and infancy. Paediatr Perinat Epidemiol 2012;26(suppl 1):108–117.

31 Craciunescu CN, Brown EC, Mar MH, Albright CD, Nadeau MR, Zeisel SH: Folic acid deficiency during late gestation decreases progenitor cell proliferation and increases apoptosis in fetal mouse brain. J Nutr 2004;134:162–166.

32 Zeisel SH: Diet-gene interactions underlie metabolic individuality and influence brain development: implications for clinical practice derived from studies on choline metabolism. Ann Nutr Metab 2012;60(suppl 3):19–25.

33 Hansen-Pupp I, Hellstrom-Westas L, Cilio CM, Andersson S, Fellman V, Ley D: Inflammation at birth and the insulin-like growth factor system in very preterm infants. Acta Paediatr 2007;96:830–836.

Michael K. Georgieff, MD
Division of Neonatology, Department of Pediatrics
2450 Riverside Avenue, East Building MB-630
Minneapolis, MN 55454 (USA)
E-Mail georg001@umn.edu

Ramel · Georgieff

Koletzko B, Poindexter B, Uauy R (eds): Nutritional Care of Preterm Infants: Scientific Basis and Practical Guidelines.
World Rev Nutr Diet. Basel, Karger, 2014, vol 110, pp 201–214 (DOI: 10.1159/000358468)

Practice of Enteral Nutrition in Very Low Birth Weight and Extremely Low Birth Weight Infants

Thibault Senterre

Department of Neonatology, University of Liège, CHU de Liège, CHR de la Citadelle, Liège, Belgium

Reviewed by Christoph Fusch, Department of Pediatrics, McMaster University, Hamilton, Ont., Canada;
Johannes B. van Goudoever, Department of Pediatrics, Free University Medical Center, Amsterdam,
The Netherlands

Abstract

The perinatal period is critical for human development. The brain of very low birth weight (VLBW, <1,500 g) infants is particularly vulnerable to undernutrition. Enteral nutrition is of major importance for the growth and the development of the gastrointestinal tract, which depends on the amount and composition of feeds. Feeding intolerance and the risk of necrotizing enterocolitis (NEC) are key concerns with enteral nutrition in VLBW infants. Controversies exist on how to feed VLBW infants during the first weeks of life, particularly in extremely low birth weight (ELBW, <1,000 g) infants. Unreasonable concerns lead to iatrogenic malnutrition, gastrointestinal atrophy, and parenteral nutrition-related complications. Many studies in the field of nutrition during the past decade demonstrated that some feeding regimens have significant benefits. There is strong evidence that the use of human milk (HM) reduces the risk of NEC and provides major advantages in VLBW infants. The feeding of fortified HM should be promoted and HM banking should be further developed to allow access to pasteurized donor HM for VLBW infants with an insufficient intake of their own mother's milk. Early enteral feeding should be promoted soon after birth to enhance gastrointestinal maturation, growth and functional development. Continuous- or short-interval intermittent feeding seems to provide better gastrointestinal tolerance and faster achievement of full enteral feeding. Feeding advancements of 20–30 ml/kg/day in VLBW infants ≥1,000 g and of 15–25 ml/kg/day in ELBW infants are reasonable strategies. Any suspicion of feeding intolerance implies short-interval evaluation to decide whether interruption of enteral feeding or its restart after a transient interruption are appropriate. One should always strive for maintaining at least minimal enteral feeding, rather than complete interruption of enteral feeding.   © 2014 S. Karger AG, Basel

The objective of postnatal nutrition in very low birth weight (VLBW, <1,500 g) infants is to achieve a postnatal growth that is similar to fetal growth and coupled with adequate long-term developmental outcomes [1]. Unfortunately, postnatal growth restriction (PNGR) is frequently observed in many VLBW infants in neonatal intensive care units (NICUs) during the first few weeks and months of life [2, 3]. PNGR is mainly due to insufficient nutritional intakes during postnatal hospitalization [4–6]. The perinatal period corresponds to a highly critical window of development in which undernutrition can have a permanent effect throughout life, and especially on the developing brain. The correlation between poor postnatal nutrition, PNGR, and later adverse developmental outcomes has been widely documented in premature infants [5–10].

Enteral nutrition in VLBW is challenging, especially in extremely low birth weight (ELBW, <1,000 g) infants [11, 12]. Suspected feeding intolerance and the potential risk of necrotizing enterocolitis (NEC) are common problems encountered in NICUs. These fears frequently lead to delayed introduction of enteral feeding, slow advancement of feeds, and insufficient nutritional intakes. The poor use of the gastrointestinal (GI) tract increases the need for parenteral nutrition (PN) and associated complications like sepsis, thrombosis, liver failure and inflammatory diseases [13, 14]. It also induces GI mucosal atrophy with insufficient protective mucus, increased permeability, decreased regenerative capabilities, and, finally, GI dysfunction and increased risk of feeding intolerance and NEC [15, 16].

NEC is a major postnatal complication that typically occurs in 5% of VLBW infants, but its incidence may sometimes be as high as up to 15%. NEC is associated with increased mortality and later neurodevelopmental disabilities and is discussed in another chapter of this book [see Neu, pp. 253–263]. GI tract maturation is essential to allow adequate postnatal transition from placental nutrition via the umbilical cord to enteral nutrition via the gut. Many studies have demonstrated the crucial role of enteral feeding for normal GI development [15, 16]. Postnatal enteral nutrition is essential to promote GI growth and development by providing nutrients to the mucosal epithelial cells, stimulating the secretion of local growth factors and GI hormones, and activating GI neural pathways [15, 16].

Several feeding regimens have been developed for VLBW infants. Practices are often determined by local knowledge, experiences and traditions [11, 12]. Enteral feeding practices significantly influence the incidence of NEC and the maturation of the GI tract. The exclusive use of human milk (HM) and the standardization of feeding practices may significantly improve feeding tolerance and reduce the incidence of NEC in VLBW infants [17–19]. Optimized feeding regimens can also improve postnatal growth and neurodevelopment up to adolescence [8, 9]. This chapter discusses the main issues concerning the provision of optimized enteral feeding support in VLBW infants.

Human Milk

A detailed review on the use of HM in VLBW infants and on its varying composition are presented in another chapter of this book [see Ziegler, pp. 215–227]. HM is considered as the standard for the nutrition of healthy infants born at term. HM provides many bioactive factors that can contribute to improving growth and development. There are many advantages in feeding VLBW infants with HM for both short- and long-term outcomes [20, 21]. The benefits on the infant's immunity and host defenses are well recognized. The use of HM in premature infants has been reported to decrease the incidence of late-onset sepsis, NEC, and hospital readmission for illnesses after discharge. HM also improves feeding tolerance and decreases the need for PN. It is also associated with an improvement of mother infant bonding, a reduction of the severity of retinopathy of prematurity, higher long-term neurodevelopmental scores, and lower risk to develop later metabolic syndrome [20, 21]. Some concerns exist about administrating HM to VLBW infants from cytomegalovirus seropositive mothers due to the risk of postnatal infection [22]. However, as HM-acquired cytomegalovirus disease is not frequent and because few long-term neurodevelopmental sequelae have been reported, several authors consider that the value of routinely feeding fresh HM to preterm infants may outweigh the risks of postnatal infection [20].

HM is the recommended source of nutrients for VLBW infants [1, 20, 23]. Providing information and encouragement to parents is essential to promote breastfeeding in perinatology. However, due to many conditions associated with preterm delivery, mothers frequently encounter some difficulties in initiating lactation. They should be informed about all the advantages of breastfeeding and be encouraged to express breast milk. After initial manual milk expressions during the first days after delivery, a double electric breast pump appears preferable. Even small amounts of colostrum are useful. Lactation will progressively improve after several days of stimulation. Nurses and neonatologists should regularly evaluate maternal efforts and encourage the mother to achieve an adequate breast milk collection within 1 week after delivery. Skin to skin contacts, daily encouragements and treatment with domperidone may be additionally useful tools to increase lactation in mother of VLBW infants [20, 21, 24].

Donor Human Milk

The existence of wet nurses exists for many centuries, but the necessity for pediatric hospitals to have access to donor HM has become apparent more recently. There are several rules and guidelines that determine how donor HM should be collected, screened, stored, and dispensed to newborns [25, 26]. Donors are screened to avoid the risk of infection (HIV, CMV, hepatitis, syphilis) or toxic contamination (medicines, drugs, alcohol, tobacco). Donor HM is also checked microbiologically and pasteurized to avoid any bacterial or viral contamination. Holder pasteurization (62.5°C for 30 min) provides microbiological safety but alters the nutritional and biological quality of donor HM compared to fresh mother's breast milk [27, 28]. Some new techniques of heat treatment of HM are under investigation to improve the bioactivity of pasteurized HM components while maintaining the safety concerns of donor HM [27, 28]. Several systematic reviews have demonstrated the important advantages to use donor HM instead of formula in VLBW infants, particularly to reduce the incidence of NEC [29–31]. Therefore, when own mother's breast milk is not available for VLBW infants, pasteurized donor HM is a good alternative [20, 29–31].

Human Milk Fortification

Despite higher protein and energy content, HM nutrients content of mothers who delivered prematurely does allow providing the high nutritional requirements of VLBW infants, especially for protein, phosphorus and calcium (see Appendix). This leads to insufficient rate of growth, osteopenia and several nutritional deficits [32, 33]. Different kind of nutritional supplements may be used in VLBW infants and several standardized multicomponent HM fortifiers (HMF) have been commercialized [see Appendix and chapter by Ziegler, pp. 215–227]. A systematic review demonstrated that multicomponent HMF significantly improves postnatal weight gain, linear growth and head growth [32].

Recent studies still documented that many infants fed with standardized fortification of HM still suffered from PNGR [33, 34]. It seems that this phenomenon is mainly due to insufficient protein and energy intakes [4, 33]. Indeed, protein and energy intakes are the major driving force of growth. The protein intake from HM is frequently overestimated in clinical practices, especially when using donor HM, and the addition of HMF frequently does not allow reaching recommended protein intakes in VLBW infants [see Ziegler, pp. 215–227; 300] (see Appendix). Additionally, the processes of collection, storage and administration of HM are associated with a decrease in fat content that also reduces energy content [35]. HM analyzers may be helpful to optimize HM fortification [35, 36]. Adapted HM supplements can be added according to each infant's needs after measuring the macro- and micronutrient content in HM before administration. Such individualized fortification of HM significantly improves weight gain in VLBW infants [36]. In the absence of milk analyzers, fortification can also be adjusted to the blood urea nitrogen (BUN) concentration (target between 3.2 and 5 mmol/l) which is an intermediate marker of the adequacy of protein supply [32, 33]. However, this adjustment does not completely prevent some nutritional deficit since it is performed a posteriori.

The addition of HMF increases HM osmolarity and some concerns were raised a long time ago about a potential relationship between milk hyperosmolarity and risk of NEC [37, 38]. However, systematic reviews were not able to demonstrate any significant adverse effects with the use of HMF [32, 39]. Additionally, a recent review has demonstrated that there is no evidence to support an association between hyperosmolar feeds and intestinal injury or NEC in VLBW infants [40]. Therefore, the benefits of HMF clearly outweigh potential risks in VLBW infants and HMF should no more be introduced lately as usually reported [11]. Even if there is still some concern about when to introduce HMF, it is well recognized that adequate fortification must be performed when enteral feeding with HM has reached 100 ml/kg/day. Recently, Senterre and Rigo [41] have reported that introduction of HMF when enteral feeding exceeds 50 ml/kg/day allows to improve nutritional intakes and to improve postnatal growth. In another recent study, immediate use of HMF with the first feeds in very premature infants was well tolerated and was associated with lower incidence of elevated alkaline phosphate levels [42].

Preterm Infant Formula

Despite the significant evidence for using HM in VLBW infants, many NICUs still do not have access to HM bank and donor HM [11]. Specifically adapted formula for preterm infants (preterm formula) are available with a composition that allows to approach meeting the nutrient needs of VLBW infants [1, 23] (see Appendix).

Initiation of Enteral Nutrition

The practice of delaying introduction of enteral feeds is frequently observed in VLBW infants due to GI immaturity and fear of NEC. Among other reasons reported to delay early enteral feeding, most neonatologists report significant perinatal asphyxia with lactic acidosis and multiorgan involvement, clinically significant patent ductus arteriosus requiring indomethacin or ibuprofen therapy, the presence of umbilical arterial catheter, and postnatal hemodynamic instability requiring inotrope medications [11, 12]. However, there is little or no evidence that withholding feeding in these situations decreases NEC or improves other outcomes [17, 43–45].

The absence of enteral feeding leads to GI mucosal atrophy and dysfunction [15, 16]. A study in piglets has suggested that an enteral intake of at least 40% of the total nutrient needs is necessary to maintain normal GI growth [46]. Therefore, unreasonable fear of GI intolerance and NEC leading to delayed introduction of enteral feeding may be considered as deleterious because it leads to GI mucosal atrophy and dysfunction, and therefore to potential iatrogenic GI diseases like NEC and nosocomial sepsis as a consequence of increased bacterial translocation [19, 47]. A recent systematic review in VLBW infants has demonstrated that there is no evidence that delaying enteral feeding after 4 days of life reduces the risk of NEC in VLBW infants [48]. This study also demonstrated that delaying introduction of enteral feeding significantly increases the time to establish full enteral feeding and therefore PN needs and PN-associated morbidities [48].

Minimal enteral feeding (MEF) represents the administration of small feeds, ≤24 ml/kg/day, during a prolonged period of time to promote postnatal GI maturation and to reduce mucosal atrophy [15, 16]. It is also called 'trophic feeding' or 'gut priming'. Compared to MEF during the first week of life, delayed enteral feeding has been associated with lower energy intakes, lower weight gain, lower head growth, higher nonconjugated hyperbilirubinemia, more episodes of nosocomial sepsis, longer needs for PN, more metabolic disturbances, later full enteral feeding achievement, more cholestasis, increased oxygen needs, more metabolic bone disease, and later discharge, without any advantages for VLBW infants [13, 49–51]. Recently, a systematic review demonstrated that early MEF beginning before 4 days of life in VLBW infants does not increase the risk of severe GI diseases like NEC [52]. Moreover, some authors have suggested that early enteral feeding with HM may be protective against NEC [19].

Feeding Administration

Due to neurological immaturity, oral feeding is generally delayed in premature infants, and VLBW infants require a prolonged period of tube feeding after birth. Feeding policies and the modes of feeds delivery vary greatly among NICUs [11]. A feeding tube may be inserted in the stomach before each feed or left in place. Leaving the feeding tube in the stomach may favor gastroesophageal reflux but in-and-out movements may induce vagal stimulation and apnea. In VLBW infants, small feeding tubes are usually inserted either via the nostril (nasogastric tube) or via the mouth (orogastric tube). Nasogastric tubes are easier to secure while orogastric tube are more easily displaced by the movements of the tongue. On the other hand, nasogastric tubes may increase work of breathing and the energy expenditure by partially obstructing nasal airways [53, 54]. A systematic review has compared nasal and oral route for placing feeding tube in premature infants but insufficient data were available to recommend a specific practice [53]. A recent study in very premature infants could not confirm an advantage of one of the two routes with respect to the incidence of bradycardia and desaturation [54].

Positioning the feeding tube in the duodenum or jejunum by transpyloric tube placement is an approach that might theoretically reduce the complications associated with gastroesophageal reflux. However, a systematic review has demonstrated that transpyloric tube feeding in preterm infants may be associated with greater incidence of GI disturbances and increased mortality [55]. This may be explained by the fact that transpyloric tube feeding bypasses the gastric phase of digestion and it also does not allow the destruction of feeding bacteria by the acidity of gastric secretions [55].

The accurate position of a feeding tube in the stomach and the length of the inserted tube are generally guided by the measure of the distances from the nose to the ear lobe and from there to the xyphoid appendix, by the appearance of feeding tube aspirates, and by auscultation of insufflated air in the stomach. Inadequate positioning may lead to potential complications like gastroesophageal reflux, lung aspiration, and gastroesophageal mucosal injury. Radiograph is the gold standard to identify correct feeding tube position but ultrasound may also be used. Few studies have evaluated the incidence of complications associated with inadequate tube position, but a recent study in neonates has estimated that nearly 60% of tube placements may be inadequately positioned [56].

The 'conventional' tube feeding method consists of delivering intermittent bolus gavage by gravity over 10–30 min every 2 or 3 h [57]. A recent retrospective study has suggested that short-interval feeding every 2 h improves feeding tolerance and decreases the time to reach full enteral feeding compared to a 3 h feeding interval [58]. Newborns have a very small gastric capacity, therefore large feeding volume may be stressful and favor gastroesophageal reflux [59]. Continuous feeding is also used in VLBW infants to reduce gastroesophageal reflux, to reduce energy expenditure, to improve postnatal GI maturation, and to improve feeding tolerance. Continuous feeding may accelerate the achievement of full enteral feeding and may also improve linear growth, especially in ELBW infants [19]. Short-interval feeding methods are also used in many NICUs, e.g. 1-hourly intermittent gavage and slow intermittent gavage over 1 or 2 h [11]. In a recent systematic review comparing continuous versus intermittent bolus feeding in VLBW infants, there was no difference in time to achieve full oral feeds, postnatal growth, hospitalization duration, and incidence of NEC [60]. However, despite clear evidence, the authors suggested that continuous feeding may be beneficial in <1,250 g infants, with improved weight gain and earlier discharge [60].

Enteral Nutrition Advancement

A variety of enteral nutrition regimens are described in the literature [11, 12]. Depending on body weight and clinical conditions, feeds are generally progressively advanced by 10–35 ml/kg/day. The major reported criteria to evaluate the adequacy of feeding regimens are time to achieve full enteral feeding, postnatal growth, and postnatal morbidities like NEC. Some studies have suggested that slow feeds advancement might be protective for NEC in VLBW infants [61, 62]. However, this has not been confirmed and slow advancement of feeds implies a greater need for PN, increases PN-associated complications like bloodstream infections and length of stay hospital stay [14, 63]. Additionally, fear of GI intolerance and slow feeds advancement leads to frequent feeding interruption, malnutrition, poor growth and adverse long-term outcomes [7, 47]. A recent systematic review has demonstrated that slow feeds advancement (<24 ml/kg/day) does not reduce the incidence of NEC in VLBW infants, compared to faster rates between 25 and 35 ml/kg/day [64]. This study also confirmed that a faster increase of feeds is associated with a shorter time to achieve full enteral feeding and to regain birth weight [64].

Feeding Tolerance

Feeding intolerance in VLBW infants is not well defined. Abdominal distension is frequently observed during non-invasive ventilation, and antegrade peristalsis with bilious aspirates is also commonly described during the first week of life in VLBW infants

[65]. In certain circumstances, feeding intolerance may be obvious when severe GI manifestations are identified (emesis, vomiting, severe abdominal distension, ileus with visible intestinal loops, blood in the stools) or when GI manifestations are associated with systemic symptoms like apnea, bradycardia, poor perfusion, and/or hemodynamic instabilities. In these cases, NEC should be suspected and will require a complete clinical evaluation. However, intermediate situations are frequent in VLBW infants and require adequate decisions whether or not to interrupt enteral feeding.

The aspiration of gastric residuals is common practice to evaluate GI tolerance while tube feeding. Many clinicians consider gastric residuals suspect if they are >3–4 ml/kg, >30–50% of the previous feed or bilious-stained. However, studies evaluating these concepts demonstrated little if any predictive value of such gastric residuals for feeding intolerance [65, 66]. Therefore, in the absence of significant clinical signs or symptoms, the presence of gastric residuals <4 ml/kg or <50% of 3 h previous feed is not a valid reason to interrupt or reduce enteral feeding [44]. Maintaining sufficient enteral feeding can in fact improve GI maturation and feeding tolerance [15, 16, 46]. However, other signs of feeding intolerance require a complete clinical examination to determine subsequent care. An abdominal radiograph is sometimes necessary to rule out NEC diagnosis but non-irradiated techniques like abdominal ultrasounds are also useful to evaluate abdominal condition in VLBW infants [67, 68]. When feeding intolerance is suspected or confirmed, feeds need to be adapted to each infant's evolution. If enteral feeding has been interrupted but clinical evolution rules out NEC or another disease, enteral feeding should be restarted as soon as possible, even after a few hours. Some concerns also exist about an association between NEC and blood transfusion, patent ductus arteriosus and treatment with cyclooxygenase inhibitors in VLBW infants. However, there is no evidence that in these situations withholding feeding decreases NEC or improves outcomes [44].

Feeding Logistics

While it is important to consider the nutrient composition of the feedings provided to the preterm infant, there are several additional issues that one should also be aware of. These include the practice of concentrating feedings and handling feedings.

One aspect of the management of infants with chronic lung disease or congenital heart disease may include fluid restriction, with concentrating feeds to 85–100 kcal/dl (26–30 kcal/oz). These practices may include some risks. First, these recipes often require the use of powders that are added to HM or liquid formula or the mixing of powdered formulas with less water than indicated on the label. This latter practice may result in osmotic loads in excess of 500 mosm/l, depending on the powdered product that is used. Similarly, the administration of medications or electrolytes supplements with milk products may also lead to high feed osmolarity [69]. Although there is no conclusive evidence for a causal relationship between osmolarity of feeds and the de-

Table 1. Reasonable strategy to optimize enteral feeding practices in ELBW (<1,000 g) and VLBW (1,000–1,499 g) infants

	ELBW	VLBW
Preferred milk	HM*	HM*
First feeding	between 6 and 48 h of life	between 6 and 48 h of life
Initial feeding (MEF)	0.5 ml/kg/h or 1 ml/kg q2h	1 ml/kg/h or 2 ml/kg q2h
Duration of MEF	1–4 days	1–4 days
Feeding advancement	15–25 ml/kg/day	20–30 ml/kg/day
If continuous feeding	+0.5 ml/kg/h q12h	+1 ml/kg q8h
If q2h intermittent feeding	+1 ml/kg q12h	+1 ml/kg q8h
HM fortification	before 100 ml/kg/day	before 100 ml/kg/day
Target energy intakes	110–130 kcal/kg/day	110–130 kcal/kg/day
Target protein intakes	4–4.5 g/kg/day	3.5–4.0 g/kg/day

* Own mother's breast milk or donor HM, but adapted preterm infant formula may also be used if there is no access to HM.

velopment of NEC, the normal physiological response to an increase in feed osmolarity is an increase in gastric secretions that will lead to a delay in gastric emptying [40]. Even if this should not be considered as feeding intolerance, it may be prudent to minimize these practices by diluting additives in the largest possible volume of feed and by using multicomponent fortifiers in preference to multiple individual supplements.

One should also be mindful that manipulations during preparation and/or storage of preterm powdered formulas or fortified HM may alter its nutrient content. In an attempt to comply with WHO recommendations to use boiled water, one should permit the water to cool before adding to prepare preterm formulations, as the direct exposure of powder to boiling water will cause the breakdown of many water-soluble nutrients, particularly vitamins. In some regions where fortified HM is pasteurized due to concerns for the bacterial counts of breast milk, such practices may also result in the destruction of the nutrient content of HM. Thus the benefit of this practice should be weighed against the use of enhanced training and attention of personnel to hygienic preparation techniques such as careful hand washing.

Some hospitals are using glass-fronted refrigerators that are also used for storing drugs. This practice can constantly expose breast milk HM or formula to the oxidizing properties of light.

Reasonable Recommendations for Optimizing Enteral Feeding Practices

There is no consensus about ideal feeding practices, but it has been demonstrated that standardized feeding regimens may be a very important tools to prevent and minimize NEC in preterm neonates [18]. Table 1 synthesizes a reasonable and optimized feeding strategy based on current knowledge. Enteral nutrition should be rapidly initiated in all VLBW infants after birth to avoid GI atrophy and dysfunction. Even if some uncertainties remain on the clinical benefit of MEF in VLBW infants, MEF has been demonstrated to be safe, and many studies demonstrated its benefits. As soon as the infant's cardiorespiratory function is stabilized after a few hours, initiation of MEF should be considered. Unreasonable delay in feeding initiation must be avoided to improve GI maturation, development and function.

There is strong evidence demonstrating that exclusive feeding of fortified HM provides major advantages for short- and long-term outcomes of VLBW infants. HM feeding should be considered as standard feeding practices for VLBW infants, and mothers should be supported in effectively stimulating lactation after delivery. Pasteurized donor HM is a favorable alternative to initiate enteral feeding in VLBW infants if own mother's milk is not available, especially in ELBW infants that are more prone to adverse later outcomes. HM needs to be rapidly fortified with protein, energy, minerals and vitamins. HM fortification can be reasonably introduced when enteral feedings exceed 50 ml/kg/day and adequate fortification must be achieved when enteral feedings reach 100 ml/kg/day, in order to provide sufficient nutritional intakes.

Uncertainties remain regarding the optimal tube feeding method for VLBW and ELBW infants. Short-interval feeding, q2 hours or continuous, regimens appear preferable in VLBW infants as they improve feeding tolerance and reduce the need for PN. Feeding tubes may be inserted either by the nose (nasogastric) or by the mouth (orogastric) until further studies demonstrate the optimal tube feeding position. Transpyloric tube feeding should not be recommended as a routine for feeding neonates.

Feeding tolerance should be regularly assessed in VLBW infants. The measurement of gastric residuals is of little value. In the absence of any significant clinical signs or symptoms of feeding intolerance, solely gastric residuals <4 ml/kg or <50% of 3 h previous feed should not be considered abnormal. Any suspicion of feeding intolerance requires a complete clinical examination before deciding to interrupt or not enteral feeding. Thereafter, repeated evaluation in short intervals should be performed to decide upon continued interruption or restarting enteral feeding. Feeding advancement of 20–30 ml/kg/day is reasonable in 1,000–1,499 g VLBW infants. In ELBW infants, the safety of such feeding advancement is not clear and advancement of 15–25 ml/kg/day might be recommended until further studies will be performed. According to premature infant needs, target feeding intake is 110–130 kcal/kg/day with 3.5–4.5 g/kg/day of protein (see Appendix). However, infant's growth parameters should be regularly assessed to adapt nutritional supply.

Such a strategy is feasible and is currently applied in several NICUs associated with significant improvements of postnatal growth [41, 70]. Figure 1a and b illustrates feeding results in all ELBW and 1,000–1,499 g VLBW infants consecutively admitted to our NICU [unpubl. data]. It demonstrates that full enteral nutrition may be achieved in most VLBW infants during the first 2 weeks of life, even if full enteral nutrition is more slowly achieved in ELBW infants (median 12 days in ELBW compared to 6 days in 1,000–1,499 g VLBW infants, p < 0.05). When combined with an optimized PN

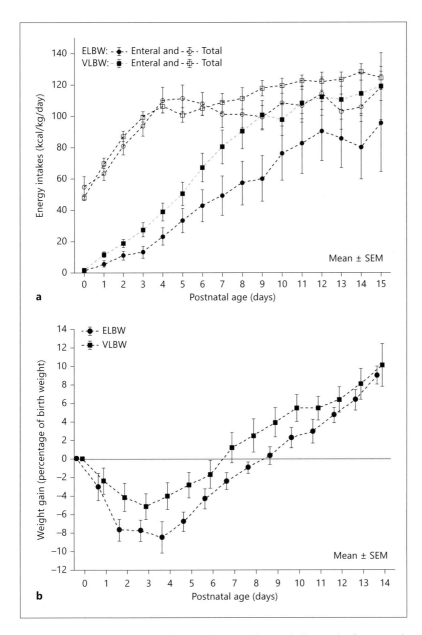

Fig. 1. a, b Early nutritional intakes and postnatal growth during the first 2 weeks of life in consecutively admitted ELBW (470–980 g, n = 8) and VLBW (1,010–1,460 g, n = 15) infants after optimizing nutritional policy to recent recommendations.

regimen, postnatal weight gain may be rapidly adequate, allowing birth weight to be regained after 7 days in average in both ELBW and 1,000–1,499 g VLBW infants (p = 0.34). Such a policy has demonstrated the potential to reduce the risk of PNGR in most VLBW infants [41]. Further studies are necessary to improve our knowledge and enteral feeding practices in VLBW infants.

References

1 Agostoni C, Buonocore G, Carnielli VP, De Curtis M, Darmaun D, Decsi T, et al: Enteral nutrient supply for preterm infants: commentary from the European Society of Paediatric Gastroenterology, Hepatology and Nutrition Committee on Nutrition. J Pediatr Gastroenterol Nutr 2010;50:85–91.

2 Martin CR, Brown YF, Ehrenkranz RA, O'Shea TM, Allred EN, Belfort MB, et al: Nutritional practices and growth velocity in the first month of life in extremely premature infants. Pediatrics 2009;124:649–657.

3 Ehrenkranz RA, Younes N, Lemons JA, Fanaroff AA, Donovan EF, Wright LL, et al: Longitudinal growth of hospitalized very low birth weight infants. Pediatrics 1999;104:280–289.

4 Senterre T, Rigo J: Reduction in postnatal cumulative nutritional deficit and improvement of growth in extremely preterm infants. Acta Paediatr 2012; 101:e64–e70.

5 Embleton NE, Pang N, Cooke RJ: Postnatal malnutrition and growth retardation: an inevitable consequence of current recommendations in preterm infants? Pediatrics 2001;107:270–273.

6 Senterre T, Rigo J: Recent advances in nutritional support and postnatal growth in premature infants (in French). Rev Med Liege 2013;68:79–85.

7 Ehrenkranz RA, Dusick AM, Vohr BR, Wright LL, Wrage LA, Poole WK: Growth in the neonatal intensive care unit influences neurodevelopmental and growth outcomes of extremely low birth weight infants. Pediatrics 2006;117:1253–1261.

8 Lucas A, Morley R, Cole TJ: Randomised trial of early diet in preterm babies and later intelligence quotient. BMJ 1998;317:1481–1487.

9 Isaacs EB, Gadian DG, Sabatini S, Chong WK, Quinn BT, Fischl BR, et al: The effect of early human diet on caudate volumes and IQ. Pediatr Res 2008;63:308–314.

10 Latal-Hajnal B, von Siebenthal K, Kovari H, Bucher HU, Largo RH: Postnatal growth in VLBW infants: significant association with neurodevelopmental outcome. J Pediatr 2003;143:163–170.

11 Klingenberg C, Embleton ND, Jacobs SE, O'Connell LA, Kuschel CA: Enteral feeding practices in very preterm infants: an international survey. Arch Dis Child Fetal Neonatal Ed 2011;97:F56–F61.

12 Hans DM, Pylipow M, Long JD, Thureen PJ, Georgieff MK: Nutritional practices in the neonatal intensive care unit: analysis of a 2006 neonatal nutrition survey. Pediatrics 2009;123:51–57.

13 Flidel-Rimon O, Friedman S, Lev E, Juster-Reicher A, Amitay M, Shinwell ES: Early enteral feeding and nosocomial sepsis in very low birth weight infants. Arch Dis Child Fetal Neonatal Ed 2004;89:F289–F292.

14 Hartel C, Haase B, Browning-Carmo K, Gebauer C, Kattner E, Kribs A, et al: Does the enteral feeding advancement affect short-term outcomes in very low birth weight infants? J Pediatr Gastroenterol Nutr 2009;48:464–470.

15 Janeczko M, Burrin DA: Trophic factors in the neonatal gastrointestinal tract; in Neu J (ed): Gastroenterology and Nutrition. Philadelphia, Saunders Elsevier, 2008, pp 121–134.

16 Neu J: Gastrointestinal development and meeting the nutritional needs of premature infants. Am J Clin Nutr 2007;85:629S–634S.

17 Neu J: Necrotizing enterocolitis. World Rev Nutr Diet. Basel, Karger, 2014.

18 Patole SK, de Klerk N: Impact of standardised feeding regimens on incidence of neonatal necrotising enterocolitis: a systematic review and meta-analysis of observational studies. Arch Dis Child Fetal Neonatal Ed 2005;90:F147–F151.

19 Dsilna A, Christensson K, Alfredsson L, Lagercrantz H, Blennow M: Continuous feeding promotes gastrointestinal tolerance and growth in very low birth weight infants. J Pediatr 2005;147:43–49.

20 American Academy of Pediatrics. Section on Breastfeeding: Breastfeeding and the use of human milk. Pediatrics 2012;129:e827–e841.

21 Tudehope DI: Human milk and the nutritional needs of preterm infants. J Pediatr 2013;162(suppl): S17–S25.

22 Lanzieri TM, Dollard SC, Josephson CD, Schmid DS, Bialek SR: Breast milk-acquired cytomegalovirus infection and disease in VLBW and premature infants. Pediatrics 2013;131:e1937–e1945.

23 Tsang RC, Uauy R, Koletzko B, Zlotkin SH (eds): Nutrition of the Preterm Infant: Scientific Basis and Practical Guidelines. Cincinnati, Digital Educating Publishing, Inc, 2005.

24 Campbell-Yeo ML, Allen AC, Joseph KS, Ledwidge JM, Caddell K, Allen VM, et al: Effect of domperidone on the composition of preterm human breast milk. Pediatrics 2010;125:e107–e114.

25 Human Milk Banking Association of North America: 2011 Best Practice for Expressing, Storing and Handling Human Milk in Hospital, Homes, and Child Care Setting, ed 3. Fort Worth, Human Milk Banking Association of North America (HMBANA), 2011.

26 Arslanoglu S, Bertino E, Tonetto P, De Nisi G, Ambruzzi AM, Biasini A, et al: Guidelines for the establishment and operation of a donor human milk bank. J Matern Fetal Neonatal Med 2010;23(suppl 2):1–20.

27 Moro GE, Arslanoglu S: Heat treatment of human milk. J Pediatr Gastroenterol Nutr 2012;54:165–166.

28 Ewaschuk JB, Unger S, O'Connor DL, Stone D, Harvey S, Clandinin MT, et al: Effect of pasteurization on selected immune components of donated human breast milk. J Perinatol 2011;31:593–598.

29 Arslanoglu S, Ziegler EE, Moro GE: Donor human milk in preterm infant feeding: evidence and recommendations. J Perinat Med 2010;38:347–351.

30 Boyd CA, Quigley MA, Brocklehurst P: Donor breast milk versus infant formula for preterm infants: systematic review and meta-analysis. Arch Dis Child Fetal Neonatal Ed 2007;92:F169–F175.

31 Quigley MA, Henderson G, Anthony MY, McGuire W: Formula milk versus donor breast milk for feeding preterm or low birth weight infants. Cochrane Database Syst Rev 2007;4:CD002971.

32 Kuschel CA, Harding JE: Multicomponent fortified human milk for promoting growth in preterm infants. Cochrane Database Syst Rev 2004;1:CD000343.

33 Arslanoglu S, Moro GE, Ziegler EE; The WAPM Working Group on Nutrition: Optimization of human milk fortification for preterm infants: new concepts and recommendations. J Perinat Med 2010;38:233–238.

34 Henriksen C, Westerberg AC, Ronnestad A, Nakstad B, Veierod MB, Drevon CA, et al: Growth and nutrient intake among very-low-birth-weight infants fed fortified human milk during hospitalisation. Br J Nutr 2009;102:1179–1186.

35 De Halleux V, Rigo J: Variability in human milk composition: benefit of individualized fortification in very-low-birth-weight infants. Am J Clin Nutr 2013 Jul 3.

36 Rochow N, Fusch G, Choi A, Chessell L, Elliott L, McDonald K, et al: Target Fortification of Breast Milk with Fat, Protein, and Carbohydrates for Preterm Infants. J Pediatr 2013;163:1001–1007.

37 American Academy of Pediatrics: Commentary on breast-feeding and infant formulas, including proposed standards for formulas. Pediatrics 1976;57:278–285.

38 De Curtis M, Candusso M, Pieltain C, Rigo J: Effect of fortification on the osmolality of human milk. Arch Dis Child Fetal Neonatal Ed 1999;81:F141–F143.

39 Martin I, Jackson L: Question 1. Is there an increased risk of necrotising enterocolitis in preterm infants whose mothers' expressed breast milk is fortified with multicomponent fortifier? Arch Dis Child 2011;96:1199–1201.

40 Pearson F, Johnson MJ, Leaf AA: Milk osmolality: does it matter? Arch Dis Child Fetal Neonatal Ed 2013;98:F166–F169.

41 Senterre T, Rigo J: Optimizing early nutritional support based on recent recommendations in VLBW infants and postnatal growth restriction. J Pediatr Gastroenterol Nutr 2011;53:536–542.

42 Tillman S, Brandon DH, Silva SG: Evaluation of human milk fortification from the time of the first feeding: effects on infants of less than 31 weeks gestational age. J Perinatol 2012;32:525–531.

43 Morgan J, Bombell S, McGuire W: Early trophic feeding versus enteral fasting for very preterm or very low birth weight infants. Cochrane Database Syst Rev 2013;3:CD000504.

44 Parker LA, Neu J, Torrazza RM, Li Y: Scientifically based strategies for enteral feeding in premature infants. Neoreview 2013;14:e350–e359.

45 Morgan J, Young L, McGuire W: Delayed introduction of progressive enteral feeds to prevent necrotising enterocolitis in very low birth weight infants. Cochrane Database Syst Rev 2011;3:CD001970.

46 Burrin DG, Stoll B, Jiang R, Chang X, Hartmann B, Holst JJ, et al: Minimal enteral nutrient requirements for intestinal growth in neonatal piglets: how much is enough? Am J Clin Nutr 2000;71:1603–1610.

47 Flidel-Rimon O, Branski D, Shinwell ES: The fear of necrotizing enterocolitis versus achieving optimal growth in preterm infants – an opinion. Acta Paediatr 2006;95:1341–1344.

48 Morgan J, Young L, McGuire W: Delayed introduction of progressive enteral feeds to prevent necrotising enterocolitis in very low birth weight infants. Cochrane Database Syst Rev 2013;5:CD001970.

49 McClure RJ, Newell SJ: Randomised controlled study of clinical outcome following trophic feeding. Arch Dis Child Fetal Neonatal Ed 2000;82:F29–F33.

50 Rochow N, Fusch G, Muhlinghaus A, Niesytto C, Straube S, Utzig N, et al: A nutritional program to improve outcome of very low birth weight infants. Clin Nutr 2012;31:124–131.

51 Dunn L, Hulman S, Weiner J, Kliegman R: Beneficial effects of early hypocaloric enteral feeding on neonatal gastrointestinal function: preliminary report of a randomized trial. J Pediatr 1988;112:622–629.

52 Bombell S, McGuire W: Early trophic feeding for very low birth weight infants. Cochrane Database Syst Rev 2009;3:CD000504.

53 Hawes J, McEwan P, McGuire W: Nasal versus oral route for placing feeding tubes in preterm or low birth weight infants. Cochrane Database Syst Rev 2004;3:CD003952.

54 Bohnhorst B, Cech K, Peter C, Doerdelmann M: Oral versus nasal route for placing feeding tubes: no effect on hypoxemia and bradycardia in infants with apnea of prematurity. Neonatology 2010;98:143–149.

55 McGuire W, McEwan P: Transpyloric versus gastric tube feeding for preterm infants. Cochrane Database Syst Rev 2007;3:CD003487.

56 Quandt D, Schraner T, Ulrich Bucher H, Arlettaz Mieth R: Malposition of feeding tubes in neonates: is it an issue? J Pediatr Gastroenterol Nutr 2009;48:608–611.

57 Dawson JA, Summan R, Badawi N, Foster JP: Push versus gravity for intermittent bolus gavage tube feeding of premature and low birth weight infants. Cochrane Database Syst Rev 2012;11:CD005249.

58 DeMauro SB, Abbasi S, Lorch S: The impact of feeding interval on feeding outcomes in very low birth weight infants. J Perinatol 2011;31:481–486.

59 Bergman NJ: Neonatal stomach volume and physiology suggest feeding at 1-h intervals. Acta Paediatr 2013;102:773–777.

60 Premji SS, Chessell L: Continuous nasogastric milk feeding versus intermittent bolus milk feeding for premature infants less than 1,500 grams. Cochrane Database Syst Rev 2011;11:CD001819.

61 Henderson G, Craig S, Brocklehurst P, McGuire W: Enteral feeding regimens and necrotising enterocolitis in preterm infants: a multicentre case-control study. Arch Dis Child Fetal Neonatal Ed 2009; 94:F120–F123.

62 Berseth CL, Bisquera JA, Paje VU: Prolonging small feeding volumes early in life decreases the incidence of necrotizing enterocolitis in very low birth weight infants. Pediatrics 2003;111:529–534.

63 Senterre T: Necrotizing enterocolitis and feeding regimen. Neonatology 2013;104:263–264.

64 Morgan J, Young L, McGuire W: Slow advancement of enteral feed volumes to prevent necrotising enterocolitis in very low birth weight infants. Cochrane Database Syst Rev 2013;3:CD001241.

65 Mihatsch WA, von Schoenaich P, Fahnenstich H, Dehne N, Ebbecke H, Plath C, et al: The significance of gastric residuals in the early enteral feeding advancement of extremely low birth weight infants. Pediatrics 2002;109:457–459.

66 Cobb BA, Carlo WA, Ambalavanan N: Gastric residuals and their relationship to necrotizing enterocolitis in very low birth weight infants. Pediatrics 2004;113:50–53.

67 Dordelmann M, Rau GA, Bartels D, Linke M, Derichs N, Behrens C, et al: Evaluation of portal venous gas detected by ultrasound examination for diagnosis of necrotising enterocolitis. Arch Dis Child Fetal Neonatal Ed 2009;94:F183–F187.

68 Epelman M, Daneman A, Navarro OM, Morag I, Moore AM, Kim JH, et al: Necrotizing enterocolitis: review of state-of-the-art imaging findings with pathologic correlation. Radiographics 2007;27:285–305.

69 Radmacher PG, Adamkin MD, Lewis ST, Adamkin DH: Milk as a vehicle for oral medications: hidden osmoles. J Perinatol 2012;32:227–229.

70 Maas C, Mitt S, Full A, Arand J, Bernhard W, Poets CF, et al: A historic cohort study on accelerated advancement of enteral feeding volumes in very premature infants. Neonatology 2013;103:67–73.

Thibault Senterre, MD, PhD, FRCPC
Service Universitaire de Néonatologie, CHR de la Citadelle
Boulevard du XII de Ligne, 1
BE–4000 Liège (Belgium)
E-Mail Thibault.Senterre@chu.ulg.ac.be

Koletzko B, Poindexter B, Uauy R (eds): Nutritional Care of Preterm Infants: Scientific Basis and Practical Guidelines.
World Rev Nutr Diet. Basel, Karger, 2014, vol 110, pp 215–227 (DOI: 10.1159/000358470)

Human Milk and Human Milk Fortifiers

Ekhard E. Ziegler

Department of Pediatrics, University of Iowa, Iowa City, Iowa, USA

Reviewed by Richard Ehrenkranz, Yale University School of Medicine, New Haven, Conn., USA; Karen Simmer,
University of Western Australia, Crawley, WA, Australia

Abstract

Human milk contains numerous immune-protective components that protect the premature infant
from sepsis and necrotizing enterocolitis. Because of these protective effects, human milk is the feeding of choice for the premature infant. However, human milk does not provide adequate amounts
of most nutrients for premature infants and must therefore be supplemented (fortified) with nutrients. Commercially available fortifiers provide energy and most nutrients in adequate amounts. The
exception is protein, which is present in expressed milk in highly variable amounts and which is not
provided in sufficient amounts by most fortifiers. Some liquid fortifiers are higher in protein content
than powder fortifiers and provide adequate amounts of protein.   © 2014 S. Karger AG, Basel

Human milk has the dual functions of supporting and complementing the preterm
infant's developing immune system, and of providing the nutrients needed for growth
and development. Because of its immune-protective function, human milk is the feeding of choice for premature infants. As a source of nutrients, however, human milk is
inadequate, necessitating nutrient supplementation (fortification) [1]. Nutrient intakes that fall short of requirements place the infant at risk of impaired neurodevelopment. The main challenge is to meet the high nutrient needs of premature infants in
the face of highly variable human milk composition. Methods of nutrient fortification
have improved over the years but have yet to reach a state where nutrient intakes are
consistently adequate.

Non-Nutritive Components of Human Milk

Many bioactive components have been identified in human milk. Table 1 provides
a select listing of these components grouped into immune-protective and trophic
components, hormones and immune cells. Their biological activity has been doc-

Table 1. Anti-infectious and other bioactive substances and cells in human milk

Anti-infectious compounds
Immunoglobulins (predominantly sIgA)
Lactoferrin
Lysozyme
Lactadherin
Nucleotides
Defensins
Mucins
Oligosaccharides
Toll-like receptors
Cytokines
Substances with trophic effects
Epidermal growth factor
Transforming growth factor-α
Transforming growth factor-β
Lactoferrin
Trefoil factors
Insulin-like growth factor (IGF)-I and -II
Nerve growth factor
Hormones
Pituitary hormones
Thyroid hormones
Steroid hormones
Cells
Neutrophils
Macrophages
T-lymphocytes

umented experimentally to varying degrees. Immune-protective components exert anti-bacterial, anti-viral and anti-inflammatory effects. The abundant oligosaccharides exert important anti-adhesive as well as prebiotic effects promoting a healthy microbiota and limiting gut inflammatory responses and growth of pathogenic bacteria. Clinical correlates associated with the use of human milk include lower rates of bacterial sepsis and necrotizing enterocolitis (NEC). These effects are attributed collectively to the bioactive components of human milk but cannot be linked to any one specific component. Other substances exert maturational, anti-inflammatory and trophic effects on the gastrointestinal tract. As with the immune components, the known clinical effects are attributed collectively to the trophic substances. Most likely it is the interplay of these multiple components that brings about beneficial clinical effects. For example, the protective effect against NEC is likely to be brought about by the synergy of gut maturational (trophic) effects with anti-infectious, anti-adhesive, anti-inflammatory as well as prebiotic effects.

Protective Effects of Human Milk

Protection against sepsis and NEC are the main reasons why human milk is fed to preterm infants. The protection of preterm infants against sepsis is widely appreciated and has been well documented over the years [2–8]. A recent study has shown that the protective effect of human milk against sepsis is strongly dose-dependent [9]. It is of interest that these findings point to the gastrointestinal tract as the portal of entry for bacteria causing late-onset sepsis. This is consistent with the notion that trophic factors in human milk play an important role in sepsis prevention by advancing maturation of the immature gastrointestinal tract.

Protection by human milk against NEC in dose-dependent fashion was first documented by Schanler et al. [4, 5]. It was confirmed subsequently by Sisk et al. [8] and most recently by Meinzen-Derr et al. [10] who demonstrated a strong and dose-dependent protective effect in a large cohort of extremely low birth weight infants. For each 100 ml/kg increase of human milk intake during the first 2 weeks of life, the risk of NEC or death after 2 weeks was decreased by a factor of 0.87.

Trophic Effects of Human Milk

Trophic components of human milk enhance and facilitate maturation of the immature gastrointestinal tract. Clinical correlates of maturational effects pertain mostly to motility of the gastrointestinal tract. Human milk leads to smaller gastric residuals (often referred to as improved 'tolerance') which are indicative of more rapid gastric emptying and which enable more rapid feeding advancement [5, 11, 12]. Improved gut motility reduces the propensity to abdominal distension [5]. Human milk decreases intestinal permeability [13, 14]. As indicated earlier, the maturational effects of human milk are thought to be key contributors to the protection it affords against sepsis and NEC.

Nutrient Requirements of Preterm Infants

Nutrient requirements of preterm infants are defined as intakes that enable the infant to grow at the same rate and with the same body composition (except for water) as the fetus. Requirements for most nutrients have been derived from accretion rates of protein, fat and minerals derived from analysis of fetal body composition at various stages of gestation. In addition, empirical methods have been employed to define requirements including those for nutrients such as vitamins [15]. As shown in table 2, requirements for protein and energy show a clear dependence on body weight, such that protein needs are highest in the least mature and smallest infants and decrease with increasing body weight, whereas energy needs increase with increasing body weight due to increasing energy deposition in the form of fat. Estimates of needs for major minerals, electrolytes and some trace minerals derived from fetal body composition are summarized in table 3. Required intakes of most nutrients are presumed

Table 2. Requirements for protein and energy; best estimates by factorial and empirical methods

	Body weight, g			
	500–1,000	1,000–1,500	1,500–2,200	2,200–3,000
Weight gain of fetus, g/kg/day	19.0	17.4	16.4	13.4
Protein, g/kg/day	4.0	3.9	3.7	3.4
Energy, kcal/kg/day	106	115	123	130
Protein/energy, g/100 kcal	3.8	3.4	3.0	2.6

Table 3. Nutrient requirements of infants weighing <1,000 g (expressed per kg/day and per 100 kcal) versus typical composition (per 100 kcal) of unfortified human milk at 4 weeks of lactation, and typical milk fortified with a powder fortifier that adds 1.0 g of protein per 100 ml of milk

	Required per kg/day	Required per 100 kcal	Human milk per 100 kcal	Fortified human milk per 100 kcal
Energy, kcal	108			
Protein, g	4.0	3.8	1.8	2.75
Ca, mg	184	170	37	156
P, mg	126	116	21	94
Mg, mg	6.9	6.4	4.8	6.6
Na, mmol	3.3	3.0	1.8	2.4
K, mmol	2.4	2.2	1.9	2.6
Cl, mmol	2.8	2.6	2.4	2.9
Fe, mg	2.0	1.85	0.13	1.9
Zn, mg	1.5	1.4	0.54	1.5
Cu, µg	120	111	56	102

to decrease with increasing body weight since growth rates per unit of body mass decrease with advancing postnatal age. Requirements for iron have been established empirically. They are dictated mainly by high needs for the expanding hemoglobin pool. However, for most micronutrients, requirements are known only approximately. This explains the wide variation in micronutrients provided by human milk fortifiers.

The consequences of intakes falling short of requirements vary from nutrient to nutrient. For the great majority of nutrients, small shortfalls are inconsequential, especially if they are temporary. Energy intakes below requirements mean that less energy is going into storage without an effect on growth of lean body mass as long as intake remains at least 90–100 kcal/kg/day. With protein, however, any shortfall is prone to affect growth, and, since growth and neurocognitive development are so closely linked [16], inadequate protein intake carries the risk of neurocognitive impairment. This is why special attention must be paid to the protein supply in early life and why intakes below requirements must be avoided.

Ziegler

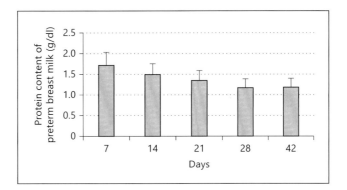

Fig. 1. Protein concentration of milk expressed by mothers of premature infants. Drawn from data of Lemons et al. [17]. Means and SD. Data represent true protein.

Nutrient Content of Human Milk

Some basic facts regarding the nutrient composition of human milk are relevant for effective nutritional support for the preterm infant. Although for very low birth weight infants all nutrients are present at inadequate concentrations, shortfalls range from slight to very large. In table 3, typical human milk composition (per 100 kcal) is juxtaposed with nutrient requirements (per 100 kcal). The shortfall is modest for some nutrients, for example chloride, but is quite large for other nutrients, notably protein, calcium and phosphorus.

Facts that need special attention:

(1) The concentration of protein decreases markedly with the duration of lactation (only zinc shows a similarly marked decrease). The changing protein content is illustrated in figure 1. Whereas the mean protein concentration of expressed milk is 1.7 g/dl on day 7 postpartum, it decreases rapidly to 1.2 g/dl ml after about 28 days [17].

(2) Milk expressed by mothers of preterm infants has a higher content of protein and of some minerals than milk of women who are breastfeeding term infants [17, 18]. The higher nutrient concentration is thought to be related to the fact that milk is expressed and that milk volume is low compared to that of mothers nursing term infants. Although the concentrations of some nutrients are increased in preterm milk, the daily supply is still insufficient to meet the needs of preterm infants.

(3) Expressed milk is highly variable in protein and energy content [19]. Figure 2 illustrates this point. Shown are protein concentrations of milk (pools fed in 24 h) expressed by mothers of preterm infants. It is evident that variation in protein concentration is greatest in the early weeks of lactation, with concentrations ranging from 0.8 g/dl all the way to 1.6 g/dl. Variation decreases with time from delivery and after 42 days protein concentration stabilizes at around 0.8–1.0 g/dl. Thus, after 42 days protein content is similar to that in term milk.

(4) Human milk contains appreciable amounts of non-protein nitrogen (about 24% of total N) while true protein accounts for 76% of total nitrogen [20]. Since about 27% of the non-protein nitrogen is considered available for protein synthesis, 83% of

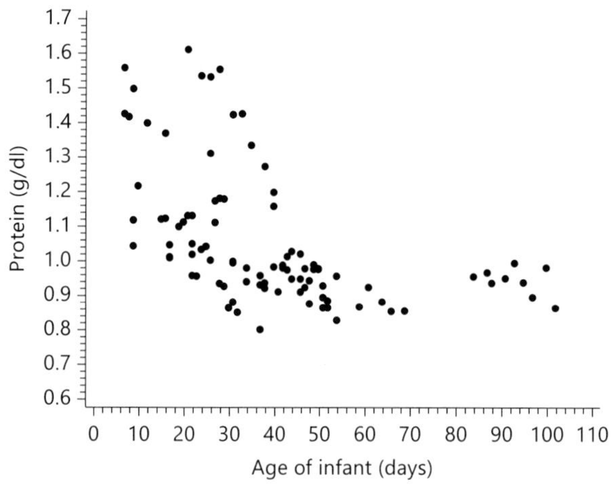

Fig. 2. Protein concentration of milk expressed by mothers of premature infants. Each symbol represents protein concentration of a pool of milk intended for consumption over 24 h. Protein obtained as total nitrogen × 0.83 × 6.25 [pers. unpubl. data].

total nitrogen is biologically available. Values presented in figure 1 represent true protein (76% of total nitrogen) whereas values in figure 2 are based on 83% of total nitrogen. Unfortunately, most bedside milk analyzers are calibrated to 100% of total nitrogen and therefore overestimate actual protein supply by about 17%.

(5) Donor milk is relatively constant in composition, with protein averaging 0.85 ± 0.08 g/dl and fat 3.9 ± 0.4 g/dl [21].

Human Milk Fortification

Principles of Fortification
The aim of fortification is to raise the concentrations of specific nutrients in relation to energy to such levels that nutrient needs are met whenever energy needs are met. This task can be achieved with relative ease for the great majority of nutrients which can safely be added to human milk in generous amounts so that intakes are always adequate, even when the concentration of a nutrient in milk should be low; fortifiers are designed according to this principle. Fortification also increases the caloric density of milk, which helps to keep feeding volumes low. Fortifiers achieve this by including carbohydrate(s) and/or lipids.

The key nutrient is protein. Because it is limiting for growth (and neurodevelopment) and there is no protein storage, needs for protein must be met at all times. However, intakes must not exceed needs by more than a modest margin because of the possibility of adverse metabolic effects. But what makes the task of protein fortification really difficult is the fact that the protein content of expressed milk provided by the mother is not only highly variable but is usually not known to the caregiver. The solutions that are being applied to solve this problem differ in their capacity to achieve

Ziegler

satisfactory protein intakes. Most widely used are generalizing approaches that add a fixed amount of fortifier to human milk. Most fortifiers provide modest amounts of protein so that unduly high protein intakes are avoided if and when the protein content of human milk is high. Thus, protein intakes are too low most of the time. If the generalizing approach uses a fortifier with a sufficiently high protein level, protein intakes are adequate even when protein content of the milk is low. In contrast, customizing methods aim to achieve adequate protein intakes for each infant using metabolic feedback from the infant, or milk analysis with adjustments of nutrient content so that nutrient intakes match closely the infant's needs.

Composition of Fortifiers

Commercial fortifiers have undergone considerable modifications since they first appeared in the 1980s (although reference is made here to publications using earlier fortifier versions, compositional data are presented for currently available fortifiers only). Available fortifiers differ considerably in their composition [22].

Powder fortifiers as well as liquid fortifiers are provided in premeasured quantities whereby the content of one sachet or one vial is added to a specified volume of human milk, commonly 25 ml. Contrary to powder fortifiers, addition of liquid fortifiers involves dilution of human milk. In the case of standard addition of liquid fortifiers, the dilution is 1 part fortifier to 4 parts human milk. The degree of dilution increases with higher fortification levels. In the case of the human milk-based fortifier, the highest fortification level results in a 1:1 dilution of human milk. The key ingredient is protein. With the exception of the human milk-based fortifier, protein is derived from cow milk fractions. Some fortifiers use partially hydrolyzed and some use intact cow milk protein. Powder fortifiers provide 1.0–1.1 g protein/dl milk. Liquid fortifiers based on bovine milk protein add 1.0–1.8 g protein/dl milk. The human milk-based liquid fortifier adds 0.6 g/dl protein when used at 80 kcal/dl, but the amount added rises as the proportion of fortifier to milk is increased and can reach 1.5 g/dl when a 1:1 ratio is used (1 part of fortifier added to 1 part milk) resulting in a caloric density of 100 kcal/dl.

As table 3 indicates, the addition of 1.0 or 1.1 g protein/dl of human milk is not sufficient to meet the protein needs of very preterm infants. Why is the protein content so low? At the time when powder fortifiers were developed, an overriding concern was to avoid 'high' protein intakes. Given the variability of the protein content of expressed human milk, only fortifiers with a suitably low protein content could guarantee that protein intake would never be 'high'. Concern about adverse effects of 'high' protein intakes was, and still is, common. This concern has its origin in the 1974 study of Goldman et al. [23] where infants fed a formula providing exceedingly high intakes of 6.0–7.2 g/kg/day of a poor quality protein (casein-predominant cow milk protein) were found on follow-up to show an increased rate of neurodevelopmental impairment. Although the details of the study [23] have faded from memory and 'high' protein intake is not defined in quantitative terms, the concern lingers on and has influenced the design of powder fortifiers. All fortifiers provide energy from varying amounts of carbohydrates and/or fat, raising the energy density of milk from 67 to 80 kcal/dl. It is customary to identify fortified human milk by its caloric density. Non-standard regimens are similarly identified by their caloric density. For example, milk fortified with 6 instead of the standard 4 packets is identified as 90 kcal/dl.

All fortifiers provide electrolytes, macrominerals, microminerals and vitamins in amounts intended to augment the nutrient content of human milk so that it provides adequate amounts of all nutrients. Table 3 shows the composition of human milk fortified with a typical powder fortifier. Amounts of nutrients other than protein vary considerably from fortifier to fortifier, the explanation is that requirements for most nutrients are not well defined. Table 3 shows that fortified milk provides most nutrients in amounts that approach or slightly exceed requirements. Some fortifiers provide selenium and iodine while others do not. Most fortifiers provide docosahexaenoic (DHA) and arachidonic (ARA) acids. Fortifiers increase the osmolality of feeds by 36–95 mosm/kg H_2O. If fortified milk is let stand, as is the practice in units that make up 24-hour supplies of fortified milk, there can be a further rise in osmolality by up to 64 mosm/kg H_2O in 24 h [24]. The rise is attributed to hydrolysis of carbohydrates by amylase activity of human milk.

For the sake of completeness, protein supplements must be mentioned here, even though they are not fortifiers in the usual sense. Protein supplements come as powders or as liquids. They are most commonly used to increase the protein content of fortified human milk. Their use requires careful weighing in the case of powders or volume measurement in the case of liquid supplements.

Is Fortification Effective?

When fortifiers were introduced in the 1980s a substantial number of studies were conducted to assess their effectiveness. Collectively these studies conducted between 1987 and 1999 showed that fortifiers improved growth and various indicators of nutritional status [25]. The largest of the studies [26], while not finding a significant growth effect overall, did find a marked effect on growth among infants who received predominantly human milk (as opposed to predominantly formula). More recent studies have evaluated new fortifiers in comparison with older ones. Thus, Porcelli et al. [27] compared a newly developed fortifier with an existing fortifier with lower protein content. Reis et al. [28] and Berseth et al. [29] evaluated newly developed fortifiers in comparison with earlier versions and found that growth was improved. In the study by Moya et al. [30] a newly developed liquid fortifier with higher protein content was compared with a powder fortifier with lower protein content. Use of the new fortifier was associated with greater attained weight and greater length gain.

The acquisition of bone mineral has been receiving little attention in recent years and the impression is that fortifiers, notwithstanding the large differences in calcium and phosphorus content [22], are reasonably effective in preventing at least gross undermineralization of the skeleton.

It is unequivocal that fortification improves growth and other outcomes. However, there is yet no evidence that outcomes such as growth are optimal and in particular that neurocognitive function is unimpaired in premature infants fed fortified human milk.

Side (Adverse) Effects of Fortification

In clinical practice, the introduction of fortifier is often accompanied by an increase in the size of gastric residuals, or by reappearance of residuals if they had ceased earlier. Moody et al. [31] documented that fortification leads to larger and more frequent gastric residuals. Increased residuals suggest a slowing of gastric emptying. The study by Ewer and Yu [32] indeed found that addition of a fortifier significantly slowed gastric emptying. However, two other studies found no such effect [33, 34]. The discrepancy in findings may have its explanation in compositional differences between fortifiers, especially with regard to the carbohydrate component. The latter is thought to be the source of a rise in intragastric osmolality, which in turn slows gastric emptying.

The possibility that fortifiers may interfere with the antibacterial activity of human milk has received a fair amount of attention. Chan [35] and Chan et al. [36], using a test system with incubation at 37°C for 24 h, found that a fortifier with added iron diminished the antibacterial action of human milk, which was left intact by a fortifier without added iron. Similar findings were reported by Ovali et al. [37] using a different test system. However, using incubation at room temperature for 6 h, Telang et al. [38] found no effect of fortifier with or without iron on antibacterial activity, and Santiago et al. [39] using incubation at refrigerator temperature similarly found no effect with or without iron. Clinical experience over the years does not suggest adverse effects due to fortifier iron.

It is sometimes suggested, based on the results of the study by Sullivan et al. [40], that bovine milk protein may have adverse effects, in particular that it may increase the risk of NEC. This is based on a misinterpretation of the results of the study [40] in which infants whose mothers had insufficient milk were randomized to formula and a bovine milk protein fortifier or to donor human milk and a human milk-based fortifier. It was the paucity or absence of human milk in the formula group that is presumed to have been the decisive difference between groups and not the use of a bovine protein-based fortifier. There is no evidence in preterm infants of any adverse effect from the addition of intact bovine milk protein to human milk.

Methods of Human Milk Fortification

The Practice of Fortification

Fortification of human milk is most commonly initiated when milk intake reaches 100 ml/kg/day. Earlier initiation would seem to be advantageous from a nutritional point of view. Tillman et al. [41] evaluated initiation of fortification with the first feed and found it to be well tolerated. Some units practice early initiation and the experience is generally favorable. Sometimes fortification is started at half strength and later advanced to full strength, but most commonly fortification is started at full strength.

Generalizing Fortification Methods
By far the most widely used fortification method is the basic generalizing method in which a powder fortifier is added in standard fixed amount. Neither the size nor the condition of the infant are taken into account with this method. The method delivers most nutrients in amounts that meet or exceed the needs of the infant, with the exception of protein where, as table 3 shows, intakes fall short of needs. Although it is well documented that fortification by this method leads to increased growth [25], it is improbable that optimal growth is often achieved. When measured, intakes of protein are considerably less than required [42]. Powder fortifiers with higher protein content (1.4 g/dl) have been studied [43] but are not commercially available.

Adequacy of the achieved protein intake depends on the needs of the infant (table 2) and the amount of protein provided by the fortifier. Generally, the higher the amount protein provided, the greater is the likelihood of protein intake being adequate. The newly available high-protein liquid fortifier adds 1.8 g of protein to each 100 ml of human milk, an amount that is sufficient to raise protein intakes to satisfactory levels in almost all situations. Protein content of milk fortified with the liquid fortifier may exceed the required level by a modest margin if and when milk protein content is relatively high. Experience so far indicates that such a modest excess of protein is well tolerated [30]. The human milk-based liquid fortifier adds 0.6 g per 100 ml milk at 80 kcal/dl, which is less protein than the powder fortifiers add. However, the ratio of fortifier to human milk can be increased and at the highest caloric density (100 kcal/dl) the human milk-based fortifier increases protein content by 1.5 g/dl.

Modifications of the basic generalizing fortification scheme are used to achieve adequate protein intakes. One modification is the use, in addition to standard amounts of the fortifier, of measured amounts of supplemental protein (powder or liquid). The method is not widely used, probably because of the cumbersome need for exact measurement of the protein supplement. Another modification consists in the addition of greater than standard amounts of fortifier. For example, 6 sachets of powder fortifier may be used instead of the standard 4 sachets. With this 'superfortification' more adequate protein intakes are achieved, but greater than intended amounts of all other nutrients are also provided, if unintentionally. To safeguard against hypercalcemia, some units perform weekly determinations of serum calcium and phosphorus.

The advantage of generalizing approaches is their relative simplicity. Because of that, generalizing approaches are assumed to be less prone to errors than other approaches.

Customizing Fortification Methods

Unsatisfactory protein intakes achieved with powder fortifiers have led to the development of customizing methods. Their aim is to achieve protein intakes that are closer to needs. One customizing approach utilizes the metabolic response of the infant to guide stepwise increases of protein content [44]. In this method the amount of fortifier is increased as a first step, followed by additions of graded amounts of protein guided by determinations of blood urea nitrogen. The method was shown to increase protein intake to close to requirements and to lead to increased weight and head circumference gain. It is not known how many units are using the Arslanoglu et al. [44] approach, but the number is thought to be modest. The biggest obstacle almost surely is that the additional fortifier and protein have to be measured precisely, a process that is cumbersome and susceptible to errors.

A different customizing approach uses periodic analysis of milk to guide the addition of protein and energy to human milk in order to meet intake targets. The targeted fortification approach was used by Polberger et al. [45] and was shown to achieve protein intakes within 10% of the target level of 3.5 g/kg/day which led to improved growth. Although anecdotal reports indicate that targeted fortification with the use of bedside milk analyzers is being used in some neonatal units, there is only one published report about this method [46]. There does not seem to be consensus regarding how frequently milk should be analyzed, nor whether pools or individual samples should be analyzed. A concern is that bedside analyzers are calibrated to total nitrogen and therefore overestimate human milk protein content by about 17%. The advantage of customizing approaches is that they bring protein intakes close to needs and at the same time safeguard against excessive protein intakes. A disadvantage is that they are labor-intensive and that their use requires time and attention to detail.

Conclusion

Human milk is the preferred feeding for preterm infants because of its immune-protective effects. As human milk is nutritionally inadequate for preterm infants, it must be fortified with nutrients. Current fortification methods are adequate to meet the needs of infants for most nutrients except protein. Fortification is a challenging task because the protein content of expressed human milk is variable and at the same time not known to the caretaker. The most widely used fortification method is one in which a standard amount of fortifier is added to human milk. Powder fortifiers are used most widely and, because their protein content is too low, protein intakes are mostly inadequate. Fortifiers with higher protein content are available. Although customizing methods achieve better protein intakes, they are not used widely because of their demanding nature. With fortifiers that provide higher protein intakes than current powder fortifiers, adequate protein intakes are possible even when using a generalizing approach. The state of the art of human milk fortification is such that satisfactory nutrient intakes are achieved with regularity with the exception of intakes of protein. Progress will depend largely on the availability of better fortifiers.

References

1 Ziegler EE: Breast-milk fortification. Acta Paediatr 2001;90:720–723.

2 El-Mohandes AE, Picard MB, Simmens SJ, Keiser JF: Use of human milk in the intensive care nursery decreases the incidence of nosocomial sepsis. J Perinatol 1997;17:130–134.

3 Hylander MA, Strobino DM, Dhanireddy R: Human milk feedings and infection among very low birth weight infants. Pediatrics 1998;102:3/e38:106.

4 Schanler RJ, Shulman RJ, Lau C, Smith EO, Heitkemper MM: Feeding strategies for premature infants: randomized trial of gastrointestinal priming and tube-feeding method. Pediatrics 1999;103:434–439.

5 Schanler RJ, Shulman RJ, Lau C, Smith EO: Feeding strategies for premature infants: beneficial outcomes of feeding fortified human milk versus preterm formula. Pediatrics 1999;103:1150–1157.

6 Furman L, Taylor G, Minich N, Hack M: The effect of maternal milk on neonatal morbidity of very low-birth-weight infants. Arch Pediatr Adolesc Med 2003;157:66–71.

7 Schanler RJ, Lau C, Hurst NM, Smith EO: Randomized trial of donor human milk versus preterm formula as substitutes for mothers' own milk in the feeding of extremely premature infants. Pediatrics 2005;116:400–406.

8 Sisk PM, Lovelady CA, Dillard RG, Gruber KJ, O'Shea TM: Early human milk feeding is associated with a lower risk of necrotizing enterocolitis in very low birth weight infants. J Perinatol 2007;27:428–433.

9 Patel AL, Johnson TJ, Engstrom JL, Fogg LF, Jegier BJ, Bigger HR, Meier PP: Impact of early human milk on sepsis and health-care costs in very low birth weight infants. J Perinatol 2013;33:514–519.

10 Meinzen-Derr J, Poindexter B, Wrage L, Morrow AL, Stoll B, Donovan EF, for the NICHHD Neonatal Research Network: Role of human milk in extremely low birth weight infants' risk of necrotizing enterocolitis or death. J Perinatol 2009;29:57–62.

11 Simmer K, Metcalf R, Daniels L: The use of breast milk in a neonatal unit and its relationship to protein and energy intake and growth. J Pediatr Child Health 1997;33:55–60.

12 Sisk PM, Lovelady CA, Gruber KJ, Dillard RG, O'Shea TM: Human milk consumption and full enteral feeding among infants who weigh <1,250 grams. Pediatrics 2008;121:e1528–e1533.

13 Shulman RJ, Schanler RJ, Lau C, Heitkemper M, Ou C-N, Smith EO: Early feeding, antenatal glucocorticoids, and human milk decrease intestinal permeability in preterm infants. Pediatr Res 1998;44:519–523.

14 Taylor SN, Basile LA, Ebeling M, Wagner CL: Intestinal permeability in preterm infants by feeding type: mother's milk versus formula. Breastfeed Med 2009;4:11–15.

15 Ziegler EE: Meeting the nutritional needs of the low-birth-weight infant. Ann Nutr Metab 2011;58(suppl 1):8–18.

16 Ehrenkranz RA, Dusick AM, Vohr BR, Wright LL, Wrage LA, Poole WK: Growth in the neonatal intensive care unit influences neurodevelopmental and growth outcomes of extremely low birth weight infants. Pediatrics 2006;117:1253–1261.

17 Lemons JA, Moye L, Hall D, Simmons M: Differences in the composition of preterm and term human milk during early lactation. Pediatr Res 1982;16:113–117.

18 Atkinson SA, Anderson GH, Bryan MH: Human milk: comparison of the nitrogen composition in milk from mothers of premature and full-term infants. Am J Clin Nutr 1980;33:811–815.

19 Weber A, Loui A, Jochum F, Bührer C, Obladen M: Breast milk from mothers of very low birth weight infants: variability in fat and protein content. Acta Paediatr 2001;90:772–775.

20 Lönnerdal B, Forsum E, Hambraeus L: A longitudinal study of the protein, nitrogen, and lactose contents of human milk from Swedish well-nourished mothers. Am J Clin Nutr 1976;29:1127–1133.

21 Colaizy TT, Ziegler EE: Protein content of pooled pasteurized donor human milk. Unpublished data.

22 Arslanoglu S, Moro GE, Ziegler EE, WAMP Working Group on Nutrition: Optimization of human milk fortification for preterm infants: new concepts and recommendations. J Perinat Med 2010;38:233–238.

23 Goldman HI, Goldman JS, Kaufman I, Liebman OB: Late effects of early dietary protein intake on low-birth-weight infants. J Pediatr 1974;85:764–769.

24 De Curtis M, Candusso M, Pieltain C, Rigo J: Effect of fortification on the osmolality of human milk. Arch Dis Child Fetal Neonat Ed 1999;81:F141–F143.

25 Kuschel CA, Harding JE: Multicomponent fortified human milk for promoting growth in preterm infants. Cochrane Database Syst Rev 2004;1:CD000343.

26 Lucas A, Fewtrell MS, Morley R, Lucas PJ, Baker BA, Lister G, Bishop NJ: Randomized outcome trial of human milk fortification and developmental outcome in preterm infants. Am J Clin Nutr 1996;64:142–151.

27 Porcelli P, Schanler R, Greer F, Chan G, Gross S, Mehta N, Spear M, Kerner J, Euler AR: Growth in human milk-fed very low birth weight infants receiving a new human milk fortifier. Ann Nutr Metab 2000;44:2–10.

28 Reis BB, Hall RT, Schanler RJ, Berseth CL, Chan G, Ernst JA, Lemons J, Adamkin D, Baggs G, O'Connor D: Enhanced growth of preterm infants fed a new powdered human milk fortifier: a randomized, controlled trial. Pediatrics 2000;106:581–588.

29 Berseth CL, Van Aerde JE, Gross S, Stolz SI, Harris CL, Hansen JW: Growth, efficacy, and safety of feeding an iron-fortified human milk fortifier. Pediatrics 2004;114:e699–e706.

30 Moya F, Sisk PM, Walsh KR, Berseth CL: A new liquid human milk fortifier and linear growth in preterm infants. Pediatrics 2012;130:e928–e935.

31 Moody GJ, Schanler RJ, Lau C, Shulman RJ: Feeding tolerance in premature infants fed fortified human milk. J Pediatr Gastroenterol Nutr 2000;30:408–412.

32 Ewer AK, Yu VYH: Gastric emptying in pre-term infants: the effect of breast milk fortifier. Acta Paediatr 1996;85:1112–1115.

33 McClure RJ, Newell SJ: Effect of fortifying breast milk on gastric emptying. Arch Dis Child Fetal Neonat Ed 1996;74:F60–F62.

34 Yigit S, Akgoz A, Memisoglu A, Akata D, Ziegler EE: Breast milk fortification: effect on gastric emptying. J Matern Fetal Neonatal Med 2008;21:843–846.

35 Chan GM: Effects of powdered human milk fortifiers on antibacterial actions of human milk. J Perinatol 2002;23:620–623.

36 Chan GM, Lee ML, Rechtman DJ: Effects of a human milk-derived human milk fortifier on the antibacterial actions of human milk. Breastfeed Med 2007;2: 205–208.

37 Ovali F, Ciftci IH, Cetinkaya Z, Bükülmez A: Effects of human milk fortifier on the antimicrobial properties of human milk. J Perinatol 2006;26:761–763.

38 Telang S, Berseth CL, Ferguson PW, Kinder JM, DeRoin M, Petschow PW: Fortifying fresh human milk with commercial powdered human milk fortifiers does not affect bacterial growth during 6 hours at room temperature. J Am Diet Assoc 2005;105: 1567–1572.

39 Santiago MS, Codipilly CN, Potak DC, Schanler RJ: Effect of human milk fortifiers on bacterial growth in human milk. J Perinatol 2005;25:647–649.

40 Sullivan S, Schanler RJ, Kim JH, Patel AL, Trawöger R, Kiechl-Kohlendorfer U, Chan GM, Blanco CL, Abrams S, Cotton CM, et al: An exclusively human milk-based diet is associated with a lower rate of necrotizing enterocolitis than a diet of human milk and bovine milk-based products. J Pediatr 2010;156:562–567.

41 Tillman S, Brandon DH, Silva SG: Evaluation of human milk fortification from time of the first feeding: effects on infants of less than 31 weeks gestational age. J Perinatol 2012;32:525–531.

42 Arslanoglu S, Moro GE, Ziegler EE: Preterm infants fed fortified human milk receive less protein then they need. J Perinatol 2009;29:489–492.

43 Miller J, Makrides M, Gibson RA, McPhee AJ, Stanford TE, Morris S, Ryan P, Collins CT: Effect of increasing protein content of human milk fortifier on growth in preterm infants born at <31 weeks' gestation: a randomized controlled trial. Am J Clin Nutr 2012;95:648–655.

44 Arslanoglu S, Moro GE, Ziegler EE: Adjustable fortification of human milk fed to preterm infants: does it make a difference? J Perinatol 2006;26:614–621.

45 Polberger S, Räihä NCR, Juvonen P, Moro GE, Minoli I, Warm A: Individualized protein fortification of human milk for preterm infants: comparison of ultrafiltrated human milk protein and a bovine whey fortifier. J Pediatr Gastroenterol Nutr 1999;29: 332–338.

46 Rochow N, Fusch G, Choi A, Chessell L, Elliott L, McDonald K, Kuiper E, Purcha M, Turner S, Chan E, et al: Target fortification of breast milk with fat, protein, and carbohydrates for preterm infants. J Pediatr 2013;163:1001–1007.

Ekhard E. Ziegler, MD
Department of Pediatrics, University of Iowa
2501 Crosspark Road
Coralville, IA 52241-8802 (USA)
E-Mail ekhard-ziegler@uiowa.edu

Koletzko B, Poindexter B, Uauy R (eds): Nutritional Care of Preterm Infants: Scientific Basis and Practical Guidelines.
World Rev Nutr Diet. Basel, Karger, 2014, vol 110, pp 228–238 (DOI: 10.1159/000358471)

Approaches to Growth Faltering

Brenda Poindexter

Indiana University School of Medicine, Section of Neonatal-Perinatal Medicine, Riley Hospital for Children at
Indiana University Health, Indianapolis, Ind., USA

Reviewed by Teresa Murguia-Peniche, Foege Fellow at Rollins School of Public Health, Hubert Department of
Global Health, Emory University, Atlanta, Ga., USA; Gert Francois Kirsten, Tygerberg Children's Hospital and
University of Stellenbosch, Cape Town, South Africa

Abstract

Postnatal growth failure remains a nearly universal complication of extreme prematurity. The incidence of postnatal growth failure is inversely related to gestational age. Unfortunately, by the time
growth faltering is recognized, the nutrient deficits that have accumulated can be difficult, if not
impossible, to recover. The perceived severity of illness in the first week can significantly impact decisions made related to early nutritional support. It is becoming increasingly clear that optimizing
nutrient intake in the first few weeks of life is critical to reduce growth faltering. In order to promote
growth and reduce growth faltering, a goal of 120 kcal/kg/day and 3.8 g/kg/day of protein should
be supplied to very low birth weight infants by the end of the first week. A combined strategy of both
parenteral and enteral nutrition is necessary to ensure that adequate protein and energy intake is
delivered and that nutrient deficits are minimized. Finally, careful monitoring of growth – including
both linear and head circumference growth – is necessary to achieve optimal outcomes.

© 2014 S. Karger AG, Basel

Over the past few decades, there has been increased recognition of the incidence and
significance of postnatal growth failure among extremely low birth weight (ELBW)
infants. Despite awareness of the importance of early nutrition, postnatal growth failure remains a nearly universal complication of extreme prematurity. Unfortunately,
by the time growth failure is recognized, the nutrient deficits that have accumulated
can be difficult, if not impossible, to recover. It is becoming increasingly clear that
optimizing nutrient intake in the first few weeks of life is critical to achieving optimal
growth outcomes. Given the challenges inherent in provision of optimal nutritional
support to extremely premature infants, the best approach to growth faltering in this
population is to prevent it altogether. This chapter will review the incidence and definition of growth failure and will discuss strategies to prevent growth faltering.

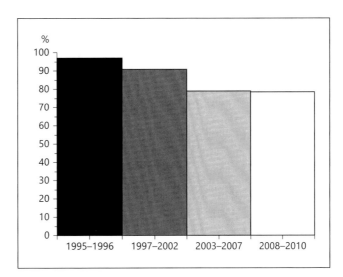

Fig. 1. Incidence of postnatal growth failure in extremely premature infants at 36 weeks' PMA reported by the Eunice Kennedy Shriver Neonatal Research Network.

Incidence of Postnatal Growth Failure

At birth, only 17% of ELBW infants are small for gestational age (GA) [1, 2]. However, after spending several months in the neonatal intensive care unit (NICU), the majority of these infants experience postnatal growth failure, which has typically been defined as an anthropometric parameter <10th percentile for GA. Figure 1 shows the incidence of postnatal growth failure at 36 weeks' postmenstrual age (PMA) for extremely premature infants as reported by investigators in the Eunice Kennedy Shriver NICHD Neonatal Research Network (NRN) over the past two decades. Lemons and colleagues [2] first reported outcomes from a large cohort of very low birth weight (VLBW) infants born in the United States between 1995 and 1996 at centers participating in the NRN. In this cohort, 99% of ELBW and 97% of VLBW infants were found to have postnatal growth failure at 36 weeks' PMA. Among more recent cohorts reported by the NRN, the incidence of growth failure has decreased, presumably due to increased use of early parenteral nutrition and a decrease in use of postnatal steroids, but remains unacceptably high at 79% [1, 3, 4]. Using a large administrative database, Clark et al. [5] reported the incidence of extrauterine growth restriction at the time of hospital discharge as 28% for weight, 34% for length, and 16% for head circumference in a cohort of more than 20,000 premature infants with a GA of 23–34 weeks. The overall incidence of growth failure at 36 weeks' PMA is inversely related to GA [4]. In a large population-based study of extremely premature infants <27 weeks' GA born in Sweden between 2004 and 2007, Sjöström et al. [6] similarly observed severe growth failure for weight, length, and head circumference during the first 28 days after birth.

Risk Factors for Growth Faltering/Postnatal Growth Failure

The first consideration in improving growth outcomes in extremely premature infants is to recognize factors associated with growth failure. Clark et al. [5] reported factors associated with growth restriction at hospital discharge to include male gender, need for assisted ventilation on the first day of life, necrotizing enterocolitis, need for respiratory support at 28 days, and receipt of postnatal steroids. It is also important to recognize the influence of perceived severity of illness on decisions made related to early nutritional support. In order to evaluate this, Ehrenkranz et al. [7] performed a secondary analysis of the cohort of infants enrolled in a randomized clinical trial of parenteral glutamine supplementation. Infants were classified as being more or less 'critically ill' by whether or not they received mechanical ventilation for the first 7 days of life. Less critically ill infants received significantly more nutritional support (both parenteral and enteral) during each of the first 3 weeks of life, started enteral feeds earlier, and achieved enteral feeds sooner than those who were more critically ill. Although critical illness was only defined by mechanical ventilation in the first week, the differences in provision of nutritional support between the groups persisted for several weeks later. There certainly is no evidence to support limiting nutritional support (either parenteral or enteral) simply because the infant is receiving mechanical ventilation.

Consequences of Postnatal Growth Failure

Although the consequences of growth failure have been the focus of many recent studies, the idea that provision of early nutrition plays an important role in outcome of premature infants is not new. Several observational studies have confirmed the strong influence of nutritional practices on growth; these studies are also reviewed in the chapter on 'Nutrition, Growth, and Clinical Outcomes'. Ehrenkranz et al. [8] reported faster weight gain in infants who received parenteral nutrition for shorter periods of time, started on enteral feeds earlier, or achieved full enteral nutrition sooner. Olsen et al. [9] conducted an observational study in premature infants <30 weeks' GA at six different NICUs and found that differences in caloric and protein intake accounted for the largest difference in growth. However, observational studies such as these have the potential to be flawed by differences in management of infants thought to be more or less critically ill.

Ehrenkranz et al. [10] demonstrated the relationship between in-hospital growth velocity and neurodevelopmental and growth outcomes in a cohort of 600 ELBW infants who participated in the NRN growth observational study between 1994 and 1995. These infants were divided into quartiles of in-hospital weight gain and head circumference growth velocity. Infants in the lowest quartile gained an average of 12 g/kg/day while those in the highest quartile gained an average of 21 g/kg/day. After adjusting for confounders and center, in-hospital growth velocity rates exerted a significant and possibly independent effect on neurodevelopmental and growth outcomes at 18 months' corrected age. Infants in the lowest quartile of in-hospital growth had significantly greater odds of cerebral palsy (OR 8.00; 95% CI 2.07–30.78), Bayley Mental Developmental Index (MDI) <70 (OR 2.25; 95% CI 1.03–4.93), and neurodevelopmental impairment at 18 months' corrected age (OR 2.53; 95% CI 1.27–5.03). Similar relationships were observed between in-hospital head circumference growth and neurodevelopmental outcome.

Ramel et al. [11] have recently demonstrated an association between poor linear growth adverse neurodevelopmental outcomes. In this study, growth was evaluated in 62 VLBW infants throughout their initial hospitalization and at 4, 12, and 24 months' corrected age. In this cohort, the mean length z-score was related with illness severity and was associated with lower cognitive function scores at 2 years of age. Although clinicians typically focus on weight gain during the NICU stay, it is likely that linear growth is also an important marker of long-term developmental outcomes.

Definition of Growth Faltering

The vast majority of investigators that have reported postnatal growth failure as an outcome have done so towards the end of the stay in the NICU, typically at 36 weeks' PMA or at the time of hospital discharge. Although this approach is useful from a research standpoint, clinicians must recognize that growth must be assessed over time if growth faltering is to be recognized and reversed.

The reference fetal weight curves published by Alexander et al. [12] have been utilized in many observational studies to determine the percentage of babies whose weight is <10th percentile at 36 weeks' PMA. It is clear that evaluation of weight alone does not give a complete assessment of postnatal growth. Linear growth, head circumference growth, and some index of body composition are also important to assess. Linear growth is closely associated with lean body mass and therefore may also have important prognostic implications for other long-term outcomes such as risk of diabetes and adult-onset cardiovascular disease. Head circumference growth has also been associated with neurodevelopmental outcomes in this population.

Identification of Growth Faltering in the NICU

Principles related to monitoring of postnatal growth in the NICU are discussed extensively in the chapter on 'Nutrition, Growth and Clinical Outcomes'. To reinforce the importance of following growth, the infant's growth curve should also be reviewed with the parents during rounds whenever possible. Weight should be measured daily and length and head circumference weekly. Olsen et al. [13] have recently validated new gender-specific intrauterine weight, length, and head circumference growth curves using a contemporary, large sample of infants from the United States. Fenton et al. [14] have also published intrauterine curves for weight, length, and head circumference, but it is important to note that different populations were utilized to create the weight curves and the length/head circumference curves. Growth faltering may be identified not only in those infants with an anthropometric parameter <10th percentile for GA, but also in those who growth trajectory falls to a lower percentile than that established once birth weight has been regained.

The rate of growth velocity should be evaluated on a weekly basis as an important in order to identify growth faltering and to review goals of nutritional support. Most clinicians have generally accepted a goal of 15 g/kg/day for weight gain. This goal, however, likely underestimates the growth velocity necessary to achieve optimal growth and outcomes. In a large, multicenter cohort study of 1,187 extremely premature infants (23–27 weeks' GA), Martin et al. [15] observed extrauterine growth restriction in 75% of the infants at 28 days of age despite a weight gain velocity of 15 g/kg/day. The mean growth velocity from the Olsen curves was 16 g/kg/day for weight, 1.4 cm/week for length, and 0.9 cm/week for head circumference growth [13].

Goals of Early Nutritional Support

The goals of early nutritional support in extremely premature infants are to promote growth and nutrient accretion comparable to that of the fetus at the same GA, minimize the risk of necrotizing enterocolitis, and to optimize neurodevelopment and long-term health outcomes. Numerous observational and randomized clinical trials have demonstrated the benefits of early parenteral and enteral nutritional support on short-term outcomes such as protein balance and in-hospital weight gain, but the extent to which changes in early parenteral and enteral nutritional support practices will result in further improvements in growth and neurodevelopmental outcomes merits further study.

Extreme prematurity should be viewed as a nutritional emergency. The ELBW infant has glucose stores of only 200 kcal at birth and will lose 1–2% of body protein per day with intravenous glucose alone [16]. In contrast, the fetus at the same GA is supplied with upwards of 3.5 g/kg/day of amino acids by the placenta – an amount that is in excess of needs of protein accretion. Embleton et al. [17] have calculated the cumulative protein deficit in infants <31 weeks' GA at birth for postnatal days 0 through 13. The cumulative protein deficit by the end of the second postnatal week was estimated to be approximately 18 g/kg, assuming a protein requirement of 3 g/kg/day and the cumulative energy deficit was 600 kcal/kg, assuming a requirement of 120 kcal/kg/day [17]. If requirements are estimated using Ziegler's factorial method [18], then even greater deficits occur.

Optimizing Early Nutritional Support Is the Best Strategy to Reduce Growth Faltering

If growth faltering is to be prevented it is clear that clinicians must focus on ensuring adequate intake of both protein and energy during the first few weeks of life. The body of evidence describing the association between early protein and energy intake and outcomes is growing. Protein intake in the first 2 weeks of life in ELBW infants is an independent positive prognostic determinant of growth [19]. In a multicenter observational study, Olsen et al. [13] found that differences in weight gain velocity at different NICUs could be predicted by early protein intake. In addition, Stephens et al. [20] found a correlation between protein and energy intake in the first week of life and the MDI on the Bayley Scales of Infant Development. Average protein and energy intake in the first week of life was 1.8 g/kg/day and 60 kcal/kg/day, respectively. In this observational study, every 1 g/kg/day of protein intake was associated with an 8.2-point increase in MDI and every 10 kcal/kg/day of energy intake was associated with a 4.6-point increase in MDI.

Senterre and Rigo [21] conducted a prospective observational study in premature infants with a birth weight <1,250 g. In this study, nutritional support in the first week of life was optimized based on recent recommendations, including a goal of achieving 120 kcal/kg/day and 3.8 g/kg/day of protein intake by the end of the first week. The nutritional protocol included a combined strategy of early parenteral nutrition and early introduction of minimal enteral nutrition with human milk. Remarkably, these investigators were able to demonstrate that postnatal weight loss was limited to the first 3 days of life and that the incidence of postnatal growth failure was significantly reduced.

Martin et al. [15] also found a positive association between nutritional support at day 7 and growth velocity between 7 and 28 days in extremely premature infants, further reinforcing the idea that nutrient provision in the first week is most crucial.

Early Intravenous Amino Acids

Based on the sum of currently available evidence, providing 2.0–3.0 g/kg/day of amino acids to ELBW infants as soon as possible after birth is a reasonable recommendation. In order to achieve fetal delivery rates of protein, the intravenous protein requirement for the infant born at 24–25 weeks' GA is 3.75–4.0 g/kg/day.

Several randomized clinical trials of amino acid dose and advancement strategy have evaluated the short-term tolerance, effect on protein balance, and safety of early parenteral amino acids. Early studies compared the particular amino acid dose with glucose alone, as clinical practice as recently as 10 years ago included a strategy of supplying only intravenous glucose for the first several days after birth. Despite difference in study populations and composition of the commercial amino acid solutions, all studies demonstrated positive nitrogen balance in response to parenteral amino acids and improved protein balance with higher amino acid intake [22–24]. A secondary analysis of ELBW infants enrolled in the NRN randomized clinical trial of parenteral glutamine supplementation found that infants who received early amino acids had significantly improved growth outcomes (weight, length, and head circumference) at 36 weeks' PMA with an odds ratio of 4.2 (95% CI 2.4–7.5) for weight <10th percentile for infants who did not receive early amino acids (defined as minimum of 3 g/kg/day in the first 5 days) [25]. At the 18-month follow-up visit, the percentage of infants with head circumference <10th and <5th percentile was significantly greater in male infants who did not receive early amino acids.

One of the easiest strategies to ensure adequate delivery of protein is the use of a 'stock' or 'starter' amino acid solution. These solutions can be made in advance by the compounding pharmacy and can be stored at room temperature for up to 1 week. One approach is to mix a 5% neonatal amino acid solution with 7.5% dextrose in a 250-ml bag. If the solution is run at 60 ml/kg/day, the amino acid delivery equals 3 g/kg/day. Given the often rapidly fluctuating fluid and dextrose requirements of extremely premature infants, other fluids can be co-infused with the starter solution as needed to meet total fluid, dextrose, and electrolyte needs. Caution must be taken to ensure that the starter amino acid solution delivery rate is not increased to avoid inadvertent delivery of excessive protein. Other investigators have advocated the use of premixed parenteral nutrition solutions [26].

Differences between Prescribed and Actual Intake

To troubleshoot suboptimal growth it is absolutely critical that the clinicians know what the baby is actually receiving. Clinicians must also pay close attention to differences between the prescribed and actual intake of macronutrients in neonates. Due to interruptions in delivery of parenteral and/or enteral nutrition, in some cases the actual intake can be as much as 10–20% less than what is prescribed. Factors contributing to differences between prescribed and actual intake include enteral feeds being held, interruptions in parenteral and enteral nutrition for transfusion of blood products, medications not compatible with parenteral nutrition, and the need to change fluids due to glucose or electrolyte imbalance. If unrecognized, these differences between intended and actual delivery of nutrients can add to the cumulative deficit experienced by these most vulnerable infants, especially during the first few weeks in the NICU.

During the transition to enteral feeds, there is also the potential to provide suboptimal nutrition. One of the dilemmas that the clinician faces is how to plan for the possibility of feeding intolerance. However, if parenteral nutrition is ordered based on the assumption that the infant will tolerate the increase in enteral feeds on a given day and the infant subsequently misses a feed or is made NPO, the parenteral nutrition prescription may no longer be adequate. In most institutions, new parenteral

Table 1. Comparison of protein intake for enteral nutrition at 150 ml/kg/day

	Protein, g/kg/day
Unfortified preterm human milk (assume 1.2–1.4 g/dl)	1.8–2.1
Unfortified donor human milk (assume 1.0 g/dl)	1.5
Human milk + liquid HMF*, 80 kcal/100 ml	3.2–4.2
'High protein' premature formula	4.0–4.2
Premature formula, 80 kcal/100 ml	3.6
Transition/post-discharge formula	3.1
Term formula	2.1

* HMF supplies an additional 1.0–1.4 g protein per 100 ml fortified human milk when prepared according to the manufacturer's recommendations.

nutrition cannot be compounded until the following day, resulting in several hours of inadequate nutrient delivery. One alternative approach is to write for full parenteral nutrition as the enteral volume is being advanced and simply run at a lower rate to account for the volume of enteral feeds. Using this strategy, the parenteral nutrition can be increased if the baby does not tolerate enteral feeds.

Optimizing Enteral Protein Intake

Table 1 provides a comparison of the amount of protein supplied when a variety of enteral options are provided at 150 ml/kg/day. It is important to note that only fortified human milk or 'high protein' preterm formula deliver 4 g/kg/day of protein at this enteral volume. For infants that require restriction of fluid volume, increasing the caloric density may be necessary but it is also important to recognize that sufficient protein and energy must be provided to ensure proportional and optimal growth. Compared to standard preterm formula, the use of high protein formula (3.6 g/100 kcal) has been shown to increase protein accretion and improve weight gain [27].

Protein Content of Human Milk

Despite recognition that fortification of human milk is necessary to meet the recommended goals for protein intake, fortification of human milk is often delayed until a particular feeding volume is reached, leading to further protein deficits. In addition, the makers of commercially available human milk fortifiers (HMF) assume a protein content of 1.4–1.6 g/dl in human milk and do not account for the normal decrease in the protein content of human milk over time. Consequently, clinicians may assume they are delivering more protein than they actually are.

Radmacher et al. [28] evaluated the protein and energy content of human milk at different points in lactation and also the macronutrient content of donor milk using near-infrared spectroscopy. Using standard fortification recipes, they also compared the actual versus the intended protein and energy content of the milk. At all stages of lactation, there were significant differences in protein and energy content from what was predicted, with the greatest differences being seen in samples of pooled donor human milk. Specifically, the mean protein content of donor milk that was analyzed in this study was 0.9 g/dl and the energy content was only 48.3 kcal/100 ml. Consequently, using typical presumed values for the composition of human milk has the potential to impact growth.

In a large randomized clinical trial of donor human milk and preterm formula, weight gain was lowest in the donor milk group, despite the fact that infants in the donor milk group received greater milk intakes and more nutritional supplements [29].

Multicomponent fortification of human milk is associated with short-term improvements in weight gain, linear growth, and head circumference growth in premature infants. Evidence is lacking, however, that human milk fortification has an impact on long-term growth or neurodevelopment. Nonetheless, future research should be directed toward comparisons between different fortification strategies to evaluate both short- and long-term outcomes in search of the optimal composition of fortifiers.

Arslanoglu et al. [30] have described an adjustable fortification of human milk strategy. They performed a randomized trial in which they compared fortification with HMF plus bovine whey protein to standard fortification in a group of premature infants to test the hypothesis that higher protein intake would result in improved weight gain. The intervention group received incremental increases in protein guided by twice-weekly measurements of BUN. The average protein intake in the group receiving the adjustable fortification was 3.2 g/kg/day while the control group received an average intake of 2.9 g/kg/day of protein. The infants who received the additional bovine whey protein had greater weight gain and head circumference gain and these differences in growth correlated with protein intake, making this strategy a safe and effective strategy to improve growth. This adjustable fortification regimen has recently been successfully implemented as a means to improve protein intake in several units in Italy [31]. Once attempts at the breast begin, some supplemental feeds with higher caloric density may be needed in addition to breastfeeding attempts to maintain energy and protein intake at the level needed to sustain growth.

Growth following Hospital Discharge

In addition to recognizing growth faltering in the NICU, clinicians must also focus on the growth of extremely premature infants following hospital discharge. At 18 months' corrected age, nearly half of former appropriate-for-gestational age (AGA) infants will have weight <10th percentile [32]. Factors associated with weight less <10th percentile at 30 months corrected age are lower birth weight, white race, male gender, SGA at birth, and moderate to severe cerebral palsy [33]. At preschool age (30 months' corrected age), having weight or head circumference <10th percentile was associated with lower motor and cognitive scores on the Bayley. Clearly, for those infants who do experience growth faltering in the NICU, catch-up growth is important, but the optimal rate at which this should be accomplished remains uncertain. The chapter on 'Feeding the Preterm Infant after Discharge' provides a comprehensive discussion on post-discharge nutrition.

Key Conclusions

- Postnatal growth failure remains a nearly universal complication of extreme prematurity.
- Growth faltering is associated with poor neurodevelopmental and growth outcomes at 18–24 months corrected age.
- Optimizing early nutritional support is the best strategy to reduce/prevent growth faltering.
- In order to minimize postnatal weight loss and reduce growth faltering, VLBW infants should receive 3.8 g/kg/day of protein and 120 kcal/kg/day by the end of the first week; this intake should be supplied with a combination of parenteral and enteral nutrition.
- Monitoring weight alone may give an incomplete assessment of growth faltering – proportional growth must be considered more than absolute weight gain.

References

1 Fanaroff AA, Stoll BJ, Wright LL, et al: Trends in neonatal morbidity and mortality for very low birth-weight infants. Am J Obstet Gynecol 2007;196:147. e1–e8.
2 Vohr BR, Oh W, Stewart EJ, et al: Comparison of costs and referral rates of three universal newborn hearing screening protocols. J Pediatr 2001;139:238–244.
3 Poindexter B, Hintz S, Langer J, Ehrenkranz R: Have we caught up? Growth and neurodevelopmental outcomes in extremely premature infants. E-PAS 2013;1395.2.
4 Stoll BJ, Hansen NI, Bell EF, et al: Neonatal outcomes of extremely preterm infants from the NICHD Neonatal Research Network. Pediatrics 2010;126: 443–456.
5 Clark RH, Thomas P, Peabody J: Extrauterine growth restriction remains a serious problem in prematurely born neonates. Pediatrics 2003;111:986–990.
6 Sjöström ES, Öhlund I, Ahlsson F, et al: Nutrient intakes independently affect growth in extremely preterm infants: results from a population-based study. Acta Paediatr 2013;102:1067–1074.
7 Ehrenkranz RA, Das A, Wrage LA, et al: Early nutrition mediates the influence of severity of illness on extremely LBW infants. Pediatr Res 2011;69:522–529.
8 Ehrenkranz RA, Younes N, Lemons JA, et al: Longitudinal growth of hospitalized very low birth weight infants. Pediatrics 1999;104:280–289.
9 Olsen IE, Richardson DK, Schmid CH, Ausman LM, Dwyer JT: Intersite differences in weight growth velocity of extremely premature infants. Pediatrics 2002;110:1125–1132.

10 Ehrenkranz RA, Dusick AM, Vohr BR, Wright LL, Wrage LA, Poole WK: Growth in the neonatal intensive care unit influences neurodevelopmental and growth outcomes of extremely low birth weight infants. Pediatrics 2006;117:1253–1261.

11 Ramel SE, Demerath EW, Gray HL, Younge N, Boys C, Georgieff MK: The relationship of poor linear growth velocity with neonatal illness and two-year neurodevelopment in preterm infants. Neonatology 2012;102:19–24.

12 Alexander GR, Himes JH, Kaufman RB, Mor J, Kogan M: A United States national reference for fetal growth. Obstet Gynecol 1996;87:163–168.

13 Olsen IE, Groveman SA, Lawson ML, Clark RH, Zemel BS: New intrauterine growth curves based on United States data. Pediatrics 2010;125:e214–e224.

14 Fenton TR, Nasser R, Eliasziw M, Kim JH, Bilan D, Sauve R: Validating the weight gain of preterm infants between the reference growth curve of the fetus and the term infant. BMC Pediatr 2013;13:92.

15 Martin CR, Brown YF, Ehrenkranz RA, et al: Nutritional practices and growth velocity in the first month of life in extremely premature infants. Pediatrics 2009;124:649–657.

16 Hertz DE, Karn CA, Liu YM, Liechty EA, Denne SC: Intravenous glucose suppresses glucose production but not proteolysis in extremely premature newborns. J Clin Invest 1993;92:1752–1758.

17 Embleton NE, Pang N, Cooke RJ: Postnatal malnutrition and growth retardation: an inevitable consequence of current recommendations in preterm infants? Pediatrics 2001;107:270–273.

18 Ziegler EE: Protein requirements of very low birth weight infants. J Pediatr Gastroenterol Nutr 2007; 45(suppl 3):S170–S174.

19 Berry MA, Abrahamowicz M, Usher RH: Factors associated with growth of extremely premature infants during initial hospitalization. Pediatrics 1997;100: 640–646.

20 Stephens BE, Walden RV, Gargus RA, et al: First-week protein and energy intakes are associated with 18-month developmental outcomes in extremely low birth weight infants. Pediatrics 2009;123:1337–1343.

21 Senterre T, Rigo J: Optimizing early nutritional support based on recent recommendations in VLBW infants and postnatal growth restriction. J Pediatr Gastroenterol Nutr 2011;53:536–542.

22 Ibrahim HM, Jeroudi MA, Baier RJ, Dhanireddy R, Krouskop RW: Aggressive early total parental nutrition in low-birth-weight infants. J Perinatol 2004;24: 482–486.

23 Te Braake FW, van den Akker CH, Wattimena DJ, Huijmans JG, van Goudoever JB: Amino acid administration to premature infants directly after birth. J Pediatr 2005;147:457–461.

24 Thureen PJ, Melara D, Fennessey PV, Hay WW Jr: Effect of low versus high intravenous amino acid intake on very low birth weight infants in the early neonatal period. Pediatr Res 2003;53:24–32.

25 Poindexter BB, Langer JC, Dusick AM, Ehrenkranz RA: Early provision of parenteral amino acids in extremely low birth weight infants: relation to growth and neurodevelopmental outcome. J Pediatr 2006; 148:300–305.

26 Rigo J, Senterre T: Intrauterine-like growth rates can be achieved with premixed parenteral nutrition solution in preterm infants. J Nutr 2013;143:2066S–2070S.

27 Cooke R, Embleton N, Rigo J, Carrie A, Haschke F, Ziegler E: High protein pre-term infant formula: effect on nutrient balance, metabolic status and growth. Pediatr Res 2006;59:265–270.

28 Radmacher PG, Lewis S, Adamkin DH: Variability in preterm and donor human milk macronutrients affects fortification. E-PAS 2012;1335.5.

29 Schanler RJ, Lau C, Hurst NM, Smith EO: Randomized trial of donor human milk versus preterm formula as substitutes for mothers' own milk in the feeding of extremely premature infants. Pediatrics 2005;116:400–406.

30 Arslanoglu S, Moro GE, Ziegler EE: Adjustable fortification of human milk fed to preterm infants: does it make a difference? J Perinatol 2006;26:614–621.

31 Arslanoglu S, Bertino E, Coscia A, Tonetto P, Giuliani F, Moro GE: Update of adjustable fortification regimen for preterm infants: a new protocol. J Biol Regul Homeost Agents 2012;26(suppl):65–67.

32 Dusick AM, Poindexter BB, Ehrenkranz RA, Lemons JA: Growth failure in the preterm infant: can we catch up? Semin Perinatol 2003;27:302–310.

33 Dusick A, Poindexter B, Ehrenkranz R, Langer J, Vohr B: Catch-up growth in extremely low birth weight infants in early childhood. E-PAS 2005;1450.

Brenda Poindexter, MD, MS
Indiana University School of Medicine, Section of Neonatal-Perinatal Medicine
Riley Hospital for Children at Indiana University Health
699 Riley Hospital Dr. RR208, Indianapolis, IN 46202 (USA)
E-Mail bpoindex@iu.edu

Koletzko B, Poindexter B, Uauy R (eds): Nutritional Care of Preterm Infants: Scientific Basis and Practical Guidelines.
World Rev Nutr Diet. Basel, Karger, 2014, vol 110, pp 239–252 (DOI: 10.1159/000358473)

Preterm Nutrition and the Lung

Fernando Moya

Betty Cameron Women and Children's Hospital, Wilmington, N.C., USA

Reviewed by Francis B. Mimouni, Dana Dwek Children's Hospital and Lis Maternity Hospital, Tel Aviv Medical
Center, Tel Aviv, Israel; Josef Neu, Department of Pediatrics, University of Florida, Gainsville, Fla., USA

Abstract

Experimental and clinical evidence show that fetal and neonatal nutrition and metabolism can markedly modulate pulmonary growth, development, and function, as well as long-term lung health and disease risks. Intrauterine growth restriction has been linked to an increased risk for respiratory distress syndrome and chronic lung disease, while excessive fetal growth reduced forced expiratory volume. Postnatal undernutrition adversely affected pulmonary function in animal models and was associated to a higher risk of chronic lung disease in very low birth weight infants. The supply of specific nutrients to very low birth weight infants, including fluids, protein, carbohydrates, inositol, docosahexaenoic acid, calcium, phosphorus and the vitamins A and E has been associated with lung development and function and deserves further evaluation. In infants with evolving or established chronic lung disease, excess fluid administration and high intravenous glucose infusion rates should be avoided and the provision of vitamin A be considered. Opportunities exist for further research relating to neonatal nutrition and lung health, for example exploring optimal strategies and effects of providing vitamin A, docosahexaenoic acid and intravenous lipid emulsions.

© 2014 S. Karger AG, Basel

Nutrition is a key factor for normal development of all fetal organs and their function. In this chapter we will describe what is known about fetal and neonatal nutrition and pulmonary growth, development, function and health from a preventive perspective, and also once pulmonary function is abnormal, i.e. bronchopulmonary dysplasia (BPD). Even though there is abundant animal experimentation about the role of nutrition in pulmonary growth and function, less is known in the clinical arena about this relationship. Moreover, there is a relative paucity of large, well-controlled clinical trials in which a nutritional intervention has had any aspect of neonatal pulmonary function as its primary outcome. This notwithstanding, more recent experimental and clinical research is bridging the gap between nutrition and pulmonary function. The role of nutrition in the prevention and management of BPD has been reviewed recently [1–3].

Influence of Nutrition during Pregnancy, Fetal and Neonatal Periods on Neonatal Lung Function

Normal lung development occurs in distinct stages, all of which can be affected by impaired availability of oxygen and other nutrients. Lung growth accelerates during the third trimester of pregnancy, but in humans most alveolar growth still occurs after birth. Increasing evidence, mostly in animal models but also in humans, clearly demonstrates the short- and long-term impact of prenatal nutritional deficiencies and intrauterine growth restriction (IUGR) on lung growth and function [4]. IUGR in fetal sheep results in decreased alveolarization and pulmonary vascular growth via complex mechanisms involving vascular endothelial growth factors, endothelial nitric oxide synthase and insulin [5]. Other reported alterations of lung structure and function after IUGR include decreases in lung weight, protein and DNA content and abnormalities of the surfactant system and type II pneumocytes. Some of these effects may be due in part to epigenetic mechanisms. Recent studies in fetal rats have suggested that IUGR alone may make the lung more vulnerable to other postnatal insults and also that these effects may be different depending on fetal sex [6]. In rats some of the fetal lung alterations brought about by IUGR may be modifiable with nutritional interventions such as maternal supplementation of docosahexaenoic acid (DHA) [7]. Also, administration of an oral DHA supplement to pregnant mice increases the amount of surfactant in amniotic fluid and the lungs of their preterm fetuses [8]. This opens the door for examining this question in clinical trials. Clinically, preterm infants with IUGR seem to be at higher risk for respiratory distress syndrome and chronic lung disease [9–11].

Other micronutrients play a major role in normal fetal and neonatal lung growth and susceptibility to postnatal pulmonary infection. Vitamin A deficiency in pregnant rats is associated with abnormal fetal/neonatal lung morphology and differentiation of critical cell lines as well as altered expression of key developmental lung genes [12]. In this animal model, some of these abnormalities can be restored with early postnatal supplementation of vitamin A [13]. The possibility of decreasing respiratory morbidity in neonates by administering vitamin A has been studied clinically (see later sections). Recent data have related low cord blood serum levels of 25(OH) vitamin D to a higher risk of lower respiratory tract infections [14].

Not only IUGR, but also excessive fetal growth can affect lung function. Recently, a 14% lower forced expiratory volume was shown among term infants born to mothers with a history of asthma who had a higher BMI compared with their normally proportioned counterparts. This effect was much larger than the 7% observed among term neonates from mothers who smoked from the same study, although it remains unclear whether this was due to maternal nutrition during pregnancy or other factors [15].

Postnatal undernutrition also has distinct effects on several aspects of neonatal lung function. These have been characterized well in animal models [for reviews, see

Table 1. Effect of restricted versus liberal water intake in selected neonatal outcomes [from 20]

Outcome	Studies n	Participants n	Risk ratio (95% CI)
PDA	4	526	0.52 (0.37–0.73)
NEC	4	526	0.43 (0.21–0.87)
BPD	4	526	0.85 (0.63–1.14)
Death	5	582	0.81 (0.54–1.23)

1, 2]. In neonatal piglets, mild postnatal undernutrition brought about by reduced food intake changes the oxidative capacity and the expression of myosin heavy chain isoforms in the diaphragm [16]. To what extent this occurs in human infants is not known.

Clinically, very low birth weight (VLBW) infants that grow along the lower quartiles during their neonatal stay are at higher risk for neurodevelopmental problems as well as chronic pulmonary problems [17]. More recent data derived from a large randomized trial of parenteral glutamine supplementation have linked early nutrition with the severity of illness on extremely low birth weight (ELBW) infants. In this trial, less critically ill infants received more total nutritional support during the first 3 weeks after delivery and had less moderate/severe BPD. Moreover, the influence of critical illness on adverse outcomes seemed to be related to total daily energy intake [18].

Importance of Nutrition for Preservation or Sustenance of Normal Neonatal Lung Function

Use of Fluids
Although water is not considered a nutrient, it is the most abundant component of the fetal and neonatal body. Moreover, it serves as the vehicle for enteral and parenteral administration of nutrients. Water homeostasis is particularly important in more immature infants in which the enteral route is often not available and most nutritional support is provided parenterally. Pulmonary edema due to fluid overload can contribute to decreases of pulmonary compliance and increased airway resistance. Also, a relationship between a high fluid intake and an increased risk of cardiorespiratory morbidity as well as necrotizing enterocolitis (NEC) has been reported [19, 20]. A recent systematic review of five randomized controlled trials of restricted versus liberal fluid intake during the neonatal period showed a considerable reduction in patent ductus arteriosus (PDA) and NEC, but only a trend towards less BPD (table 1). These studies, however, differed in terms of the populations enrolled, the duration of the intervention and the target volumes for restricted or liberal fluid intake. This notwithstanding, from the aforementioned studies included in this systematic review, for

infants <1,750–2,000 g initial fluid intakes in the 60–80 ml/kg/day and progressive increases to a maximum of 120–140 ml/kg/day by days 5–7 may confer clinical advantages over starting with higher intakes and reaching total volumes above those values during the first week after birth. These recommendations cannot be extended to infants weighing <750 g at birth since very few of them were enrolled in these trials. Indeed, neonatal lung function can be best preserved by avoiding free water overload and by close monitoring of weight, urine output and electrolytes [21].

Role of Specific Nutrients in Neonatal Lung Function

Carbohydrates

They are the primary source of energy for neonates. Because in ELBW and VLBW infants the parenteral route is used preferentially during the first several days after birth, glucose is the main source of carbohydrates utilized. The oxidation of glucose results in higher production of carbon dioxide (CO_2) than fat oxidation. Thus, when energy generation is derived mainly from oxidation of carbohydrates the respiratory quotient (RQ), the ratio between generated CO_2 and consumed oxygen (O_2), is higher than if fats predominate as the energy source. These aspects have been studied well in adults.

Normal O_2 consumption of preterm infants without respiratory distress is around 6–7 ml/kg/min and resting energy expenditure (REE) oscillates around 50–60 kcal/kg/day. This can be elevated among infants with signs of severe respiratory distress during the first several days after birth [22]. However, given that there is a lesser need for energy destined for growth at that time, these increased requirements can be met with the current approach to maximize early parenteral and enteral nutrition. Administration of enough intravenous glucose to correct hypoglycemia results in increases of O_2 consumption and RQ in small for gestational age infants and those born to diabetic women [23]. A hypermetabolic state with increased O_2 consumption and RQ seems to persist in small for gestational age infants beyond correction of the low glucose. The impact of changes in intravenous glucose administration on O_2 consumption, CO_2 production and REE has also been studied among infants evolving to or with established BPD [24, 25]. In these infants, loading with up to 12 mg/kg/min of intravenous glucose results in about a 20% increase in O_2 consumption and REE; however, in one study these changes were not readily observed among control infants of similar gestation but without BPD [24]. Avoidance of high glucose infusion rates >10–12 mg/kg/min may be of importance among infants who have restrictions to eliminate CO_2 due to lung disease. Infants with BPD exhibit an elevated REE that may be responsible for their commonly observed growth failure [26, 27]. Among these infants, respiratory rate is the single most important determinant of energy expenditure [28]. How this needs to be managed among infants evolving to or with established BPD is discussed later in this chapter.

Inositol

This is a six-carbon sugar alcohol found mostly as part of phosphatidylinositol and is provided in high amounts with human milk. This phospholipid is involved in surfactant synthesis [29]. Changes in fetal rat lung surfactant correlate with plasma inositol levels [29]. Moreover, infants with a more significant drop in serum inositol levels after delivery have a more severe course of respiratory distress syndrome [30]. Several small trials have ascertained whether inositol administration started after birth can decrease or ameliorate neonatal morbidity in preterm infants. These have been summarized in a recent systematic review [31]. Cumulative data suggest a decrease in neonatal death (risk ratio 0.53, 95% CI 0.31–0.91), severe retinopathy of prematurity (risk ratio 0.09, 95% CI 0.01–0.67) and severe intraventricular hemorrhage (risk ratio 0.53, 95% CI 0.31–0.80), but no effect on BPD at 28 days or 36 weeks corrected gestational age (risk ratio 0.78, 95% CI 0.54–1.13 and 1.30, 0.64–2.64, respectively). Nonetheless, there is a need for a larger randomized trial of this intervention to determine whether it should be recommended for wide use in neonates. While first data on the pharmacokinetics and safety of intravenous inositol application in immature preterm infants have been reported [32], currently no intravenous preparation is available for use in VLBW infants.

Protein

It is abundantly clear that provision of parenteral or enteral protein sources soon after birth to newborn infants is critical to prevent a negative nitrogen balance and stimulate protein accretion [33]. This is especially true for more preterm neonates. Several authors have characterized changes in ventilatory responses of preterm infants after administration of specific amino acids. Parenteral administration of solutions enriched with branched amino acids like leucine can modulate respiration [34]. This intervention also results in short-term increases in compliance and decreases in total pulmonary resistance [35]. There may also be a beneficial effect in reducing apneic episodes. However, these findings have yet to be corroborated in large clinical trials. Porcelli et al. [36] reported less BPD in a small cohort of ELBW infants given up to 4 g/kg/day of parenteral protein compared with historical controls that received a lesser intake. However, in a previous randomized trial of an aggressive nutritional regimen, which included a protein intake up to 3.5 g/kg/day, Wilson et al. [37] failed to demonstrate improvements in pulmonary outcomes among preterm infants. Supplementation of the amino acid glutamine in parenteral nutrition solutions was studied in a large randomized trial of ELBW infants [38]. No beneficial effects on pulmonary outcomes or infectious morbidity were reported. However, among all participants in that trial, less moderate and severe BPD was seen among those infants who received more total nutritional support during the first 3 weeks after birth [18].

Trials comparing protein supplementation of breast milk with protein alone or with multiple components including protein versus no supplementation (lower protein intake) have not shown benefits in terms of pulmonary morbidity [39]. Moreover, more recent trials comparing protein supplementation of breast milk versus driving protein

Table 2. High-dose supplementation of DHA and pulmonary outcomes of preterm infants [from 45]

Outcome	High/standard DHA, n	High DHA, n (%)	Standard DHA, n (%)	Adjusted RR (95% CI)[1]	Adjusted p
Oxygen at 36 weeks	319/334	60 (18.8)	84 (25.1)	0.77 (0.59–1.02)	0.07
Birth weight <1,250 g	145/149	50 (34.5)	70 (47.0)	0.75 (0.57–0.98)	0.04
Birth weight ≥1,250 g	174/185	10 (5.7)	14 (7.6)	0.81 (0.37–1.80)	0.61
Male infants	171/182	32 (18.7)	51 (28.0)	0.67 (0.47–0.96)	0.03
Female infants	148/152	28 (18.9)	33 (21.7)	0.94 (0.64–1.39)	0.76

[1] Adjusted for gestational age at delivery and gender except in gender subgroup analysis.

supplementation to a higher protein intake of up to 4.5 g/kg/day also have not shown improvements in pulmonary problems, although these interventions usually started past 2 weeks after birth and enrolled infants at lower risk for pulmonary morbidity [40–42].

Triglycerides and Fatty Acids

Triglycerides and fatty acids are not only critical components of the diet as sources of non-protein energy, but some long-chain polyunsaturated fatty acids (LC-PUFA) also serve critical functions in development of the brain and retina. In addition, they play important pro-inflammatory (n–6) or anti-inflammatory (n–3) roles and can act as immune modulators [43]. However, less is known about their role in lung growth or function. In a rat model of IUGR, alterations of the lung are modifiable with maternal supplementation of DHA [7]. In mice, addition of DHA to the maternal diet at critical times of pregnancy increases surfactant in amniotic fluid and the fetal lung [8]. DHA activates one of the key enzymes involved in surfactant synthesis and increasing its intake improves surfactant lipid concentrations in preterm baboons [44].

In a randomized trial of maternal DHA supplementation using tuna oil as a way to increase this LC-PUFA in breast milk (mothers consumed six 500-mg DHA-rich tuna oil capsules per day), a lower risk of BPD was seen among infants with birth weight <1,250 g and in male infants (table 2) [45]. Infants in this trial received the enriched human milk feedings, which achieved about 1% of total fatty acids as DHA, only several days after delivery; therefore, it is likely that their DHA levels were either low due to their prematurity or dropped from birth given that parenteral sources of DHA were not readily available. Recent data have shown that ELBW infants have low levels of DHA after birth and that those levels drop further during the first several weeks, especially with prolonged administration of lipid solutions that do not contain DHA [46]. Moreover, DHA levels drop further among infants that go on to develop BPD versus those that do not [47].

The standard intravenous source of lipids in the USA is based on soybean oil and does not provide any appreciable amounts of DHA. In contrast, lipid emulsions with part of the triglycerides comprised of marine oil are used in neonatal units in many other countries around the world. Lipid emulsions based on soybean oil as the only triglyceride source lead to high blood and tissue levels of n–6 PUFAs, which are precursors of potent pro-inflammatory mediators. An older randomized study of early administration of a soybean oil lipid emulsion to preterm infants <1,000 g suggested an increased risk of death for infants between 600 and 800 g birth weight and no improvements on the incidence of BPD [48]. Moreover, an additional study of early parenteral lipid administration in preterm infants suggested an increased severity of chronic lung disease with this practice [49]. A systematic review of parenteral lipid administration did not show evidence of benefit on neonatal respiratory outcomes with early (within the first several days after birth) versus delayed initiation of intravenous lipid solutions [50]. However, most of these studies utilized lipid preparations devoid of DHA. Newer mixed parenteral lipid emulsions with fish oils (e.g. SMOF Lipid™, Lipidem™, Lipoplus™) do provide preformed EPA and DHA; however, it is unclear whether their use will benefit in any way neonatal lung function. It is plausible to think that preventing the postnatal drop in DHA until an adequate enteral supply of LC-PUFAs are established may benefit neonatal lung function, especially in view of the aforementioned findings by Manley et al. [45]. However, this hypothesis has not been tested appropriately in clinical trials.

There have been many trials examining the role of supplementing LC-PUFAs in preterm and term infants, however they have focused primarily on brain- and retina-related outcomes, not pulmonary function [43]. Moreover, in those studies involving preterm infants, the addition of LC-PUFAs was started many days or even weeks after birth, thereby skipping a critical time period when pulmonary outcomes may have been impacted.

Administration of intravenous lipids based only on soybean oil has been associated with elevations of pulmonary artery pressure in newborns with respiratory failure [51]. Recent experimental data in fetal lambs have demonstrated that administration of intravenous lipid solutions that contain n–3 LC-PUFA results in improvements of pulmonary blood flow, which is not seen when linoleic acid-rich lipid solutions are infused [52]. These effects involve vasoactive mediators produced by CYP450 epoxygenase and potassium channel activation. Even though this issue has not been carefully examined among infants with persistent pulmonary hypertension, these findings suggest that the use of intravenous lipid solutions should be very cautious among infants with evidence of pulmonary hypertension, especially if emulsions based only on soybean oil are used.

Parenteral or enteral administration of lipids serves as an important energy source during the early neonatal period and can prevent deficiency of essential fatty acids. Depending on the intravenous lipid source used, the postnatal fall of DHA might be avoided or ameliorated. Whereas definitive data is still lacking, there are strong suggestions that sustaining and supplementing levels of n–3 LC-PUFAs, especially DHA, during the neonatal period may lower the risk of chronic pulmonary problems. Furthermore, n–3-based intravenous lipid solutions may be able to play a role in the management of infants with pulmonary hypertension. These clinical goals may be able to be accomplished using new parenteral lipid formulations that provide n–3 LC-PUFAs followed by enteral administration of feedings that contain n–3 LC-PUFAs like breast milk of women with an adequate DHA status, although this needs to be ratified by controlled clinical trials.

Calcium and Phosphorus

These elements are not only critical for bone health but also participate in key physiologic and metabolic functions of the cardiovascular and respiratory systems. There is a large body of information about their homeostasis during the perinatal period (reviewed elsewhere in this book). Calcium (Ca) is key for normal function of the cardiovascular system and both hypocalcemia and hypercalcemia can affect myocardial contractility and rhythm. In addition, hypocalcemia has been associated with apnea in preterm infants [53] and laryngospasm is mentioned as a clinical sign of severe hypocalcemia. Chronic alterations of bone mineralization seen with inadequate calcium, phosphorus or vitamin D intake may alter thoracic stability and, therefore, contribute to ventilatory problems. However, these abnormalities need to be marked to be of clinical significance. Recent relatively small clinical trials examining provision of extra calcium to preterm infants did not demonstrate reductions in the incidence of BPD, although this intervention may prevent a short-term decline in bone strength [54, 55].

Phosphorus (P) is needed for the formation of ATP and phosphocreatine, both forms of intracellular energy storage. Measurements of ATP and phosphocreatine using nuclear magnetic resonance showed that VLBW infants have limited energy reserves [56]. Recent data have shown that VLBW infants, particularly those with IUGR, often develop significant hypophosphatemia soon after delivery or during the first week after birth [57, 58]. This in turn has been associated with higher risks for sepsis, prolonged ventilation and BPD [58, 59]. Phosphorus is also part of the phospholipids that compose pulmonary surfactant. However, it is not known whether the higher risks for prolonged ventilation and BPD shown in infants with early hypophosphatemia are the result of decreased muscle performance or a direct impact to the surfactant system.

Based on these findings it appears that monitoring the concentrations of Ca and P as well as providing an adequate supply of these elements may be the best approach for sustaining neonatal lung function. Administering higher amounts of these elements above normal requirements may afford no benefits and potentially lead to side effects. This notwithstanding, when there is a high likelihood of abnormalities of these elements, as is the case in preterm infants with IUGR, they should be prevented or corrected promptly.

Vitamin A

There is abundant animal and clinical data that show that a deficiency of vitamin A is associated with decreased lung growth and repair (see previous section). Very immature infants exhibit lower concentrations of retinol in serum and various tissues.

Table 3. Systematic review of vitamin A to prevent morbidity and mortality in preterm infants [from 61]

Outcome	Studies, n	Participants, n	Risk ratio (95% CI)
Death before 1 month	5	1,011	0.86 (0.66–1.11)
Death before 36 weeks' postmenstrual age	2	847	1.06 (0.77–1.47)
Chronic lung disease (oxygen use at 1 month in survivors)	5	884	0.93 (0.86–1.01)
Chronic lung disease (oxygen use at 36 weeks' postmenstrual age in survivors)	2	724	0.84 (0.73–0.97)
Death or chronic lung disease (oxygen use at 1 month)	5	1,011	0.93 (0.86–1.00)
Death or chronic lung disease (oxygen use at 36 weeks' postmenstrual age)	2	847	0.89 (0.79–0.99)

Only studies using the intramuscular route to give vitamin A are included in the table.

In preterm infants, lower plasma retinol levels are associated with increased risk for long-term respiratory morbidity [60]. Preterm infants also have lower levels of retinol-binding protein. Fortunately, the addition of higher doses of vitamin A to the diet of preterm infants has been studied in a relatively large number of infants. Data from a large randomized trial of vitamin A supplementation in ELBW infants as well as a systematic review including several additional trials suggest that postnatal supplementation with intramuscular, not enteral, administration of 5,000 IU started within a few days after birth and given three times a week for 4 weeks reduces the risk of BPD by about 7%. This modest reduction translates into a number needed to treat with vitamin A to prevent one case of BPD of about 14 infants [61, 62]. No specific measures of lung function have been performed in infants supplemented or not with vitamin A from these or other studies (table 3). Therefore, the functional mechanisms whereby administration of vitamin A reduces BPD are unclear. Whereas there may be other dosing schemes that may provide additional benefit, those studies have yet to be conducted. Nonetheless, this intervention is worthy of being considered in the management of ELBW infants given its low cost and relative safety in the doses studied.

Vitamin E

It has antioxidant properties that protect cell membranes. Extensive animal data suggest that a deficiency of vitamin E exacerbates O_2 toxicity. Earlier trials of vitamin E supplementation given to infants with deficient levels of this vitamin suggested a beneficial effect in decreasing chronic respiratory morbidity [63]. However, subsequent studies when a deficiency of vitamin E was less prevalent did not show benefit [64]. Moreover, excessive administration of vitamin E has been associated with a higher risk of sepsis in neonates [65]. This notwithstanding, there is still a strong correlation between plasma levels of vitamin E and selenium determined in cord blood and day 3 after birth and BPD [66].

Current recommendations for vitamin E during the neonatal period do not call for additional supplementation over and above intake obtained from a regular diet, unless there is a demonstrated deficiency state.

Nutritional Management of Infants with Evolving or Established BPD

As mentioned previously, infants who develop BPD often have had lower total daily energy intake after birth and less enteral feedings than infants those with a lower risk of BPD [17, 67]. These infants have been shown to have variable increases of energy demands, O_2 consumption, CO_2 production and REE [24, 26]. Their total energy expenditure is associated with their respiratory status [28]. Moreover, they often exhibit growth failure that seems to correlate with higher rates of REE [27].

Early nutritional management of high-risk infants aimed at preventing BPD should start by avoiding excess fluid administration and provision of a minimum of 50–60 kcal/kg/day during the first few days after birth. This energy intake needs to be increased progressively in following days. Although using the enteral route would be ideal, parenteral nutrition with a combination of glucose and protein plus intravenous lipid solutions is frequently the only initial alternative. High glucose infusion rates may lead to hyperglycemia but generally do not have a major impact on respiratory morbidity in early stages of respiratory disease. However, providing high glucose infusion rates over 10–12 mg/kg/min can become a problem for infants with limitations for CO_2 elimination. Protein intake should be advanced as per current recommendations. Likewise, the use of intravenous lipids is critical as a source of additional energy. If available, lipid solutions that provide LC-PUFAs are preferable given the postnatal decrease in their levels, especially DHA [46, 47]. There is no benefit of adding extra quantities of Ca or P parenterally. However, one must anticipate a higher risk of particularly hypophosphatemia in preterm infants with IUGR, which increases the risk for BPD [58]. It has been suggested that exposure of parenteral nutrition solutions to ambient light generates peroxides that can overload the antioxidant capacity of high-risk infants and increase the risk of BPD, although this evidence has not been consistent [68, 69]. However, to date there has not been a randomized trial with enough power to answer this question definitively.

Special consideration should be given to the use of vitamin A in doses that have been shown to effectively reduce the risk of BPD [61, 62]. At this time, the use of additional vitamin E is not recommended. However, if the local epidemiology of the population suggests a frequent deficiency in cord blood levels of this vitamin, this must be diagnosed and prevented/treated appropriately.

The enteral route should be used as soon as possible, ideally by feeding breast milk of the infant's own mother (which provides LC-PUFAs) or preterm formulas enriched with LC-PUFAs. Given that DHA supplementation of lactating mothers who provide human milk to their preterm infants resulted in a lower risk of chronic lung disease, this practice may need to be encouraged [45]. Among infants with respiratory instability, continuous feedings may be of benefit since intermittent feeds can decrease tidal volume, minute ventilation and dynamic compliance [70]. There may be some advantages to feeding in the prone position even though these benefits may be offset by the tendency of these infants to exhibit a higher body temperature while in this position [71].

For infants with established BPD, special emphasis needs to be placed on continuing some fluid restriction while still supply enough free water for growth. Also, continuous feeds for more unstable infants may be preferable. If the oral route needs to be avoided, special efforts must be placed on maintaining non-nutritive sucking. Due to their relatively high REE and O_2 consumption, these infants often have a need for more energy than other preterm infants. Short-term studies have demonstrated that administration of a high-fat diet decreases CO_2 production while maintaining adequate growth [72]. Among infants that were O_2-dependent at 28 days, a moderate size randomized trial (total n = 60) of a high nutrient density formula (100 kcal/100 ml with higher CHO, protein and fat content) compared with feeding a regular preterm formula (80 kcal/100 ml) did not show advantages in terms of respiratory outcomes or growth [73]. Nonetheless, almost two thirds of infants in both groups received a dexamethasone course during the study period. Administration of steroids is known to decrease the rate of growth and induce protein catabolism [74]. For selected infants with established BPD, energy intake may need to be increased beyond 120–130 kcal/kg/day [75]. There is limited information on what is the best method to do this. However, increasing energy intake using easily digestible sources is preferable as opposed to concentrating feeds even further due to concerns about osmolality and excess administration of other solutes. All of these nutritional interventions often need to be continued way past the neonatal period as infants with BPD are at high risk for growth failure for weeks or months.

Opportunities for Further Research

The following areas of clinical research related to nutrition and neonatal lung disease are potentially very promising and need to be pursued in clinical trials:
- Different dosing schemes of vitamin A to prevent BPD
- Further studies of maternal and early neonatal supplementation of DHA to reduce the risk of BPD
- Use of intravenous solutions that provide DHA and their impact on neonatal lung function
- Prevention of early neonatal hypophosphatemia and its effects on neonatal pulmonary morbidity

References

1 Biniwale MA, Ehrenkranz RA: The role of nutrition in the prevention and management of bronchopulmonary dysplasia. Semin Perinatol 2006;30:200–208.

2 Bhatia J, Parish A: Nutrition and the lung. Neonatology 2009;95:362–367.

3 Dani C, Poggi C: Nutrition and bronchopulmonary dysplasia. J Matern Fetal Neonatal Med 2012;25(suppl 3):37–40.

4 Pike K, Pillow JJ, Lucas JS: Long-term respiratory consequences of intrauterine growth restriction. Semin Fetal Neonatal Med 2012;17:92–98.

5 Rozance PJ, Seedorf GJ, Brown A, et al: Intrauterine growth restriction decreases pulmonary alveolar and vessel growth and causes pulmonary artery endothelial cell dysfunction in vitro in fetal sheep. Am J Physiol Lung Cell Mol Physiol 2011;30:L860–L871.

6 Joss-Moore L, Carroll T, Yang Y, et al: Intrauterine growth restriction transiently delays alveolar formation and disrupts retinoic acid receptor expression in the lung of female rat pups. Pediatr Res 2013;73:612–620.

7 Joss-Moore L, Wang Y, Baack M, et al: IUGR decreases PPAR-γ and SETD8 Expression in neonatal rat lung and these effects are ameliorated by maternal DHA supplementation. Early Hum Dev 2010;86:785–791.

8 Blanco PG, Freedman SD, Lopez MC, et al: Oral docosahexaenoic acid given to pregnant mice increases the amount of surfactant in lung and amniotic fluid in preterm fetuses. Am J Obstet Gynecol 2004;190:1369–1374.

9 Tyson JE, Kennedy K, Broyles S, Rosenfeld CR: The small for gestational age infant: accelerated or delayed pulmonary maturation? Increased or decreased survival? Pediatrics 1995;95:534–538.

10 Bardin C, Zelkowitz P, Papageorgiou A: Outcome of small-for-gestational age and appropriate-for-gestational age infants born before 27 weeks of gestation. Pediatrics 1997;100:e4.

11 Bose C, Van Marter LJ, Laughon M, O'Shea TM, et al: Fetal growth restriction and chronic lung disease among infants born before 28th week of gestation. Pediatrics 2009;124:e450–e458.

12 Antipatis C, Ashworth CJ, Grant G, et al: Effects of maternal vitamin A status on fetal heart and lung: changes in expression of key developmental genes. Am J Physiol 1998;275:L1184–L1191.

13 Wei H, Huang HM, Li TY, et al: Marginal vitamin A deficiency affects lung maturation in rats from prenatal to adult state. J Nutr Sci Vitaminol (Tokyo) 2009;55:208–214.

14 Maxwell CS, Carbone ET, Wood RJ: Better newborn vitamin D status lowers RSV-associated bronchiolitis in infants. Nutr Res 2012;70:548–552.

15 Bisgaard H, Loland L, Holst KK, Pipper CB: Prenatal determinants of neonatal lung function in high-risk newborns. J Allergy Clin Immunol 2009;123:651–657.

16 White P, Cattaneo D, Dauncey MJ: Postnatal regulation of myosin heavy chain isoform expression and metabolic enzyme activity by nutrition. Br J Nutr 2000;84:185–194.

17 Ehrenkranz RA, Dusick AM, Vohr BR, et al: Growth in the neonatal intensive care unit influences neurodevelopmental and growth outcomes of extremely low birth weight infants. Pediatrics 2006;117:1253.

18 Ehrenkranz RA, Das A, Wrage LA, et al: Early nutrition mediates the influence of severity of illness on extremely LBW infants. Pediatr Res 2011;69:522–529.

19 Van Marter LJ, Leviton A, Allred EN, Pagano M, Kuban KC: Hydration during the first days of life and the risk of bronchopulmonary dysplasia in low birth weight infants. J Pediatr 1990;116:942–949.

20 Bell EF, Acarregui MJ: Restricted versus liberal water intake for preventing morbidity and mortality in preterm infants. Cochrane Database Syst Rev 2008;1:CD000503.

21 Oh W: Fluid and electrolyte management of very low birth weight infants. Pediatr Neonatol 2012;53:329–333.

22 Hazan J, Chessex P, Piedboeuf B, Bourgeois M, et al: Energy expenditure during synthetic surfactant replacement therapy for neonatal respiratory distress syndrome. J Pediatr 1992;120:S29–S33.

23 Kinnala A, Manner T, Nuutila P, et al: Differences in respiratory metabolism during treatment of hypoglycemia in infants of diabetic mothers and small-for-gestational-age infants. Am J Perinatol 1998;15:363–367.

24 Yunis KA, Oh W: Effects of intravenous glucose loading on oxygen consumption, carbon dioxide production, and resting energy expenditure in infants with bronchopulmonary dysplasia. J Pediatr 1989;115:127–132.

25 Chessex P, Belanger S, Piedboeuf B, Pineault M: Influence of energy substrates on respiratory gas exchange during conventional mechanical ventilation of preterm infants. J Pediatr 1995;126:619–624.

26 Weinstein MR, Oh W: Oxygen consumption in infants with bronchopulmonary dysplasia. J Pediatr 1981;99:958–961.

27 Kurzner SI, Garg M, Bautista DB, et al: Growth failure in infants with bronchopulmonary dysplasia: nutrition and elevated resting metabolic expenditure. Pediatrics 1988;81:379–384.

28 De Meer K, Westerterp KR, Houwen RHJ, Brouwers R, et al: Total energy expenditure in infants with bronchopulmonary dysplasia is associated with respiratory status. Eur J Pediatr 1997;156:299–304.

29 Hallman M, Gluck L: Formation of acidic phospholipids in rabbit lung during perinatal development. Pediatr Res 1980;14:1250–1259.

30 Hallman M, Saugstad OD, Porreco RP, Epstein BL, Gluck L: Role of myoinositol in regulation of surfactant phospholipids in the newborn. Early Hum Dev 1985;10:245–254.

31 Howlett A, Ohlsson A, Plakkal N: Cochrane Database Syst Rev 2012;3:CD000366.

32 Phelps DL, Ward RM, Williams RL, Watterberg KL, Laptook AR, Wrage LA, Nolen TL, Fennell TR, Ehrenkranz RA, Poindexter BB, Michael Cotten C, Hallman MK, Frantz ID 3rd, Faix RG, Zaterka-Baxter KM, Das A, Bethany Ball M, Michael O'Shea T, Backstrom Lacy C, Walsh MC, Shankaran S, Sanchez PJ, Bell EF, Higgins RD: Pharmacokinetics and safety of a single intravenous dose of myo-inositol in preterm infants of 23–29 weeks. Pediatr Res 2013;74:721–729.

33 Poindexter B, Denne S: Nutrition and metabolism in the high-risk neonate. Fanaroff and Martin's Neonatal-Perinatal Medicine. Missouri: Elsevier, 2011, pp 643–668.

34 Manner T, Wiese S, Katz DP, Skeie B, Askanazi J: Branched-chain amino acids and respiration. Nutrition 1992;8:311–315.

35 Blazer S, Reinersman GT, Askanazi J, et al: Branched-chain amino acids and respiratory pattern and function in the neonate. J Perinatol 1994;14:290–295.

36 Porcelli PJ, Sisk PM: Increased parenteral amino acid administration to extremely low-birth weight infants during early postnatal life. J Pediatr Gastroenterol Nutr 2002;34:174–179.

37 Wilson DC, Cairns P, Halliday HL, et al: Randomised controlled trial of an aggressive nutritional regimen in sick very low birth weight infants. Arch Dis Child 1997;77:F4–F11.

38 Poindexter BB, Ehrenkranz RA, Stoll BJ, Wright LL, et al: Parenteral glutamine supplementation does not reduce the risk of mortality or late-onset sepsis in extremely low birth weight infants. Pediatrics 2004;113:1209–1215.

39 Kuschel CA, Harding JE: Multicomponent fortified human milk for promoting growth in preterm infants. Cochrane Database Syst Rev 2004;1:CD000343.

40 O'Connor DL, Jacobs J, Hall R, Adamkin D, et al: Growth and development of premature infants fed predominantly human milk, predominantly premature infant formula, or a combination of human milk and premature formula. J Pediatr Gastroenterol Nutr 2003;37:437–446.

41 Sullivan S, Schanler RJ, Kim JH, Patel AL, et al: An exclusively human milk-based diet is associated with a lower rate of necrotizing enterocolitis than a diet of human milk and bovine milk-based products. J Pediatr 2010;156:562–567.

42 Moya F, Sisk PH, Walsh KR, Berseth CL: A new liquid human milk fortifier and linear growth in preterm infants. Pediatrics 2012;130:e928–e935.

43 Lapillonne A, Groh-Wargo S, Gonzalez C, Uauy R: Lipid needs of preterm infants: updated recommendations. J Pediatr 2013;162:S37–S47.

44 Chao AC, Ziadeh BI, Diau GY, et al: Influence of dietary long-chain PUFA on premature baboon lung FA and dipalmitoyl PC composition. Lipids 2003;38:425–429.

45 Manley BJ, Makrides M, Collins CT, et al: High-dose docosahexaenoic acid supplementation of preterm infants: respiratory and allergy outcomes. Pediatrics 2011;128:e71–e77.

46 Robinson DT, Carlson SE, Murthy K, et al: Docosahexaenoic and arachidonic acid levels in extremely low birth weight infants with prolonged exposure to intravenous lipids. J Pediatr 2013;162:56–61.

47 Martin CR, Dasilva DA, Cluette-Brown JE, Dimonda C, et al: Decreased postnatal docosahexaenoic and arachidonic acid blood levels in premature infants are associated with neonatal morbidities. J Pediatr 2011;159:743–749.

48 Sosenko IRS, Rodriguez-Pierce M, Bancalari E: Effect of early initiation of intravenous lipid administration on the incidence and severity of chronic lung disease in premature infants. J Pediatr 1993;123:975–982.

49 Hammerman C, Aramburo MJ: Decreased lipid intake reduces morbidity in sick premature neonates. J Pediatr 1988;113:1083–1088.

50 Simmer K, Rao SC: Early introduction of lipids to parenterally-fed preterm infants. Cochrane Database Syst Rev 2005;2:CD005256.

51 Prasertsom W, Phillipos EZ, Van Aerde JE, Robertson M: Pulmonary vascular resistance during lipid infusion in neonates. Arch Dis Child Fetal Neonatal Ed 1996;74:F95–F98.

52 Houeijeh A, Aubry E, Coridon H, Montaigne K, et al: Effects of n–3 polyunsaturated fatty acids in the fetal pulmonary circulation. Crit Care Med 2011;39:1431–1438, 1587–1589.

53 Gershanik JJ, Levkoff AH, Duncan R: The association of hypocalcemia and recurrent apnea in premature infants. Am J Obstet Gynecol 1972;113:646–652.

54 Pereira-da-Silva L, Costa AB, Pereira L, Filipe AF, et al: Early high calcium and phosphorus intake by parenteral nutrition prevents short-term bone strength decline in preterm infants. J Pediatr Gastroenterol Nutr 2011;52:203–209.

55 Carroll WF, Fabres J, Nagy TR, Frazier M, et al: Results of extremely-low-birth-weight infants randomized to receive extra enteral calcium supply. J Pediatr Gastroenterol Nutr 2011;53:339–345.

56 Bertocci LA, Mize CE, Uauy R: Muscle phosphorus energy state in very-low-birth-weight infants: effect of exercise. Am J Physiol 1992;262:E289–E294.

57 Ichikawa G, Watabe Y, Suzumura H, Sairenchi T, et al: Hypophosphatemia in small for gestational age extremely low birth weight infants receiving parenteral nutrition in the first week after birth. J Pediatr Endocrinol Metab 2012;25:317–321.

58 Ross JR, Finch C, Ebeling M, Taylor SN: Refeeding syndrome in very-low-birth-weight intrauterine growth-restricted neonates. J Perinatol 2013;33:717–720.

59 Moltu SJ, Strommen K, Blakstad EW, Almaas AN, et al: Enhanced feeding in very-low-birth-weight infants may cause electrolyte disturbances and septicemia – a randomized, controlled trial. Clin Nutr 2013; 32:207–212.

60 Spears K, Cheney C, Zerzan J: Low plasma retinol concentrations increase the risk of developing bronchopulmonary dysplasia and long-term respiratory disability in very-low-birth-weight infants. Am J Clin Nutr 2004;80:1589–1594.

61 Tyson JE, Wright LL, Oh W, et al: Vitamin A supplementation for extremely-low-birth-weight infants. A national institute of child health and human development neonatal research network. N Engl J Med 1999;340:1962–1968.

62 Darlow BA, Graham PJ: Vitamin A supplementation for preventing morbidity and mortality in very low birth weight infants. Cochrane Database Syst Rev 2002;4:CD000501.

63 Ehrenkranz RA, Bonta BW, Ablow RC, et al: Amelioration of bronchopulmonary dysplasia after vitamin E administration. A preliminary report. N Engl J Med 1978;299:564–569.

64 Ehrenkranz RA, Ablow RC, Warshaw JB: Effect of vitamin E on the development of oxygen-induced lung injury in neonates. Ann NY Acad Sci 1982;393: 452–466.

65 Brion LP, Bell EF, Raghuveer TS: Vitamin E supplementation for prevention of morbidity and mortality in preterm infants. Cochrane Database Syst Rev 2003;4:CD003665.

66 Falciglia HS, Johnson JR, Sullivan J, et al: Role of antioxidant nutrients and lipid peroxidation in premature infants with respiratory distress syndrome and bronchopulmonary dysplasia. Am J Perinatol 2003; 20:97–107.

67 Wemhoner A, Ortner D, Tschirch E, Strasak A, Rudiger M: Nutrition of preterm infants in relation to bronchopulmonary dysplasia. BMC Pulm Med 2011;11:1–6.

68 Sherlock R, Chessex P: Shielding parenteral nutrition from light: does the available evidence support a randomized, controlled trial. Pediatrics 2007;123: 1529–1533.

69 Bassiouny MR, Almarsafawy H, Abdel-Hady H, Naset N, et al: A randomized controlled trial on parenteral nutrition, oxidative stress, and chronic lung diseases in preterm infants. J Pediatr Gastroenterol Nutr 2009;48:363–369.

70 Blondheim O, Abbasi S, Fox WW, Bhutani VK: Effect of enteral gavage feeding rate on pulmonary functions of very low birth weight infants. J Pediatr 1993;122:751–755.

71 Ammari A, Schulze KF, Ohira-Kist K, Kashyap S, et al: Effects of body position on thermal, cardiorespiratory and metabolic activity in low birth weight infants. Early Hum Dev 2009;85:497–501.

72 Pereira GR, Baumgart S, Bennett MJ, Stallings VA, et al: Use of high-fat formula for premature infants with bronchopulmonary dysplasia: metabolic, pulmonary, and nutritional studies. J Pediatr 1994;124: 605–611.

73 Fewtrell MS, Adams C, Wilson DC, Cairns P, et al: Randomized trial of high nutrient density formula versus standard formula in chronic lung disease. Acta Paediatr 1997;86:577–582.

74 Leitch CA, Ahlrichs J, Karn C, Denne SC: Energy expenditure and energy intake during dexamethasone therapy for chronic lung disease. Pediatr Res 1999; 46:109–113.

75 Brunton JA, Saigal S, Atkinson SA: Growth and body composition in infants with bronchopulmonary dysplasia up to 3 months corrected age: a randomized trial of a high-energy nutrient-enriched formula fed after hospital discharge. J Pediatr 1998;133:340–345.

Fernando Moya, MD
Betty Cameron Women and Children's Hospital
2131 S. 17th Street
Wilmington, NC 28401 (USA)
E-Mail Fernando.Moya@ccneo.net

Moya

Koletzko B, Poindexter B, Uauy R (eds): Nutritional Care of Preterm Infants: Scientific Basis and Practical Guidelines.
World Rev Nutr Diet. Basel, Karger, 2014, vol 110, pp 253–263 (DOI: 10.1159/000358474)

Necrotizing Enterocolitis

Josef Neu

Department of Pediatrics/Neonatology, University of Florida, Gainesville, Fla., USA

Reviewed by Nicholas B. Embleton, Neonatal Service, Newcastle Hospitals, Institute of Health and Society,
Newcastle University, Newcastle upon Tyne, UK; Brenda Poindexter, Riley Hospital for Children at Indiana
University Health, Indianapolis, Ind., USA

Abstract

Necrotizing enterocolitis (NEC) is the most common severe neonatal gastrointestinal emergency that
predominantly affects premature infants. Its morbidity and mortality is similar to other severe childhood
diseases such as meningitis and leukemia, and is becoming increasingly recognized as a major cause of
neurodevelopmental delays. The etiology of NEC remains obscure despite over 40 years of research,
partly because it is more than one disease and databases including NEC have been diluted by these
different entities. Furthermore, good animal models that represent the most classic form of the disease
seen in preterm human infants are lacking. This chapter provides an overview of the pathophysiology,
diagnosis, treatment and prevention of what has been termed 'NEC'.   © 2014 S. Karger AG, Basel

Necrotizing enterocolitis (NEC) is the most common severe neonatal gastrointestinal emergency that predominantly affects premature infants. The mortality of NEC ranges between 20 and 30%, with the greatest mortality among those requiring surgery [1].

What is termed 'NEC' is likely to be more than one entity. Although the final outcome in NEC is necrosis of the bowel, different cases are preceded by different triggering events and pathophysiologic mechanisms, which is one of the factors that makes this such an elusive disease to diagnose, prevent and manage. In this chapter, the author will review some of the current ideas about pathogenesis of the most common form of NEC seen in preterm infants, discuss diagnosis, current treatment modalities, and preventative strategies.

Pathogenesis

While it is well known that NEC primarily affects premature infants, 7–15% of NEC cases occur in term or late preterm infants [2, 3]. In term infants, bowel necrosis is commonly associated with congenital heart diseases, such as hypoplastic left heart syn-

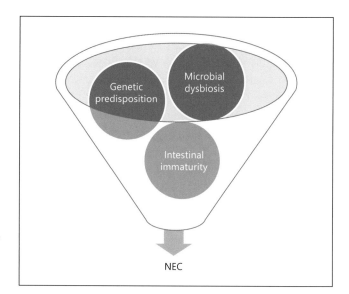

Fig. 1. Genetic predisposition, intestinal immaturities and microbial dysbiosis combine to induce NEC.

drome and coarctation of the aorta, which result in intestinal ischemic necrosis [4, 5]. NEC has also been associated with other anomalies, including aganglionosis [6] and gastroschisis [7]. Most of the cases of NEC in term infants present within the first few days after birth. More than 85% of all NEC cases occur in very low birth weight premature infants (<1,500 g, <32 weeks of gestation) [8]. In preterms, the age of onset is inversely related to gestational age at birth [3, 9, 10]. This late presentation suggests causes other than acute stress-related primary ischemic injury to the bowel as a major component in the pathophysiologic cascade that leads to intestinal necrosis in these infants.

The pathophysiology of NEC in babies with congenital heart disease is primarily caused by hypoxic-ischemic injury [11]. A NEC-like illness can also occur with cow milk protein allergy [12]. The pathophysiology of 'classic NEC' seen in most preterms is incompletely understood but primary hypoxia-ischemia in the intestine does not appear to play a major etiologic role [13]. Epidemiologic observations strongly suggest a multifactorial etiology [14]. The concurrence of intestinal immaturity, imbalanced microvascular tone, an abnormal microbial intestinal colonization and a highly dysregulated immunoreactive intestinal mucosa present a confluence of predisposing factors that provide a tenable explanation for some of the features associated with NEC (fig. 1). Here the intestinal immaturity and microbial colonization will be discussed in more detail.

Intestinal Immaturity
Immature motility, digestion, absorption, immune defenses, barrier function, and circulatory regulation predispose the preterm infant to an increased risk of intestinal injury [15]. Certain interventions may exacerbate the preexisting immaturities. For example, since gastric acid secretion is not yet fully developed and relatively low in the

preterm infant, this is associated with an increased risk of NEC, who receive H_2 blockers [16, 17].

Pathology of the bowel in infants with NEC shows an excessive inflammatory response to luminal microbial stimuli. This has been implicated in the development of intestinal injury [18, 19]. The high serum levels of several cytokines and chemokines that recruit inflammatory cells are higher in patients with NEC than in unaffected preterm infants. For example, interleukin-8 [18], which is produced by epithelial cells and attracts neutrophils to the site of inflammation and their activation, is known to cause necrosis and in the gut [20].

Microbial Colonization

Another hypothesis is that inappropriate initial microbial colonization in preterm infants is an important risk factor for NEC [21], particularly since the disease most often does not occur until at least 8–10 days after birth, at a time when microbes from the extrauterine environment have colonized the gut. Although specific microbes have been cultured in outbreaks of NEC in single institutions, no single organism has consistently been implicated and this may have been due to limitations in our previous capability to cultivate many of the microorganisms that reside in the intestine.

New technologies that are not based on the cultivation of microbes are providing potential insights into a microbial origin of NEC. The Human Microbiome Project was initiated in 2007 [22, 23] in conjunction with technological advances that allow for the molecular identification of a vast array of microbes that are difficult or impossible to culture from the intestine. The findings of this project are just beginning to provide the evidence supporting the colonization hypothesis in the pathogenesis of NEC [24]. For example, molecular methods to evaluate fecal microbiota from affected and unaffected preterm infants, from whom samples were obtained before and during the disease [25, 26], suggest the involvement of unusual intestinal microbial species, blooms of phyla such as Proteobacteria, and lower diversity of microbiota, especially when there has been prolonged preceding antibiotic therapy, which is also supported by epidemiologic data [27, 28]. The excessive immature inflammatory response associated with abnormal intestinal microbiota is currently considered to be a very likely component in the pathogenesis of NEC [2].

Clinical Signs

The clinical presentation of NEC can range from non-specific signs that progress insidiously over several days to a fulminant onset of gastrointestinal signs, multiorgan system dysfunction, and shock over a few hours. Clinical signs include both intestinal and systemic perturbations. NEC can present as feeding intolerance, emesis, abdominal distension, and bloody stools. However, many of these are commonly seen in preterm infants in the neonatal intensive care unit and the majority of occurrences do

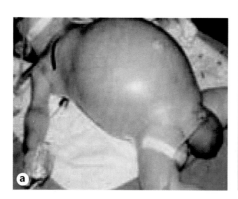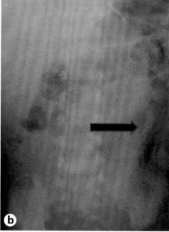

Fig. 2. a Distended, shiny abdomen associated with advanced NEC. **b** Radiograph with the arrow pointing to an intestine with pneumatosis intestinalis.

not represent necrotic bowel, but rather signs of an immature intestinal tract. During the advanced stages of NEC, the abdomen may appear shiny, distended, and erythematous (fig. 2a).

An early presentation suggestive of NEC can be visibly bloody stools but occult hematochezia diagnosed by a hemoccult test correlates poorly with NEC [29]. Emesis, increased gastric residuals, and/or abdominal distension can also be initial clinical signs but these are also highly variable and are seen in most very preterm infants who do not go on to develop NEC. Hence, what has been termed Bell's stage 1 NEC [30] is so non-specific, it is a term that probably should no longer be used.

Once NEC develops, systemic signs include lethargy, hypotension, poor perfusion and pallor, increased episodes of apnea and bradycardia, worsening of respiratory function, temperature instability, tachycardia, hyperglycemia, or hypoglycemia. These signs are indistinguishable from systemic inflammatory response associated with sepsis and need to be correlated to radiographic and laboratory findings.

Laboratory Evaluation
Abnormal laboratory tests include anemia, left shift of neutrophils, neutropenia, thrombocytopenia, metabolic acidosis, raised C-reactive protein and hyponatremia. These commonly used tests are clinically available in most hospitals, but have poor sensitivity, specificity and predictive value for the diagnosis of NEC. Better diagnostic as well as predictive biomarkers are needed. Diagnostic biomarkers should help in differentiating those babies who show some signs and symptoms suggestive of NEC, but do not exhibit the classic pneumatosis intestinalis, portal venous gas or pneumoperitoneum. Recent studies suggest diagnostic biomarkers with high sensitivity, specificity and predictive value include intestinal fatty acid-binding proteins, claudin-3,

and fecal calprotectin. Intestinal fatty acid-binding protein and claudin-3 can be measured in the blood or urine (which has the advantage of being non-invasive). Calprotectin, measured in feces, is dependent on the ability to obtain fecal specimens that are not always readily available [31, 32].

Radiographs

Intramural gas or pneumatosis and portal venous gas are pathognomonic signs of NEC (fig. 2b). Pneumatosis is caused by gas within the bowel wall and may appear linear or circular if gas is subserosal or bubbly if gas is submucosal [33]. Bubbly lucencies could also indicate air within fecal material, which can mimic pneumatosis intestinalis and make the diagnosis more challenging. The amount of pneumatosis does not always relate to the severity of disease, and its disappearance does not necessarily imply pathologic or clinical improvement [33].

A pneumoperitoneum is diagnostic of a perforated viscus and when small may be difficult to visualize on a single plain film. A left lateral decubitus film will allow free air to rise to the top over a non-dependent surface, facilitating visualization of an abnormal lucency [33].

Ultrasound

Radiographs expose preterm infants to irradiation. In situations when radiographic signs are non-specific, the abdominal ultrasound is another modality that can identify even small volumes of free gas without such exposures. Ultrasound is also the preferred modality for visualization of abdominal fluid and ascites. Thickness and echogenicity of the bowel wall and qualitative assessment of peristalsis can be visualized best by color Doppler ultrasound. Portal venous gas can be more readily seen using abdominal sonography than plain film [33]. Color Doppler sonography demonstrates 100% sensitivity for free air and absent blood flow (necrotic gut) compared with 40% sensitivity by radiography [34]. The use of computed tomography is not advocated for the diagnosis of NEC [33].

Management

Medical
When an infant is suspected of having NEC, all enteral feedings and medications should be discontinued. Prompt gastric and intestinal decompression is aided by the placement of a large lumen gastric tube with either the institution of low, constant suction or regular intermittent aspiration. If the abdomen continues to distend, the

tube should be checked for proper placement and for blockage and consideration should be given for discontinuation of nasal continuous positive airway pressure. Intravascular volume must be monitored to ensure adequate tissue perfusion and may be partially gauged by frequent assessment of urine output, serum electrolytes, and hematocrit. Hemodynamic support with inotropes is often needed. Parenteral nutrition should be started with adequate protein (3.5–4.0 g/kg/day) to maintain positive nitrogen balance and to allow the repair of injured tissue. Adequate energy intake necessitates the use of lipids usually at approximately 3 g/kg/day. Following blood culture, broad-spectrum intravenous antibiotics are usually initiated.

Surgical identification of a pneumoperitoneum caused by bowel perforation and relentless systemic deterioration despite conservative medical management are two absolute indications for surgical intervention. Without surgical intervention, it has been difficult to diagnose dead gut in infants with NEC [3]. Worsening of metabolic, hematologic and hemodynamic status often is associated with continued or worsening necrosis and may help guide the need for surgical intervention. These metabolic derangements include severe metabolic acidosis, progressive or persistent thrombocytopenia, hypotension, hyponatremia, neutropenia, left shift of neutrophils, and positive blood culture.

The choice of primary peritoneal drainage (PPD) or laparotomy as a primary surgical intervention remains controversial despite two randomized controlled trials that showed no differences with respect to mortality and duration for total parenteral nutrition between the drainage and laparotomy [35, 36]. However, these studies did not distinguish between isolated perforation and NEC.

One of these two trials (Necrotizing Enterocolitis Trial (NET) from the United Kingdom) found that 74% of infants initially treated with PPD required a rescue laparotomy [36]. A study of neurodevelopmental outcome in extremely low birth weight infants (<1,000 g) suggested that laparotomy had an advantage over PPD with respect to the likelihood of survival and better neurodevelopmental outcome at 18–22 months of age [37]. Whether this is due to earlier cessation of inflammatory cytokines by more complete drainage after laparotomy is speculative, but may be answered with additional studies that are currently being done.

With respect to the type of surgery, PPD has thus emerged as an alternative to laparotomy in infants with bowel perforation and may serve as a definitive treatment of some patients and as a temporizing measure for unstable sick infants until laparotomy can be performed after their stabilization. Acute decompression of a tense abdomen secondary to perforation using a simple cannula may enable stabilization where access to surgical support is not immediately available.

Prevention

Table 1 shows several strategies that have been studied for the prevention of NEC. The use of human milk appears to provide the greatest benefit, while the others either have not undergone adequate study or still are unproven.

Table 1. Prevention of NEC

Measures that are known to be effective in prevention
Human milk
Careful advancement of feedings
Questionable measures
Formula acidification
IgG-IgA
Oral antibiotics
Glucocorticoids
Anticytokine therapy
Pre-, pro-, and postbiotics

Human Milk

Providing human milk to premature infants has been shown to decrease the incidence of NEC [38, 39]. Whether donor milk provides the same preventive benefits as babies' own mothers' milk remains debatable, but a recent meta-analysis suggests potential benefit [40].

An immature enteric nervous system and intestinal dysmotility warrants gradual and cautious increments in enteral feedings. Aggressive and improper enteral feeding may be a risk factor associated with NEC [41, 42]. This has, in many cases, caused neonatologists to institute an overly cautious approach in which they withhold enteral feedings for prolonged periods, which is equally inappropriate because of bowel atrophy, increased risk of sepsis, and other complications of not using the gastrointestinal tract. Prolonged periods of nulla per os (NPO) are known to cause atrophy of the intestinal mucosa and result in delayed development of absorptive function, motility, and exocrine hormone secretion, and shift the intestinal inflammatory response to one that favors the pro-inflammatory cytokines and chemokines over the anti-inflammatory mediators [43]. Initiating low-volume feedings and increasing them gradually appears to be a safe approach even in infants receiving ventilator support, using umbilical catheters, or receiving drugs such as indomethacin or dopamine [44]. It has been recommended that feedings should be advanced 'carefully' but the exact advancement that is optimal for an individual baby is not known. The lack of any enteral feeding may be very detrimental because of intestinal atrophy, increased bacterial translocation and inflammation of the intestine. This is discussed further in the enteral feeding chapter of this book [see Senterre, pp. 201–214].

Controversies

Transfusion-Associated NEC and Feeding

Several publications including a meta-analysis have reported and summarized NEC associated with transfusions [45, 46]. It is one of the most severe forms of

NEC in preterm infants with a high rate of surgery and mortality. The timing of this entity is typically within 48 h of transfusion and commonly within 12 h. However, there remains controversy about the causality of transfusions for NEC and confounding factors may be at play in these epidemiologic studies [46]. There has been controversy about whether feedings should be withheld when a baby receives a transfusion, but the evidence for this practice is not very well substantiated [47, 48].

Withholding Feedings While on Indomethacin
Indomethacin is commonly used for prophylaxis of intraventricular hemorrhage and for medical closure of a patent ductus arteriosus. Concern has been raised about indomethacin causing decreased intestinal blood flow, hence increasing the risk for NEC. This relationship has never been substantiated. If fact, holding feedings may actually further decrease mesenteric arterial blood flow [49] and a large trail of feeding and indomethacin has not shown that enteral feeding while on indomethacin increases the risk of NEC [50].

Probiotics
Several trials over the past decade have evaluated the effects of various probiotics to prevent NEC [51]. Meta-analyses across the available randomized trials have prompted recent commentaries suggesting the routine use of probiotics. Whilst caution in the adoption of probiotics has been advised [25, 52, 53] they are already used in several countries. Another chapter in this book addresses this controversy in more detail.

Microbial Components That Modulate Inflammation
Studies in epithelial cells and in an infant-formula-fed rodent model suggest that dead microbes may be as effective as live microbes in modulating excessive inflammatory stimuli [54]. This is supported by a study of preterms that showed a decreased incidence of NEC with inactivated probiotics [55].

Outcomes and Complications

In addition to death, complications of NEC include intestinal strictures, enterocutaneous fistula, intra-abdominal abscess, cholestasis, and short-bowel syndrome.

Strictures typically occur 3–8 weeks after the acute episode but can also present several months later [56]. Contrast enema is indicated if signs of subacute intestinal obstruction appear several weeks after the acute episode of NEC. The colon is the most common site for stricture development, but strictures can also occur in the ileum or jejunum. Risks of all comorbidities of prematurity increase with NEC, including neurodevelopmental, motor, sensory, and cognitive problems [57–59].

Future Directions

Prediction

Because of the fulminant nature of NEC, it is unlikely that new treatment strategies will provide major breakthroughs in alleviating its mortality and morbidity. Preventive approaches are more likely to yield the best results. The multifactorial etiology of NEC suggests that there will be no magic bullet for the prevention of all cases of NEC. The prediction of infants at an increased risk of NEC may be possible through the use of methods that are currently available at a few research facilities. These methods use non-invasive indicators, such as profiling of the fecal microbiome [26], and the identification of the expression of inflammatory proteins from buccal epithelium using buccal swab collection [60, 61].

Key Points

(1) The multifactorial etiology of NEC and the fact that NEC is more than one disease makes it a difficult target for uniform preventative therapies.

(2) Human milk feedings appear to be protective against NEC, but it remains unclear whether use of donor milk or supplementation with human milk-based fortifiers are protective against NEC.

(3) The pathophysiology of the classic form of NEC seen in preterms that involves intestinal inflammation is likely due to a combination of dysbiosis of the intestinal microbial ecology and an exaggerated inflammatory response to these alterations in intestinal microbial ecology.

(4) There is a very strong need for the development of both diagnostic and predictive biomarkers for NEC.

References

1 Fitzgibbons SC, Ching Y, Yu D, et al: Mortality of necrotizing enterocolitis expressed by birth weight categories. J Pediatr Surg 2009;44:1072–1076.

2 Neu J, Walker WA: Necrotizing enterocolitis. N Engl J Med 2011;364:255–264.

3 Sharma R, Hudak ML, Tepas JJ III, et al: Impact of gestational age on the clinical presentation and surgical outcome of necrotizing enterocolitis. J Perinatol 2006;26:342–347.

4 De La Torre CA, Miguel M, Martínez L, et al: The risk of necrotizing enterocolitis in newborns with congenital heart disease. A single institution-cohort study. Cir Pediatr 2010;23:103–106.

5 Martinez-Tallo E, Claure N, Bancalari E: Necrotizing enterocolitis in full-term or near-term infants: risk factors. Biol Neonate 1997;71:292–298.

6 Raboei EH: Necrotizing enterocolitis in full-term neonates: is it aganglionosis? Eur J Pediatr Surg 2009; 19:101–104.

7 Snyder CL: Outcome analysis for gastroschisis. J Pediatr Surg 1999;34:1253–1256.

8 Thompson AM, Bizzarro MJ: Necrotizing enterocolitis in newborns: pathogenesis, prevention and management. Drugs 2008;68:1227–1238.

9 Yee WH, Soraisham AS, Shah VS, et al: Incidence and timing of presentation of necrotizing enterocolitis in preterm infants. Pediatrics 2012;129:e298–e304.

10 Neu J: Neonatal necrotizing enterocolitis: an update. Acta Paediatr Suppl 2005;94:100–105.

11 Young CM, Kingma SD, Neu J: Ischemia-reperfusion and neonatal intestinal injury. J Pediatr 2011; 158:e25–e28.

12 Srinivasan P, Brandler M, D'Souza A, Millman P, Moreau H: Allergic enterocolitis presenting as recurrent necrotizing enterocolitis in preterm neonates. J Perinatol 2010;30:431–433.

13 Neu J: The 'myth' of asphyxia and hypoxia-ischemia as primary causes of necrotizing enterocolitis. Biol Neonate 2005;87:97–98.

14 Stoll BJ: Epidemiology of necrotizing enterocolitis. Clin Perinatol 1994;21:205–218.

15 Martin CR, Walker WA: Intestinal immune defences and the inflammatory response in necrotising enterocolitis. Semin Fetal Neonatal Med 2006;11:369–377.

16 Guillet R, Stoll BJ, Cotten CM, et al: Association of H_2-blocker therapy and higher incidence of necrotizing enterocolitis in very low birth weight infants. Pediatrics 2006;117:e137–e142.

17 Terrin G, Passariello A, De Curtis M, et al: Ranitidine is associated with infections, necrotizing enterocolitis, and fatal outcome in newborns. Pediatrics 2012; 129:e40–e45.

18 Markel TA, Crisostomo PR, Wairiuko GM, Pitcher J, Tsai BM, Meldrum DR: Cytokines in necrotizing enterocolitis. Shock 2006;25:293–337.

19 Sharma R, Tepas J Jr, Hudak ML, et al: Neonatal gut barrier and multiple organ failure: role of endotoxin and proinflammatory cytokines in sepsis and necrotizing enterocolitis. J Pediatr Surg 2007;42:454–461.

20 Mukaida N: Interleukin-8: an expanding universe beyond neutrophil chemotaxis and activation. Int J Hematol 2000;72:391–398.

21 Claud EC, Walker WA: Hypothesis: inappropriate colonization of the premature intestine can cause neonatal necrotizing enterocolitis. FASEB J 2001;15: 1398–1403.

22 Turnbaugh PJ, Ley RE, Hamady M, Fraser-Liggett CM, Knight R, Gordon JI: The human microbiome project. Nature 2007;449:804–810.

23 Hattori M, Taylor TD: The human intestinal microbiome: a new frontier of human biology. DNA Res 2009;16:1–12.

24 Torrazza RM, Neu J: The altered gut microbiome and necrotizing enterocolitis. Clin Perinatol 2013; 40:93–108.

25 Wang Y, Hoenig JD, Malin KJ, et al: 16S rRNA gene-based analysis of fecal microbiota from preterm infants with and without necrotizing enterocolitis. ISME J 2009;3:944–954.

26 Mai V, Young CM, Ukhanova M, et al: Fecal microbiota in premature infants prior to necrotizing enterocolitis. PLoS One 2011;6:e20647.

27 Cotten CM, Taylor S, Stoll B, et al: Prolonged duration of initial empirical antibiotic treatment is associated with increased rates of necrotizing enterocolitis and death for extremely low birth weight infants. Pediatrics 2009;123:58–66.

28 Kuppala VS, Meinzen-Derr J, Morrow AL, Schibler KR: Prolonged initial empirical antibiotic treatment is associated with adverse outcomes in premature infants. J Pediatr 2011;159:720–725.

29 Abramo TJ, Evans JS, Kokomoor FW, Kantak AD: Occult blood in stools and necrotizing enterocolitis. Is there a relationship? Am J Dis Child 1988;142: 451–452.

30 Bell MJ, Ternberg JL, Feigin RD, et al: Neonatal necrotizing enterocolitis: therapeutic decisions based upon clinical staging. Ann Surg 1978;187:1–6.

31 Thuijls G, Derikx JP, van Wijck K, et al: Non-invasive markers for early diagnosis and determination of the severity of necrotizing enterocolitis. Ann Surg 2010;251:1174–1180.

32 Ng EW, Poon TC, Lam HS, et al: Gut-associated biomarkers L-FABP, I-FABP, and TFF3 and LIT score for diagnosis of surgical necrotizing enterocolitis in preterm infants. Ann Surg 2013;258:1111–1118.

33 Epelman M, Daneman A, Navarro OM, et al: Necrotizing enterocolitis: review of state-of-the-art imaging findings with pathologic correlation. Radiographics 2007;27:285–305.

34 Faingold R, Daneman A, Tomlinson G, Babyn PS, Manson DE, Mohanta A, Moore AM, Hellmann J, Smith C, Gerstle T, Kim JH: Necrotizing enterocolitis: assessment of bowel viability with color Doppler ultrasound Radiology 2005;235:587–594.

35 Moss RL, Dimmitt RA, Barnhart DC, et al: Laparotomy versus peritoneal drainage for necrotizing enterocolitis and perforation. N Engl J Med 2006;354: 2225–2234.

36 Pierro A, Eaton S, Rees CM, et al: Is there a benefit of peritoneal drainage for necrotizing enterocolitis in newborn infants? J Pediatr Surg 2010;45:2117–2118.

37 Blakely ML, Tyson JE, Lally KP, et al: Laparotomy versus peritoneal drainage for necrotizing enterocolitis or isolated intestinal perforation in extremely low birth weight infants: outcomes through 18 months adjusted age. Pediatrics 2006;117:e680–e687.

38 Lucas A, Cole TJ: Breast milk and neonatal necrotising enterocolitis. Lancet 1990;336:1519–1523.

39 Meinzen-Derr J, Poindexter B, Wrage L, Morrow AL, Stoll B, Donovan EF: Role of human milk in extremely low birth weight infants' risk of necrotizing enterocolitis or death. J Perinatol 2009;29:57–62.

40 Quigley MA, Henderson G, Anthony MY, McGuire W: Formula milk versus donor breast milk for feeding preterm or low birth weight infants. Cochrane Database Syst Rev 2007;4:CD002971.

41 Anderson DM, Kliegman RM: The relationship of neonatal alimentation practices to the occurrence of endemic necrotizing enterocolitis. Am J Perinatol 1991;8:62–67.

42 Berseth CL, Bisquera JA, Paje VU: Prolonging small feeding volumes early in life decreases the incidence of necrotizing enterocolitis in very low birth weight infants. Pediatrics 2003;111:529–534.

43 Kudsk KA: Current aspects of mucosal immunology and its influence by nutrition. Am J Surg 2002;183:390–398.

44 Neu J, Zhang L: Feeding intolerance in very-low-birth-weight infants: what is it and what can we do about it? Acta Paediatr Suppl 2005;94:93–99.

45 La Gamma EF, Blau J: Transfusion-related acute gut injury: feeding, flora, flow, and barrier defense. Semin Perinatol 2012;36:294–305.

46 Mohamed A, Shah PS: Transfusion-associated necrotizing enterocolitis: a meta-analysis of observational data. Pediatrics 2012;129:529–540.

47 Wan-Huen P, Bateman D, Shapiro DM, Parravicini E: Packed red blood cell transfusion is an independent risk factor for necrotizing enterocolitis in premature infants. J Perinatol 2013;33:786–790.

48 Keir AK, Wilkinson D: Question 1: do feeding practices during transfusion influence the risk of developing necrotising enterocolitis in preterm infants? Arch Dis Child 2013;98:386–388.

49 Niinikoski H, Stoll B, Guan X, et al: Onset of small intestinal atrophy is associated with reduced intestinal blood flow in TPN-fed neonatal piglets. J Nutr 2004;134:1467–1474.

50 Clyman R, Wickremasinghe A, Jhaveri N, et al: Enteral feeding during indomethacin and ibuprofen treatment of a patent ductus arteriosus. J Pediatr 2013;163:406–411.

51 Deshpande G, Rao S, Patole S, Bulsara M: Updated meta-analysis of probiotics for preventing necrotizing enterocolitis in preterm neonates. Pediatrics 2010;125:921–930.

52 Neu J: Routine probiotics for premature infants: let's be careful! J Pediatr 2011;158:672–674.

53 Caplan MS: Probiotic and prebiotic supplementation for the prevention of neonatal necrotizing enterocolitis. J Perinatol 2009;29:S2–S6.

54 Li N, Russell WM, Douglas-Escobar M, Hauser N, Lopez M, Neu J: Live and heat-killed *Lactobacillus rhamnosus* GG (LGG): effects on pro- and anti-inflammatory cyto/chemokines in gastrostomy-fed infant rats. Pediatr Res 2009;66:203–207.

55 Awad H, Mokhtar H, Imam SS, Gad GI, Hafez H, Aboushady N: Comparison between killed and living probiotic usage versus placebo for the prevention of necrotizing enterocolitis and sepsis in neonates. Pak J Biol Sci 2010;13:253–262.

56 Schimpl G, Höllwarth ME, Fotter R, Becker H: Late intestinal strictures following successful treatment of necrotizing enterocolitis. Acta Paediatr Suppl 1994;396:80–83.

57 Pike K, Brocklehurst P, Jones D, et al: Outcomes at 7 years for babies who developed neonatal necrotising enterocolitis: the ORACLE Children Study. Arch Dis Child Fetal Neonatal Ed 2012;97:F318–F322.

58 Martin CR, Dammann O, Allred E, et al: Neurodevelopment of extremely preterm infants who had necrotizing enterocolitis with or without late bacteremia. J Pediatr 2010;157:751–756.e1.

59 Hintz SR, Kendrick DE, Stoll BJ, et al: Neurodevelopmental and growth outcomes of extremely low birth weight infants after necrotizing enterocolitis. Pediatrics 2005;115:696–703.

60 Warner BB, Ryan AL, Seeger K, Leonard AC, Erwin CR, Warner BW: Ontogeny of salivary epidermal growth factor and necrotizing enterocolitis. J Pediatr 2007;150:358–363.

61 Morrow AL, Meinzen-Derr J, Huang P, et al: Fucosyltransferase-2 non-secretor and low secretor status predicts severe outcomes in premature infants. J Pediatr 2011;158:745–751.

Prof. Josef Neu, MD
Pediatrics/Neonatology, University of Florida
1600 SW Archer Road
Gainesville, FL 32610 (USA)
E-Mail neuj@peds.ufl.edu

Koletzko B, Poindexter B, Uauy R (eds): Nutritional Care of Preterm Infants: Scientific Basis and Practical Guidelines.
World Rev Nutr Diet. Basel, Karger, 2014, vol 110, pp 264–277 (DOI: 10.1159/000358475)

Feeding the Preterm Infant after Discharge

Alexandre Lapillonne

Paris Descartes University, APHP Necker Hospital, Paris, France and CNRC, Baylor College of Medicine,
Houston, Tex., USA

Reviewed by Alison Leaf, National Institute for Health Research, University of Southampton, Southhampton,
UK; Thibault Senterre, Department of Neonatology, University of Liège, Liège, Belgium

Abstract

In recent years, much attention has been focused on enhancing the nutritional support of very preterm infants to improve both survival and quality of life. In most countries throughout the world, preterm infants tend to be discharged from hospital earlier than the expected term for economic and other reasons. The question has arisen whether such infants might require special nutritional regimens or special discharge formulas. Since nutrition during hospitalization tends to improve, thereby reducing acquired nutrition deficit, the question of the systematic use of specially designed nutrient-enriched discharge formulas should be questioned. Recommendations for feeding the preterm infant after hospital discharge are made keeping in mind that the goal in nourishing preterm infants after discharge should be to promote human milk feeding, minimize nutrient deficits, promptly address these deficits once identified, and avoid over-nourishing or promoting postnatal growth acceleration once nutrient deficits have been corrected.   © 2014 S. Karger AG, Basel

Current Practices for Feeding after Hospital Discharge

The very preterm infant at the time of discharge presents a nutritional challenge to healthcare providers beginning with the decisions on what type of milk should be given after discharge and on the need to continue to supplement mother's milk. Furthermore, establishing breastfeeding is frequently problematic and because of a certain degree of immaturity, preterm infants at the time of discharge may be sleepier and have less stamina and may have more difficulty with latch, suck, and swallow than full-term infants. Any one or a combination of these conditions places the mothers and infants at risk for difficulty in establishing successful lactation or for breastfeeding failure.

Post-discharge practices regarding breastfeeding and nutrient enrichment of feedings vary widely by country, neonatal intensive care units (NICUs) and even by the neonatologist on service. Depending on the NICU, infants could be sent home on human milk alone (breast- and/or bottle-fed), on partially or fully nutrient-fortified human milk or on nutrient-enriched or conventional term formula. Furthermore, in most countries throughout the world, preterm infants tend to be discharged from hospital earlier than the expected term for economic and other reasons. The question has arisen whether such infants might require special nutritional regimens or special discharge formulas.

At the time of discharge the volume of feeds consumed varies greatly and may reach 200 ml/kg day or more if the infants are fed ad libitum. Caloric density makes a difference as infants on less caloric-dense formulas have been shown to have increased formula intake (22–23% or more) compared with infants on higher caloric dense formulas [1]. Therefore, energy density of feeding will determine in part the intake of other nutrients including proteins and macronutrients.

Guidance on how to feed very low birth weight (VLBW) infants after hospital discharge is both scarce and conflicting. Although there is a lack of evidence to suggest a prescriptive approach to feeding all VLBW infants after discharge, there is general consensus in the literature that human milk should be fed in preference to infant formula and that subgroups of infants in the NICU are likely to be at the highest nutritional risk after discharge. However, since nutrition during hospitalization tends to improve, thereby reducing acquired nutrition deficit, the systematic use of specially designed nutrient-enriched discharge formulas should be questioned.

Ideally, the pre- and post-discharge nutritional concerns for the low birth weight infant should be a continuum, but this is generally not the case. VLBW infants are continuing to be discharged at earlier postmenstrual ages and lower body weights, and are supervised by healthcare providers not involved with their inpatient care. Close nutritional monitoring of infants after hospital discharge is frequently not accomplished since high-risk neonatal follow-up clinics have been traditionally more concerned with neurodevelopmental rather than the nutritional follow-up of infants. Therefore, it is of significant interest to establish post-discharge feeding guidelines.

Nutritional Status at Hospital Discharge

Several lines of evidence suggest that preterm infants, particularly those born of VLBW, are at greater nutritional risk at the time of hospital discharge than at birth. Extrauterine growth retardation, also called extrauterine growth restriction, postnatal growth retardation or postnatal growth failure, has been identified as a major problem secondary to suboptimal nutrition and has been reported from all over the world [2–6]. Numerous studies have also shown an altered body composition at the time of discharge including a reduced fat-free mass [7] and an increased total [7–9] or intra-abdominal adiposity [7, 10]. This predominant fat mass deposition during postnatal life among preterm infants might be speculated to be a consequence of imbalanced nutrition during hospitalization, especially the protein/energy ratio [11]. It has also become evident that assessing growth during hospitalization should include measurements of the head circumference since it predicts long-term outcomes [12–15].

As a general principle, the earlier an infant is born before his or her expected delivery date, the greater is their risk for morbidity and malnutrition and the likelihood that not all nutrient deficits will be resolved prior to hospital discharge. Therefore, preterm infants born VLBW and particularly those born extremely low birth weight have the greatest nutrient needs especially if they are discharged home much before their expected date of delivery, are predominantly fed human milk, have fallen below the 3rd or 5th percentile on growth references or have persistent morbidities that elevate nutritional requirements or limit the volume of feeds consumed, i.e. infants with chronic lung disease and those with an uncoordinated suck swallow and/or short bowel.

It should be noted that most attention has been focused on the macronutrient content of feedings that contribute to caloric intake, including protein which is very important for growth. However, attention should also be paid to other possible nutrient deficiencies which may not affect growth and hence often go undetected. Among these nutrients, specific attention should be paid to minerals, iron, long-chain polyunsaturated fatty acid, and vitamin A.

It is clear that the nutritional status of preterm infants at the time of discharge is heterogeneous and that it varies according to gestational age, postnatal age, in utero growth, nutritional management during hospitalization, associated morbidities and likely genetic factors. Therefore, it is unlikely that a standardized nutritional practice may covert the need of all preterm infants after hospital discharge and an individualized approach would best meet this goal. However, common features might be identified and should be known by physicians in order to adapt their prescription and guidelines given to parents.

Current Guidelines for Feeding the Preterm Infant after Discharge

The World Health Organization, American Pediatric Society, Canadian Pediatrics Society, European Society for Paediatric Gastroenterology Hepatology and Nutrition (ESPGHAN) and many other professional bodies globally recommend mothers' own milk for nutrition of infants for the first 6 months of life and beyond [16–18]. These endorsements have evolved from an extensive body of literature in both term and preterm infants that support many advantages to human milk over formula feeding including improved neurodevelopment, gastrointestinal function and host defense [19–21]. Despite the advantages of using human milk after hospital discharge, for a variety of reasons such as maternal illness, stress, lack of support and other factors related to preterm birth, rates of human milk feeding among preterm fall significantly below that of term-born infants and recommendations [22].

In its recent position statement, the ESPGHAN Committee on Nutrition concluded that infants discharged home with a normal weight for post-conceptional age are not at increased risk of long-term growth failure and could be fed similarly to term infants of similar gestational age. By contrast, those with a subnormal weight for post-conceptional age are at increased risk of long-term growth failure and require particular attention and follow-up [23]. Breastfeeding and fortified human milk should be promoted and if formula-fed, a preterm formula or a special post-discharge formula with a higher concentration of protein, minerals and trace elements as well as long-chain fatty acids than standard term formula should be provided until the preterm infant reaches 40 weeks' post-conceptional age but possibly until 52 weeks' post-conceptional age [23, 24].

The most recent edition of the Pediatric Nutrition Handbook of the American Academy of Pediatrics, unlike its predecessors, now supports the use of specially designed nutrient-enriched discharge formulas that may promote better linear growth, weight gain, and bone mineral content than standard term formula [17].

Evidence in Support of the Need for Nutrient-Enriched Formula after Hospital Discharge

Young et al. [25] in their Cochrane review identified 15 good quality controlled trials (n = 1,128 infants) that examined the efficacy of feeding preterm infants after hospital discharge a nutrient-enriched formula compared with a standard term formula. Nutrient-enriched formulas were either preterm formulas (energy content >75 kcal/100 ml; protein content >2.0 g/100 ml) or post-discharge formulas (energy content >72 kcal/100 ml and <75 kcal/100 ml; protein content >1.7 g/100 ml) containing additional minerals, trace elements and vitamins. Standard term formulas used in the studies contained 66–68 kcal/100 ml and 1.4–1.5 g/100 ml protein.

The authors concluded that 'current recommendations to prescribe post-discharge formula for preterm infants following hospital discharge are not supported by the available evidence'. While it is difficult to argue with their conclusions, it is important to understand that preterm infants at highest nutritional risk were either excluded or were under-represented in these analyses. For example, in 8 trials, a significant proportion of infants were born >1,500 g. Additionally, very few participants in the trials were small for gestational age at birth or enrolment. However, the analysis of the 3 trials that recruited infants growth-restricted at birth, demonstrated a statistically significant effect at 6 months corrected age on crown-heel length [8.88 (95% CI 0.94–16.83) mm] and head circumference [5.36 (95% CI 0.62–10.11) mm] suggesting that these infants may benefit from receiving a post-discharge formula. Finally, infants with additional problems at discharge, particularly inadequate independent oral feeding or receipt of supplemental oxygen secondary to chronic lung disease, were not eligible to participate in the trials although they were very likely growth-retarded at discharge from hospital.

The conclusion of the meta-analysis with regard to the effects of feeding a preterm formula after discharge is somewhat different. Indeed, there was some evidence of higher rates of growth through infancy. The infants fed the preterm formula for 2–6 months after discharge weighed ~500 g more and were 5–10 mm taller at 12–18 months corrected age compared to infants fed a term formula. Furthermore, they exhibited a 5-cm larger head circumference since 6 months corrected age which tracked up to 18 months corrected age.

Among the studies excluded from the meta-analysis, it should be noted that feeding nutrient-enriched formula without extra energy after term does not change the quantity of growth but does influence the quality of growth of preterm infants [26]. Infants fed the nutrient-enriched formula had a lower fat mass corrected for body size at 6 months corrected age than infants fed a standard formula or human milk. Similarly, preterm infants fed a preterm formula after discharge had both an increase fat-free and peripheral fat mass but not central adiposity compared to infants fed a standard term formula [27]. Similarly, another study exhibited a better weight gain, a proportional increase in fat mass and lean mass and a better bone mineral content at expected term in preterm infants fed an isocaloric preterm formula enriched with protein, calcium and phosphorus versus the control preterm formula [24]. These data provide evidence that nutrient-dense formula after discharge does not promote central adiposity in preterm infants [27] and may be beneficial in increasing immediate weight gain and mineralization.

Results with regard to outcomes other than growth or body composition showed no significant effect of feeding either a post-discharge formula or a preterm formula after discharge on development (tables 1, 2). Furthermore, there is no data allowing studying the effect of feeding an enriched formula after discharge on later blood pressure or insulin resistance [25].

Evidence in Support of the Need for Nutrient-Enriched Human Milk after Hospital Discharge

Although feeding human milk to VLBW infants is widely acknowledged as being superior to formula feeding, human milk-fed infants often accrue the greatest nutritional deficits by hospital discharge. The ESPGHAN Committee on Nutrition recommends that human milk-fed infants with subnormal weight for post-conceptional age consume milk after discharge that is supplemented to provide an adequate nutrient supply [23]. Very little work, to date, has been done to evaluate whether multinutrient fortification of human milk after hospital would be beneficial. Recently, a small study was conducted in which predominantly human milk-fed VLBW (750–1,800 g) pre-

Table 1. Nutritional needs by weeks of gestation

	Nutritional needs per kg/day GA, weeks					
	<28	28–31	32–33	34–36	37–38	39–41
Fetal growth						
Weight gain, g	20	17.5	15	13	11	10
Lean body mass gain, g	17.8	14.4	12.1	10.5	7.2	6.6
Protein gain, g	2.1	2	1.9	1.6	1.3	1.2
Requirements						
Energy, kcal/kg	125	125	130	127	115	110
Proteins, g/kg	4	3.9	3.5	3.1	2.5	1.5
Protein/energy ratio, g/100 kcal	3.2	3.1	2.7	2.4	2.2	1.4
Calcium, mg/kg	120–140	120–140	120–140	120–140	70–120	55–120
Phosphorus, mg/kg	60–90	60–90	60–90	60–90	35–75	30–75

Weight gain, lean body mass and protein gain during the last trimester of pregnancy and theoretical energy and protein requirements for enteral nutrition are indicated by gestational age (GA) group. Before 39 weeks GA, requirements are based on the fetal growth, fetal accretion rate and intestinal absorption, after 40 weeks GA, requirements are based on the composition of human milk [adapted from 11, 44]. The values indicated in this table are theoretical values per GA groups. They show that both the late preterm (i.e. 34–36 weeks GA) and the early term infant (i.e. 37–38 weeks GA) have nutritional requirements that are different than the full-term infant (i.e. 39–41 weeks GA). The values indicated do not take into account the nutrient supply needed to compensate for any nutritional deficit and therefore are not applicable as such for the very preterm infant at time of, or after, hospital discharge.

Table 2. Summary of the randomized controlled studies reporting developmental indexes at 18 months corrected age (Bayley Scales of Development) of preterm infants fed a term formula or an enriched formula (either post-discharge or preterm formula) after hospital discharge

Type of enrichment	Ref.	Enriched formula	Term formula
Mental development index			
Post-discharge formula	45	92.3 (14.7)	91.4 (13.9)
Preterm formula	32	102 (14)	103 (14)
Preterm formula	46	92 (16)	101 (17)
Psychomotor development index			
Post-discharge formula	45	91.7 (12.7)	89.8 (14.8)
Preterm formula	32	102 (8)	103 (9)
Preterm formula	46	101 (18)	111 (11)

term infants were randomly assigned at hospital discharge (38 weeks post-conceptional age) to either a control (unfortified human milk) or an intervention (1/2 human milk feeds nutrient-enriched) group [28, 29]. Intensive lactation support was provided to both groups. The authors reported a more rapid rate of growth during the 12-week feeding intervention for infants fed nutrient-enriched human milk compared to infants sent home on human milk alone. The observed differences in absolute weight and length, and in smaller babies head circumference were sustained for the first year [28]. In addition, for both groups the duration of human milk feeding was significantly longer than reported for preterm infants in the literature [22].

A second larger randomized control trial was conducted in Denmark in which human milk-fed preterm infants (535–2,255 g) were randomized to receive 20–50 ml of expressed breast milk containing a multinutrient fortifier (17.5 kcal and 1.4 g protein) each day from the time of discharge to 4 months corrected age. The control group of human milk-fed infants did not receive the nutrient-fortified supplement. Like the Canadian study, the introduction of the expressed breast milk supplement did not influence breastfeeding but in contrast it did not have a significant impact on growth. It is likely that there was considerably more formula feeding in the Danish trial and a much smaller incremental increase in the nutrition provided by the supplement versus the Canadian study accounting for the differences between the studies [30].

In the meta-analysis which pulled the results of these two studies, no significant effect of being fed with fortified breast milk was seen on weight and head circumference during the first year of life, but a small and significant effect on length at 12 months was observed [31]. Finally, one study [29] showed an improved visual acuity at 6 months corrected age in the supplemented group, but no significant effect on the developmental score at 18 months corrected age.

Nutritional Deficiencies Other than Protein/Energy Deficiency

It should be noted that most attention (see paragraphs above) has focused on the macronutrient content of feedings that contribute to caloric intake, including protein which is very important for growth. However, attention should also be paid to other possible nutrient deficiencies (e.g. minerals, iron, long-chain polyunsaturated fatty acid, vitamin A) which may not affect growth and hence often go undetected.

Feeding post-discharge preterm infants formulas or breast milk with higher concentrations of calcium and phosphorus than those found in formulas for term infants results in improved bone mineralization, particularly if the special formulas for preterm infants used during hospitalization are continued after hospital discharge [24, 32]. However, osteopenia, or rickets, of prematurity seems to be a self-resolving disease quite similar to that observed during adolescence after the initial acceleration of growth. Bone mineral content improves spontaneously in most infants and rapid catch-up mineralization is observed after discharge in VLBW infants. At 3–6 months corrected age, spine and total bone mineral density, corrected for anthropometric values, are in the range of normal term newborn infants [33, 34]. Nevertheless, potential long-term consequences on attainment of peak bone mass are not clearly known. Bone mass may be reduced at adulthood but is mainly the result of a persistent growth retardation since it is appropriate for the body size achieved. Furthermore, bone mass during childhood is not affected by early diet or human milk feeding [34, 35]. Therefore, based on the limited data available, it is likely that mineral intake after discharge should exceed that of term infants when catch-up growth occurs and is supported by enriched feeds, but it is unlikely that extra mineral supplementation is necessary when a mineral-rich post-discharge or preterm formula or enriched human milk is used. With regard to vitamin D intake, there is no evidence that the preterm infant after discharge should receive higher doses that term infants.

With regard to iron supplementation after discharge, it should be noted that the body iron store is highly variable at the time of discharge and screening for iron deficiency at hospital discharge as well as during the first year of life is warranted. Both the American Academy of Pediatrics (AAP) and ESPGHAN recommend that the preterm infant receive a supplement of iron after discharge from hospital [36, 37]. The AAP recommends that all preterm infants should have an iron intake of at least 2 mg/kg/day through 12 months of age, which is the amount of iron supplied by iron-fortified formulas. Preterm infants fed human milk should receive an iron supplement of 2 mg/kg/day by 1 month of age, and this should be continued until the infant is weaned to iron-fortified formula or begins eating complementary foods that supply the 2 mg/kg of iron. An exception to this practice would include infants who have received an iron load from multiple transfusions of packed red blood cells. On the other hand, the ESPGHAN recommend that iron supplementation should be continued after discharge from hospital, at least until 6–12 months of age depending on diet but no specific doses are indicated.

With regard to long-chain polyunsaturated fatty acid supply to preterm infants, recommendations have been revised [see chapter on 'Enteral and Parenteral Lipid Requirements of Preterm Infants', pp. 82–98]. The recommendations for DHA, AA and EPA for preterm infants should be continued until due date but thereafter there are limited data available for setting the recommendations and therefore recommendations are in line with those for term infants [38].

In formula-fed VLBW infants, suboptimal vitamin A status may occur for many months after discharge [39]. Thus, even a target intake of 1,000 IU vitamin A per day in post-discharge preterm infants is not unreasonable and may not be adequate. An observational study showed that higher vitamin A intakes may be needed [40]. Supplementation for 90 days with 3,000 IU of vitamin A per day orally did not achieve plasma vitamin A concentrations characteristic of repletion status. This observation contrasts with previous studies performed in term infants, in which a similar supplementation protocol was sufficient to replete plasma vitamin A concentrations [40]. The failure to achieve full optimal vitamin A concentrations may, in part, be explained by the immaturity of the fat digestion mechanisms at birth in premature infants, which resolves within 3–4 months of life. Although these results suggest that oral supplementation with vitamin A might be required in preterm infants after discharge, further studies are needed to determine the dose and duration of the vitamin A which allows reaching full repletion values.

How to Monitor the Post-Discharge Infant

Accurate serial measurements of weight, length and head circumference plotted precisely on validated growth charts facilitate early identification of potential nutritional or a health problem after hospital discharge. To ensure accuracy of measurements, trained measurers need to use a standardized measurement technique and quality but not necessarily expensive equipment [41].

There are two types of growth charts that can be used to monitor the growth of preterm infants after hospital discharge: those that are based on (1) fetal growth until term and then growth of a preterm population of infants thereafter and (2) growth of a term-born population of infants. Most growth charts, including those designed using preterm infants, merely describe how infants actually grow but not how they should grow to promote optimal neurodevelopment. When using charts designed for term infants, it is important to correct for the gestational age of the infant at the time of measurement. Failure to do so will result in inappropriate referrals for failure-to-thrive as it is well known that infants that plot within the normal reference range on intrauterine growth charts will fall well below the 3rd percentile on growth charts designed for term infants.

However, using two different charts that do not perfectly overlap between 36 and 46 weeks' gestational age make it difficult to monitor growth during this period. Furthermore, it has been shown that intrauterine as well as postnatal growth in term infants are gender-related. To address these issues, specific gender-related fetal-infant growth charts for preterm infants were recently designed by merging intrauterine growth curves with the World Health Organization (WHO) growth standards for term infants [42]. Since these curves are available online for unrestricted use, it is likely that they will become widely used in clinical settings. Exact z-scores and percentile have also been made available online for download (http:// ucalgary.ca/fenton).

Close monitoring of feeding and growth is recommended after hospital discharge, especially for infants that are at risk of nutritional deficit, have an uncoordinated suck swallow, have persistent co-morbidities or are predominantly breastfed. Parents should be reminded that breastfeeding is the optimal way to feed their infant. Breastfed infants may be fed every 1.5–3 h, with no more than one period of prolonged sleep of up to 5 h to keep up their mother's milk supply and ad libitum feeding is encouraged to optimize infant growth. Infants should be weighed within 48 h of discharge to allow for assessment of intake and provide reassurance to families. This is particularly important for babies that were very rapidly transitioned from nasogastric and/ or enriched feedings to feeding at the breast prior to hospital discharge. A complete feeding assessment should be completed within the first week of discharge. If not part of the early follow-up team, information should be provided to parents on how to contact a dietitian and/or lactation consultant after discharge, ideally one that has experience working with mothers of preterm infants. Finally, and as a general rule, infants including formula-fed infants should be transitioned to the feeding that they will go home consuming several days prior to discharge to assess tolerance and growth.

Research Gaps

Although poor early growth is associated with adverse neurodevelopmental outcomes, it is not clear whether rapid growth provides neurodevelopmental advantages. The utility of growth as the sole or principal indicator of nutrition status in the preterm infant is limited because we do not know what defines optimal growth and because many nutritional factors may affect development without affecting growth. Further studies are therefore needed to assess the efficacy on neurodevelopment of promoting enriched nutrition after hospital discharge.

Adults born prematurely have a significantly greater risk of developing hypertension and insulin resistance than those born at term [43]. In contrast to adults born IUGR or LBW at term, fetal growth of adults born prematurely does not seem to play a significant role in the later risk of hypertension or insulin resistance in VLBW infants [43]. Very interestingly, current data also suggest that (1) growth velocity of preterm infants between birth and expected term and/or before 12–18 months post-term has no significant effect on later blood pressure and metabolic syndrome and (2) growth during late infancy and childhood appears to be a major determinant of later health, suggesting a nutritional intervention during this period would be effective [43]. However, many epidemiological studies have shown an increased risk of developing type 2 diabetes and metabolic syndrome in adults who were born at term and who have shown, as neonates, signs of fetal growth restriction followed by rapid catch-up growth. This finding raises the possibility that catch-up growth, whilst potentially beneficial in the short term, may be detrimental to long-term survival. Research in this area should be promoted to examine if such a relationship may exist in preterm infants.

There are few published studies in the literature that have systematically evaluated whether a proactive approach to feeding VLBW infants after hospital discharge (e.g. feeding VLBW infants different than term infants), as opposed to a reactive approach (e.g. intervening if growth failure has occurred), results in improved growth and development. This gap in the literature is particularly pronounced for the predominantly human milk-fed VLBW infant after hospital discharge and those VLBW infants with persistent morbidities.

In recent years, much attention has been focused on enhancing the nutritional support of very preterm infants to improve both survival and quality of life. Significant efforts have been made to improve the provision of adequate nutrition during their in-hospital course and to avoid an accumulation of nutritional deficits. However, the effects of these changes deserve to be studied to demonstrate that they improve development and other long-term health outcomes.

Recommendations for the Infants after Hospital Discharge

The goal in nourishing preterm infants after discharge should be to promote human milk feeding, minimize nutrient deficits, promptly address these deficits once identified, and avoid over-nourishing or promoting postnatal growth acceleration once nutrient deficits have been corrected. The recommendations for feeding the preterm infant after hospital discharge are as follows:

- The importance of proactive nutritional support during hospitalization to prevent nutritional deficits and reduce the degree of growth failure is strongly emphasized. This, in turn, will limit the need for specialized feeding for preterm infants after discharge.
- Close monitoring of growth (weight-, length- and head circumference-for-age, indexes of body proportionality) and feed intake should be performed at discharge and regularly after discharge (i.e. at expected term and every 2–4 weeks after discharge) using appropriate growth curves (i.e. WHO growth curves, Fenton curves). Predominantly breastfed infants, infants with persistent morbidities, and infants who were recently transitioned to a different type/mode of feeding should be more closely monitored immediately after discharge and ideally during the first week after discharge.
- Selective biological indexes (e.g. BUN, ferritin, 25(OH) vitamin D, retinol-binding protein) may be useful in order to assess selective nutrient deficiencies but should be determined on an individual basis.
- Because of the heterogeneity in nutritional status, postnatal age and corrected age of preterm infants at the time of hospital discharge an individualized approach is highly recommended over the use of general guidelines. The individualized approach should be based on growth, quality of growth, personal history and selective nutrient deficiencies. As a rule of thumb, however, infants that are born small (i.e. <1,000 g) and/or that are discharge small (<2,000 g) most certainly will require some kind of post-discharge nutritional intervention.
- To avoid creating nutritional deficits after discharge, preterm infants should at least receive the nutrient intake of their respective corrected age (see table 1) until their reach full term (i.e. 39–41 weeks). This strategy does not take into account the nutrient supply needed to compensate for any nutritional deficit.
- The use of a human milk fortifier or formula powder or concentrate in the case of the human milk-fed infant or enriched formulas (i.e. preterm formula, post-discharge formulas) in case of formula feeding may be an effective strategy in addressing early discharge nutrient deficits and poor growth.
- A post-discharge nutritional intervention is more effective in promoting growth if performed early (i.e. before expected term). As a rule of thumb, it should be undertaken until indexes of growth are >–2 SD. However, the strategy should be limited to the period of poor feeding or poor growth and should be discontinued as soon as possible after expected term to avoid overfeeding.

- In agreement with other reports, the authors of this review strongly endorse human milk feeding as the preferred method of nourishing preterm infants after discharge and emphasize the importance of lactation support after discharge to accomplish this.
- The recommendations for DHA, AA and EPA supply for preterm infants should be continued until they reach full term. Thereafter, recommendations for term infants should be applied.
- Screening for iron deficiency is warranted. Iron supplementation should be continued after discharge for hospital, at least until 6–12 months of age depending on diet.
- Further studies are needed before routine supplementation with other vitamins or micronutrients is implemented.

Acknowledgement

The author thanks the ARFEN Association for its support.

Disclosure Statement

The author has no conflicts of interest to disclose.

References

1 Cooke RJ, McCormick K, Griffin IJ, Embleton N, Faulkner K, Wells JC, et al: Feeding preterm infants after hospital discharge: effect of diet on body composition. Pediatr Res 1999;46:461–464.

2 Bertino E, Coscia A, Mombro M, Boni L, Rossetti G, Fabris C, et al: Postnatal weight increase and growth velocity of very low birth weight infants. Arch Dis Child Fetal Neonatal Ed 2006;91:F349–F356.

3 Roggero P, Gianni ML, Amato O, Orsi A, Piemontese P, Cosma B, et al: Postnatal growth failure in preterm infants: recovery of growth and body composition after term. Early Hum Dev 2008;84:555–559.

4 Sakurai M, Itabashi K, Sato Y, Hibino S, Mizuno K: Extrauterine growth restriction in preterm infants of gestational age < or =32 weeks. Pediatr Int 2008;50:70–75.

5 Wang DH: Multicenter study of the nutritional status of premature infants in neonatal intensive care unit in China: report of 974 cases (in Chinese). Zhonghua Er Ke Za Zhi 2009;47:12–17.

6 Bertino E, Coscia A, Boni L, Rossi C, Martano C, Giuliani F, et al: Weight growth velocity of very low birth weight infants: role of gender, gestational age and major morbidities. Early Hum Dev 2009;85:339–347.

7 Cooke RJ, Griffin I: Altered body composition in preterm infants at hospital discharge. Acta Paediatr 2009;98:1269–1273.

8 Roggero P, Gianni ML, Amato O, Orsi A, Piemontese P, Morlacchi L, et al: Is term newborn body composition being achieved postnatally in preterm infants? Early Hum Dev 2009;85:349–352.

9 Ahmad I, Nemet D, Eliakim A, Koeppel R, Grochow D, Coussens M, et al: Body composition and its components in preterm and term newborns: a cross-sectional, multimodal investigation. Am J Hum Biol 2010;22:69–75.

10 Uthaya S, Thomas EL, Hamilton G, Dore CJ, Bell J, Modi N: Altered adiposity after extremely preterm birth. Pediatr Res 2005;57:211–215.

11 Rigo J: Protein, amino acid and other nitrogen compounds; in Tsang RC, Uauy R, Koletzko B, Zlotkin SH (eds): Nutrition of the Preterm Infant Scientific Basis and Practical Aspects. Cincinnati, Digital Educational Publishing, Inc, 2005, pp 45–80.

12 Ehrenkranz RA, Dusick AM, Vohr BR, Wright LL, Wrage LA, Poole WK: Growth in the neonatal intensive care unit influences neurodevelopmental and growth outcomes of extremely low birth weight infants. Pediatrics 2006;117:1253–1261.

13 Powers GC, Ramamurthy R, Schoolfield J, Matula K: Post-discharge growth and development in a predominantly Hispanic, very low birth weight population. Pediatrics 2008;122:1258–1265.

14 Cooke RW, Foulder-Hughes L: Growth impairment in the very preterm and cognitive and motor performance at 7 years. Arch Dis Child 2003;88:482–487.

15 Weisglas-Kuperus N, Hille ET, Duivenvoorden HJ, Finken MJ, Wit JM, van Buuren S, et al: Intelligence of very preterm or very low birth weight infants in young adulthood. Arch Dis Child Fetal Neonatal Ed 2009;94:F196–F200.

16 Canada H: Exclusive breastfeeding duration. http://www.hc-sc.gc.ca/fn-an/nutrition/child-enfant/infant-nourisson/excl_bf_dur-dur_am_excl_e.html. 2004.

17 Kleinman RE: Pediatric Nutrition Handbook, 6 ed. Elk Grove Village/IL, American Academy of Pediatrics, 2009.

18 Agostoni C, Decsi T, Fewtrell M, Goulet O, Kolacek S, Koletzko B, et al: Complementary feeding: a commentary by the ESPGHAN Committee on Nutrition. J Pediatr Gastroenterol Nutr 2008;46:99–110.

19 Gartner LM, Morton J, Lawrence RA, Naylor AJ, O'Hare D, Schanler RJ, et al: Breastfeeding and the use of human milk. Pediatrics 2005;115:496–506.

20 Kramer MS, Aboud F, Mironova E, Vanilovich I, Platt RW, Matush L, et al: Breastfeeding and child cognitive development: new evidence from a large randomized trial. Arch Gen Psychiatry 2008;65:578–584.

21 Morales Y, Schanler RJ: Human milk and clinical outcomes in VLBW infants: how compelling is the evidence of benefit? Semin Perinatol 2007;31:83–88.

22 Callen J, Pinelli J: A review of the literature examining the benefits and challenges, incidence and duration, and barriers to breastfeeding in preterm infants. Adv Neonatal Care 2005;5:72–88; quiz 9–92.

23 Aggett PJ, Agostoni C, Axelsson I, De Curtis M, Goulet O, Hernell O, et al: Feeding preterm infants after hospital discharge: a commentary by the ESPGHAN Committee on Nutrition. J Pediatr Gastroenterol Nutr 2006;42:596–603.

24 Lapillonne A, Salle BL, Glorieux FH, Claris O: Bone mineralization and growth are enhanced in preterm infants fed an isocaloric, nutrient-enriched preterm formula through term. Am J Clin Nutr 2004;80:1595–1603.

25 Young L, Morgan J, McCormick FM, McGuire W: Nutrient-enriched formula versus standard term formula for preterm infants following hospital discharge. Cochrane Database Syst Rev 2012;3:CD004696.

26 Amesz EM, Schaafsma A, Cranendonk A, Lafeber HN: Optimal growth and lower fat mass in preterm infants fed a protein-enriched post-discharge formula. J Pediatr Gastroenterol Nutr 2010;50:200–207.

27 Cooke RJ, Griffin IJ, McCormick K: Adiposity is not altered in preterm infants fed with a nutrient-enriched formula after hospital discharge. Pediatr Res 2010;67:660–664.

28 Aimone A, Rovet J, Ward W, Jefferies A, Campbell DM, Asztalos E, et al: Growth and body composition of human milk-fed premature infants provided with extra energy and nutrients early after hospital discharge: 1-year follow-up. J Pediatr Gastroenterol Nutr 2009;49:456–466.

29 O'Connor DL, Khan S, Weishuhn K, Vaughan J, Jefferies A, Campbell DM, et al: Growth and nutrient intakes of human milk-fed preterm infants provided with extra energy and nutrients after hospital discharge. Pediatrics 2008;121:766–776.

30 Zachariassen G, Faerk J, Grytter C, Esberg BH, Hjelmborg J, Mortensen S, et al: Nutrient enrichment of mother's milk and growth of very preterm infants after hospital discharge. Pediatrics 2011;127:e995–e1003.

31 Young L, Embleton ND, McCormick FM, McGuire W: Multinutrient fortification of human breast milk for preterm infants following hospital discharge. Cochrane Database Syst Rev 2013;2:CD004866.

32 Cooke RJ, Embleton ND, Griffin IJ, Wells JC, McCormick KP: Feeding preterm infants after hospital discharge: growth and development at 18 months of age. Pediatr Res 2001;49:719–722.

33 Lapillonne AA, Glorieux FH, Salle BL, Braillon PM, Chambon M, Rigo J, et al: Mineral balance and whole-body bone mineral content in very low-birth-weight infants. Acta Paediatr Suppl 1994;405:117–122.

34 Rigo JSJ: Nutritional needs of premature infants: current issues. J Pediatr 2006;149:S80–S88.

35 Fewtrell MS, Cole TJ, Bishop NJ, Lucas A: Neonatal factors predicting childhood height in preterm infants: evidence for a persisting effect of early metabolic bone disease? J Pediatr 2000;137:668–673.

36 Agostoni C, Buonocore G, Carnielli VP, De Curtis M, Darmaun D, Decsi T, et al: Enteral nutrient supply for preterm infants: commentary from the European Society of Paediatric Gastroenterology, Hepatology and Nutrition Committee on Nutrition. J Pediatr Gastroenterol Nutr 2010;50:85–91.

37 Baker RD, Greer FR: Diagnosis and prevention of iron deficiency and iron-deficiency anemia in infants and young children (0–3 years of age). Pediatrics 2010;126:1040–1050.

38 Lapillonne A, Groh-Wargo S, Gonzalez CH, Uauy R: Lipid needs of preterm infants: updated recommendations. J Pediatr 2013;162:S37–S47.

39 Peeples JM, Carlson SE, Werkman SH, Cooke RJ: Vitamin A status of preterm infants during infancy. Am J Clin Nutr 1991;53:1455–1459.

40 Delvin EE, Salle BL, Claris O, Putet G, Hascoet JM, Desnoulez L, et al: Oral vitamin A, E and D supplementation of pre-term newborns either breast-fed or formula-fed: a 3-month longitudinal study. J Pediatr Gastroenterol Nutr 2005;40:43–47.

41 Dietitians of Canada, Canadian Paediatric Society, The College of Family Physicians of Canada, Community Health Nurses of Canada Collaborative Statement: Promoting optimal monitoring of child growth in Canada: using the new WHO growth charts. http://www.cps.ca/english/publications/CPS10–01.htm. 2010.

42 Fenton TR, Kim JH: A systematic review and meta-analysis to revise the Fenton growth chart for preterm infants. BMC Pediatr 2013;13:59.

43 Lapillonne A, Griffin IJ: Feeding preterm infants today for later metabolic and cardiovascular outcomes. J Pediatr 2013;162:S7–S16.

44 Ziegler EE: Protein requirements of very low birth weight infants. J Pediatr Gastroenterol Nutr 2007; 45(suppl 3):S170–S174.

45 Lucas A, Fewtrell MS, Morley R, Singhal A, Abbott RA, Isaacs E, et al: Randomized trial of nutrient-enriched formula versus standard formula for post-discharge preterm infants. Pediatrics 2001;108:703–711.

46 Jeon GW, Jung YJ, Koh SY, Lee YK, Kim KA, Shin SM, et al: Preterm infants fed nutrient-enriched formula until 6 months show improved growth and development. Pediatr Int 2011;53:683–688.

Prof. Alexandre Lapillonne, MD, PhD
Department of Neonatology
Necker-Enfants Malades Hospital
149 rue de Sevres, FR–75015 Paris (France)
E-Mail alexandre.lapillonne@nck.aphp.fr

Koletzko B, Poindexter B, Uauy R (eds): Nutritional Care of Preterm Infants: Scientific Basis and Practical Guidelines.
World Rev Nutr Diet. Basel, Karger, 2014, vol 110, pp 278–296 (DOI: 10.1159/000358476)

Meeting the Challenge of Providing Neonatal Nutritional Care to Very or Extremely Low Birth Weight Infants in Low-Resource Settings

Teresa Murguia-Peniche[a] · Gert Francois Kirsten[b]

[a]Rollins School of Public Health, Hubert Department of Global Health, Emory University, Atlanta, Ga., USA;
[b]Neonatal Division, Tygerberg Children's Hospital and University of Stellenbosch, Cape Town, South Africa

Reviewed by Berthold Koletzko, Dr. von Hauner Children's Hospital, University of Munich Medical Centre,
Munich, Germany; Ricardo Uauy, Institute of Nutrition and Food Technology, University of Chile, Santiago de
Chile, Chile; Ekhard Ziegler, Department of Pediatrics, University of Iowa, Coralville, Iowa, USA

Abstract

Most infant deaths (99%) occur in developing countries. The 14.9 million infants born prematurely (>11% of all live births) carry a particularly high mortality risk. This chapter discusses strategies to improve neonatal outcome under resource-restricted conditions, with a focus on nutritional interventions. Evidence-based interventions begin before conception with strategies to prevent and treat malnutrition among women of reproductive age, and micronutrient supplementation in pregnancy. As an example, a practically feasibly strategy of feeding very low birth weight infants in South Africa is presented. The use of parenteral nutrition can be limited by feasibility and affordability, but intravenous glucose and electrolytes should generally be provided after birth. Emphasis is put on the use of expressed own mother's milk without or with pasteurization from women without or with HIV infection, respectively, which is complemented by the use of pasteurized donor milk. If human milk fortifiers are not available, calcium and phosphate should be added, and high total daily feed volumes should be strived for, e.g. by frequent feedings. With restricted resources, human milk fortifiers or preterm formula can be used for high-risk groups such as infants with poor growth. Kangaroo mother care and breastfeeding should be actively encouraged.

Quality of Neonatal Care: An Overview

Annually ~4 million babies die in the world, most (99%) of these deaths occur in developing countries. The main causes of neonatal death are sepsis, asphyxia and prematurity [1, 2]; most if not all can be prevented, this illustrates an important problem of equity in access to healthcare.

Neonatal mortality is the basic indicator to measure the quality of care of newborns; however, quality of care in neonatology means more than averting death, qual-

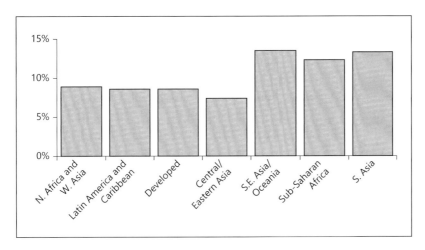

Fig. 1. Prevalence rates of preterm births (% of total number of births) in different regions in 2010. Drawn from data of Blencowe et al. [50].

ity care promotes proper nutrition and augments the potential for a healthy life years for every baby, decreasing the risk of long-term chronic disorders and also promotes an environment for emotional bonding. Prematurity and low birth weight (LBW) is on the rise in many countries. Globally an estimated 14.9 million preterm babies were born in 2010, accounting for 11.1% of all live births, with a prevalence ranging from about 5% in Europe to 18% in some African countries [2, 3] (fig. 1). Estimates of national prevalence of premature births were reported to vary from 7% (North Africa region) to 14% (South Asia region), and an estimated 32.4 million infants were born small for gestational age. The Millennium Development Goal 4 (reduce by two thirds, between 1990 and 2015, the under-five mortality rate) will not be met without important reductions in neonatal mortality. Nutritional support to extremely low birth weight (ELBW) and very low birth weight (VLBW) infants is important to improve neonatal outcomes, but is a challenge under constraint conditions.

In the following section, we discuss evidence-based strategies to improve neonatal care, focusing on nutritional issues. Given that prematurity is on the rise and maternal nutritional strategies have been shown to decrease the incidence of preterm birth, we present as a case study the regional experience (Cape Town, South Africa) to improve nutrition of VLBW infants in low-resource settings.

Nutritional Interventions in Women of Reproductive Age

To improve neonatal care and outcomes, it is important to acknowledge the continuum of care between mother and baby. Interventions to improve neonatal outcomes should begin before conception. Maternal malnutrition, defined as either undernutrition or overweight and obesity, have adverse implications for fetal and maternal health

[4, 5]. Vitamins (A and D), protein, calcium, iron, zinc, folate and iodine deficiencies are major nutritional problems in low-resource countries; deficits of these nutrients are associated with LBW, congenital malformations, cretinism, adult-onset chronic diseases and maternal complications. The Institute of Medicine and the American College of Obstetricians and Gynecologists of USA have established recommendations of weight gain during pregnancy as a function of pre-pregnancy body mass index [6]. While deviations from these recommendations may be associated with LBW, prematurity, macrosomia, and problems at delivery (ACOG, 2012), it is not generally accepted that these guidelines that are based on observational studies in the USA should serve as the basis for clinical practice in other parts of the world [7].

Another cost-effective form of care is the use of antenatal corticosteroids. Given to women in premature labor to speed up fetal lung development and prevent respiratory distress of premature babies, antenatal corticosteroid injections cost as little as USD 0.50 per dose and are routinely given to women in high-income countries. Yet only 5–10% of women in low- and middle-income countries receive this intervention. Use of antenatal corticosteroids is a key recommendation of the UN Commission on Life-Saving Commodities for Women and Children.

Greater availability of antibiotics is also important in tackling prematurity. Newborn babies with infection require immediate injectable antibiotics. Similarly, women who experience premature rupture of the membranes before 37 weeks – a major risk of preterm delivery – require access to antibiotics to reduce the risk of infections and to delay birth.

Looking at the connection between the health of women and children, better access to family planning can prevent unwanted births. This need is particularly acute for adolescent girls, who have a proportionately increased risk of having premature and LBW babies. An estimated 230,000 lives could be saved if access to family planning was scaled up to 60% coverage or to the level of achieving a total fertility rate of 2.5.

Preventing and caring for prematurity is an important part of the work that needs to be done to enhance newborn survival and health. The global Every Newborn action plan to be launched in 2014, hinges on this simple message: we can and must do better for the most vulnerable infants.

Multiple Micronutrient Supplements during Pregnancy and Birth Outcomes

Micronutrient supplementation during pregnancy has been evaluated in different trials. A recent systematic review, which included 16 randomized controlled trials from countries in Africa, Asia, Central America and Europe, concluded that supplementation with 5 or more micronutrients was more effective in reducing LBW (risk ratio (RR) 0.86; 95% CI 0.81–0.91) and small for gestational age (RR 0.83; 95% CI 0.73–0.95) (8 trials), as compared to those supplemented with three or fewer micronutrients [8]. Calcium supplementation during pregnancy has been associated with a lower risk of pregnancy-induced hypertension and LBW. It is recommended to give 1.5 g/day and if the patient's intake of calcium is low, 2 g/day, ideally before 24 weeks' gestation (Pan American Health Organization, 2011). The first 1,000 days of life (conception to 2 years) is a critical period for growth and development which has long-term effects for individual children and for populations [9, 10]. Interventions to improve nutrition during this period require pre-pregnancy, antenatal and postnatal strategies. These interventions are especially critical when dealing with LBW and ELBW infants; nutritional support needs to be strengthened in this group of patients using available resources.

Interventions during the Neonatal Period

Delayed cord clamping (DCC) increases placental transfusion, leading to an increase in neonatal blood volume at birth of approximately 30% [11]. In a recent meta-analysis, DCC (30–120 s) was associated with less need of transfusions, better circulatory stability, less intraventricular hemorrhage and lower risk of necrotizing enterocolitis (NEC) in preterm infants. In term infants, DCC seems to decrease the risk of anemia during the first months of life and to improve ferritin levels (weighted mean difference 17.89; 95% CI 16.58–19.21). DCC is a simple, safe and cheap method to improve iron status of babies, however the risk of polycythemia and jaundice may be increased [12, 13]. DCC may be useful in regions with poor resources where medical units do not have available blood banks or do not have safe transfusion practices. Children of low-resource countries with high prevalence of anemia may also benefit from this practice by improving iron status, especially in malaria-endemic regions, where iron and folic acid supplementation has been associated with adverse outcomes as suggested from the Pemba trial [14, 15].

Family Community Care

Studies in Bangladesh and India have shown substantial (34–54%) reductions in neonatal mortality when introducing packages of interventions for essential newborn care which include early home neonatal visits which promote breastfeeding and other interventions directed to the LBW infant [16, 17]. Breastfeeding decreases neonatal and post-neonatal mortality; it is important to start breastfeeding as early as possible (<1 h of life) [18]. When looking at the prevalence of breastfeeding and outcomes associated with early breastfeeding, a recent study which included the last Health Survey Data from 14 low-income countries, concluded that early breastfeeding was reported by 38% of mothers and was associated with a lower incidence of underweight in infants 0–5 months of age (odds ratio 0.83; 95% CI 0.7–0.98) [19]. Breastfeeding for a least 6 months is universally recommended [20, 21]. Many countries are still far from achieving this goal [22].

Research to understand barriers to breastfeeding needs to be urgently implemented, especially in ELBW and LBW infants. Also, the use, expression and storage of human milk are quite difficult in low-resource settings. Many strategies are implemented in different regions to overcome these problems, such as flash-heat pasteurization of human milk, cup feeding, and other strategies which will be discussed below. Early skin to skin contact in mother-LBW infant's dyads has been used for several years, mostly in developing countries. It is also known as Kangaroo Mother's Care (KMC). It was developed in Colombia in 1978 [23]. A recent meta-analysis of 34 randomized trials using skin to skin contact concluded that there seemed to be benefits in breastfeeding outcomes and cardiorespiratory stability with KMC; however, the overall methodological quality of studies was mixed with high heterogeneity [24]. Kangaroo care may also improve thermal control, although alternative methods need to be implemented. Further research, with clearly established methodologies and proper epidemiologic analysis, is needed.

Feeding the Hospitalized VLBW Infant in a Developing Country: A Regional Experience

Providing optimal medical care and nutrition during the early neonatal period remains a challenge in most of the world. The high maternal HIV infection rates in many of these countries further complicates the nutritional care of these infants, as transmission of HIV through expressed breast milk (EBM) is a continuous threat [25]. Meeting these challenges has demanded innovative solutions. The following section will present the approach used by Tygerberg Children's Hospital and University of Stellenbosch in Cape Town, South Africa, which serves communities with a very low socioeconomic status.

The availability of breast milk fortifiers, parenteral nutrition, preterm milk formula and cooling facilities for EBM are problematic as is a clean water supply at home to sterilize milk bottles. Furthermore, high care and neonatal intensive care facilities vary significantly between regions and countries.

Initial Management of VLBW Infants in an Institution with Limited Resources

Due to limited neonatal intensive care facilities, VLBW infants are managed in neonatal wards. In many resource-constrained countries, ventilator support is only offered to infants >1,000 g or even >1,500 g. Nasal continuous positive airway pressure is widely used. The initiation of colostrum and breast milk expressing is commenced as soon as possible after delivery. Parenteral nutrition is often not available or when available is limited to infants with feeding intolerance or bowel obstruction [26].

Enteral Feeding of VLBW Infants in a Resource-Constrained Setting

Colostrum, followed by breast milk, is the enteral feeding of choice. It decreases the risk of infections and NEC, and contains growth factors to stimulate gut growth and maturation. Additionally the use of breast milk reduces costs, prevents post-discharge infections and may improve long-term neurodevelopment [27–29]. The use of pre-term formula is limited in LBW infants due to the increased risk of NEC, gastrointestinal disorders and the absence of anti-infective properties; additionally it imposes an economic burden on constrained hospital budgets. Enteral nutrition is commenced as soon as colostrum is available, unless clinical condition precludes this; oropharyngeal administration of colostrum immunoglobulins, lymphoid cells, and other factors which contribute to local barrier protection are provided. Human milk oligosaccharides provide additional protection, based on their ability to inhibit the adhesion of pathogens. The administration of 0.2 ml of colostrum every 2 h to ELBW infants is well tolerated by even the sickest babies [30].

A mother should begin manual expressing of colostrum and breast milk as soon after delivery of her infant as possible. Handling colostrum requires dedicated, caring and well-trained nursing staff who must instruct the mother in manually expressing colostrum and breast milk. The first 2 days' colostrum, usually a few milliliters at a time, can be collected in a sterilized teaspoon (disposable plastic teaspoons are preferable) or a new disposable 1- or 2-ml syringe and immediately administered directly into the mouth of the infant. Mothers should express 8–12 times per day and ensure that they fully express the breasts each time. Appropriate sterile containers for storage of expressed milk must be used and milk must be refrigerated immediately after expressing. Human milk may be stored at 4°C for up to 96 h or should be frozen [31]. If cooling or freezing facilities are not available, preterm EBM may be stored for up to 4 h at room temperature [32].

EBM is used in three forms:
- Unpasteurized own mother's EBM from HIV– women
- Pasteurized own mother's EBM from HIV+ women
- Pasteurized donor EBM

A neonatal ward should have a milk kitchen with ample refrigeration and freezer facilities as well as the necessary equipment for the flash-heating method of pasteurization [33].

Nutritional Care of VLBW Infants in Developing Countries: Practical Aspects

Feeding and Precautions under Special Circumstances: Pasteurization of EBM
Due to the risk of HIV transmission through EBM, the HIV status of every mother must be known on the admission of her baby to a neonatal ward. HIV+ mothers are taught to pasteurize their breast milk immediately after expressing milk. It is important to take precautions to avoid stigmatization of HIV+ mothers. All HIV+ and po-

tentially HIV+ EBM (i.e. EBM from mothers who refuse to be tested) must be pasteurized and labelled before it can be stored in the ward's refrigerator. Flash-heating pasteurization can be used in hospital or at home after discharge. The nursing staff must demonstrate the technique to the mothers, the correct labelling of the milk bottles and the applying of a designated colored sticker (e.g. purple) to the bottle to indicate that it contains pasteurized EBM from an HIV+ mother. Jars must be labelled with the baby's name, surname, hospital number, date and time of expressing as well as date and time of pasteurization. A wall chart should be available for reference. Mothers should always be supervised when pasteurizing their breast milk for the first time.

The following equipment is needed for flash-heating pasteurization:
- Pot with approximately 1 liter capacity
- Sterilized glass jar with approximately 400 ml capacity, e.g. empty glass peanut butter jar
- A weight to hold down the jar of milk in the water, e.g. another jar with water
- Electric/gas stove/hot plate
- Insulation boards on which to place the hot pot
- Patient stickers
- A colored sticker to identify pasteurized HIV+ EBM
- Pen to write the date on the patient sticker

Fifty to 150 ml breast milk is expressed into a sterile glass jar and the lid is then closed. The jar with EBM is placed in the pot which is then placed on the stove and a weight is placed on the jar. Approximately 450 ml of tap water is poured into the pot with the water level 2 fingers (2 cm) above the level of the expressed milk. The water and milk are heated together on a high heat setting, until the water is at a rolling boil. The pot is immediately removed from the stove and the jar with EBM removed from the hot water. The pasteurized EBM is allowed to cool at room temperature. EBM from an HIV+ mother may only be placed in the refrigerator or freezer once it has been pasteurized. EBM from HIV+ and HIV– mothers is ideally stored in separate refrigerators. Milk from HIV+ mothers should be easily identified according to a specifically designated colored sticker, especially if it is stored in the same refrigerator as EBM from HIV– mothers.

Once pasteurized, the cooled EBM can be used immediately or stored in the designated milk refrigerator for up to 96 h; when stored for longer periods, it should be frozen [31]. Pasteurized EBM may be stored at room temperature for 24 h, especially if kept in the pasteurization container and is not handled [34]. Strict protocols must be followed to ensure that the correct EBM is administered to a baby. Two nurses must check the baby's name, the hospital number and the date of collection on the container of milk before it is administered to the baby and must sign the relevant nursing documentation in the infant's folder. The name of the nurse, signature, date and time that the milk was checked must be noted. Protocols must also be in place for the management of an infant after the inadvertent administration of HIV+ EBM to the wrong baby. The use of breast pumps is discouraged as sharing between mothers may result in HIV, cytomegalovirus and hepatitis B transmission [35].

Murguia-Peniche · Kirsten

Pasteurized donor EBM is used if the mother does not produce enough breast milk, if the mother is too sick to express or if she dies. Donor milk is obtained from healthy non-smoking, non-drug using HIV-, hepatitis B- and non-syphilis-infected mothers in the KMC ward and from mothers attending breastfeeding clinics in the community. If EBM has to be pasteurized in large volumes, a commercial pasteurization bath is installed in the central milk kitchen of the hospital. The Holder technique is used whereby EBM is heated to 62.5°C for 30 min, followed by rapid cooling. If a commercial pasteurizer is unaffordable, donor EBM from suitable donor mothers can be pasteurized using the flash-heating method.

Early Administration of EBM in VLBW Infants, Fortification and Alternatives to Human Milk Fortification

EBM is initially administered by orogastric tube. Breast milk intake is advanced by 15–35 ml/kg daily (depending on clinical condition) and administered to infants <1,000 g as a continuous infusion. The aim is to reach an enteral intake of 150 ml/kg/day by day 6 or 7 of life.

EBM from mothers of premature infants has certain inherent deficiencies in regions with low resources. For example, preterm expressed breast milk (PEBM) from Xhosa (ethnic group) mothers with VLBW infants in the Western Cape, South Africa, contains approximately 66 kcal/100 ml during the first week following delivery but is as low as 52 kcal/100 ml during the fourth week (table 1). As enterally fed VLBW infants require between 110 and 135 kcal/kg/day to gain at least 15 g/kg/day, these infants will need an intake of at least 200–220 ml of EBM/kg/day to attain this. Furthermore, the protein content of breast milk from these mothers progressively decreases over the first 4 weeks of life to a mean of 1.46 g/100 ml (95% CI 0.95–1.96) [E. van Wyk, pers. commun.]. Even when the intake is 200 ml/kg/day, an average of 3 g/kg/day of protein is provided instead of the required 3.5–4.5 g/kg/day.

Due to the low calcium, phosphate, protein, vitamin and caloric content of EBM for the nutritional requirements of VLBW infants, a breast milk fortifier should be added after enteral intake is well tolerated [36]. Milk fortification in infants <1,000 g is initially added at half strength for 2–3 days before it is increased to full strength. A daily weight gain of 15 g/kg is acceptable once birth weight is regained. If the weight gain on fortified EBM is still suboptimal on 200 ml/kg/day, medium chain triglycerides in the form of vegetable or coconut oil is an affordable way of increasing the energy content of EBM. Coconut or vegetable oil, which provides 7.7 kcal/ml, is administered at a dose of 2–3 ml/kg/day in four divided dosages. This will increase the caloric intake by 15–23 kcal/day.

If breast milk fortifiers are not available, coconut oil or vegetable oil can also be added to increase the caloric content of PEBM. The use of large total daily feed volumes in smaller more frequent aliquots is helpful when high-density nutrient milk

Table 1. Composition of 100 ml of EBM (mean [95% CI]) from Xhosa mothers with VLBW infants in South Africa over the first 4 weeks of life [E. van Wyk, pers. commun.]

Nutrient	Week 1	Week 2	Week 3	Week 4	p value
Energy, kcal	66.5 [57–77]	63.1 [52–74]	67.2 [51.1–83.2]	61.8 [52.1–71.6]	0.44
Protein, g	2.01 [1.5–2.5]	1.7 [1.0–2.4]	1.6 [0.99–2.3]	1.46 [0.95–1.96]	<0.001
Carbohydrate, g	6.88 [6.3–7.5]	6.7 [5.9–7.5]	6.6 [5.9–7.3]	6.56 [6–7.1]	0.15
Fat, g	3.37 [2.4–4.5]	3.2 [2.0–4.3]	3.8 [2.3–5.3]	3.30 [2.4–4.3]	0.45
Calcium, mg	27.2 [17.8–36.6]	23.8 [19.0–28.5]	23.9 [19.1–28.6]	23.69 [19.8–27.6]	0.14
Phosphorous, mg	15.7 [11.5–20.0]	15.5 [12.4–18.6]	13.9 [10.8–17.0]	13.20 [10.2–16.2]	0.10
Sodium, mg	45.8 [29.3–62.4]	35.3 [16.6–54.0]	36.4 [23.1–49.7]	38.26 [22.6–53.9]	0.21
Iron, mg	0.19 [0.12–0.26]	0.17 [0.1–0.2]	0.156 [0.1–0.2]	0.184 [0.10–0.27]	0.48

Table 2. Composition of a multivitamin syrup for premature infants (Abidec Multivitamin Drops™) compared to intakes recommended by ESPGHAN [49]

Vitamin	Requirement/day[a]	Dose/day	Abidec® 0.6 ml/day	Comment
Vitamin A	400–1,000 µg/kg	400 µg (1,333 IU)	1,333 IU vitamin A palmitate	discontinue at 12 months of age
Vitamin D	800–1,000 IU/day	400 IU	400 IU ergocalciferol	discontinue at 12 months of age
Thiamine	140–300 µg/kg	400 µg	400 µg	discontinue at 12 months of age
Riboflavin	200–400 µg	800 µg	800 µg riboflavin	discontinue at 12 months of age
Niacin	380–5,500 µg/kg	8,000 µg	8,000 µg niacin	discontinue at 12 months of age
Vitamin C	11–46 mg/kg	40 mg	40 mg vitamin C	discontinue at 12 months of age

[a] ESPGHAN [49].

preparations are not available to provide adequate nutrition at lower volumes. If preterm formula is available, breast milk feeding can be alternated with preterm formula though this should be the last option if infants are not growing and should not be done in infants born to HIV+ mothers. Alternatively the baby can be fed hindmilk as its fat and caloric content are substantially higher than foremilk [37].

The low phosphate and calcium content of breast milk can be supplemented by the nasogastric tube administration of 60–90 mg/kg/day phosphate solution and 120–140 mg/kg/day calcium solution, each divided into four dosages. The calcium and phosphate solutions cannot be administered simultaneously, but should be alternated due to the high osmotic load. The oral phosphate and oral calcium solutions can be prepared by the hospital's pharmacy.

If an iron- and vitamin-containing fortifier is not available, enteral iron at a dosage of 2–3 mg/kg/day should be commenced at 2 weeks of age. A multivitamin supplement should be commenced once the infant is on full enteral feeding (table 2). If the vitamin D content of multivitamin supplements is too low (as in this example), an additional 400 IU vitamin D should be prescribed.

Proposed advancement of feeds in stable and unstable preterm infants in resource constrained regions are presented in tables 3 and 4.

Table 3. Proposed strategy for feeding stable preterm infants in low-resource settings

	ELBW	1–1.5 kg	>1.5 kg
First feeding	human milk	human milk	human milk
Start minimal enteral feedings	day 1	not applicable	not applicable
Volume	0.5 ml/h	not applicable	not applicable
Start feeds	day 2	day 1	day 1
Advance[a]	30 ml/kg/day	30–35 ml/kg/day	full feeds
Full feeds	day 6	days 4–5	day 1
Vitamins	at full feeds	at full feeds	at full feeds
Iron[b]	2 weeks	2 weeks	3 weeks
Not growing[c]	180–200 ml/kg	180–200 ml/kg	180–200/ml/kg

[a] Try continuous feeding <1 kg. [b] See text for considerations in malaria-endemic regions. [c] Add fortifier; if not available consider 'cooking oil' and calcium and phosphate supplementation (see text).

Table 4. Proposed strategy for feeding unstable preterm infants in low-resource settings

	ELBW	1–1.5 kg	>1.5 kg
First feeding	human milk	human milk	human milk
Start minimal enteral feeding	day 2	day 2	day 2
Volume	0.5 ml/h	1 ml/h	1 ml/h
Start feeds	day 4	day 4	day 4
Advance[a]	15–20 ml/kg/day	30–35 ml/kg/day	50 ml/kg/day
Full feeds	day 14	days 8–9	day 6
Vitamins	at full feeds	at full feeds	at full feeds
Iron[b]	2 weeks	2 weeks	3 weeks
Not growing[c]	180–200 ml/kg	180–200 ml/kg	180–200 ml/kg

[a] Try continuous feeding <1 kg; carefully monitor gastrointestinal condition. Stop if intolerance. [b] See text for considerations in malaria-endemic regions. [c] Add fortifier at enteral intake of 100 ml/kg/day; if not available consider 'cooking oil' and calcium and phosphate supplementation (see text).

Parenteral Nutrition

If the preferred approach of providing all VLBW infants with an intravenous supply of glucose and amino acids (and lipids if doable) from birth cannot be realized, at least a 10% glucose-electrolyte solution should be started after birth at a volume of 80–100 ml/kg/day. If such a solution is not commercially available, 2 mmol sodium and 1.5 mmol potassium can be added to 100 ml of a 10% glucose solution for intravenous administration. Parenteral nutrition (PN) is usually not available for VLBW infants treated in low-resource institutions due to the high costs and lack of medical and nursing expertise. If there is no local expertise to provide safe PN it should not be used; other strategies to provide fluids and electrolytes (sodium, potassium, calcium and phosphate) should be implemented (see table 6) and oral feeding started and ad-

Table 5. Composition of a 3-in-1 parenteral nutrition solution/150 ml used in South Africa, compared to assumed nutrient

	3-in-1 parenteral nutrition[a]	Recommended daily intake, kg/day
Volume, ml	150	150
Protein, g	3.12	3.0–4.0
Dextrose, g	15.5	10–15
Lipid, g	3.1	3.0–4.0
Non-protein energy, kcal	94	90–100
Sodium, mmol	3.2	2–3.5
Potassium, mmol	2.5	2.5
Calcium, mmol	1.5	1.5–2.25
Magnesium, mmol	0.25	0.15–0.25
Phosphate, mmol	1.54	1.1–2.3

[a] Peditrace 1.05 ml, Soluvit Novum 0.105 ml and Vitalipid N infant 0.525 ml are added.

Table 6. Proposed progression of intravenous nutritional supply for VLBW infants

Age, days	Total volume of fluid, ml		Glucose electrolyte (GE)[a]	Parenteral nutrition (PN)[a]
	<1.0 kg	1.0–1.5 kg	uncomplicated or PN not available	complicated[b]
1	100	80	10% GE solution[c]	10% GE solution + 3-in-1 PN
2	120	100	10% GE solution	3-in-1 PN
3	140	120	10% GE solution	3-in-1 PN
4	160	140	10% GE solution	3-in-1 PN[d]
5	180	160	10% GE solution	3-in-1 PN[d]
6	200	180	10% GE solution	3-in-1 PN[d]
			until full feeds…	until feeds tolerated…

[a] Intravenous volume is decreased at the same rate as enteral feeds are advanced.
[b] Complicated, i.e. feeding intolerance, NEC, bowel obstruction (enteral feeds discontinued). PN should be given only if resources and experience available.
[c] 10% glucose with electrolytes: 2–3 mmol/kg/day of sodium and potassium, 120–140 mg calcium salt/kg/day and 60–90 mg phosphate/kg/day. Sodium and potassium may be added until adequate diuresis has been established.
[d] Recommended volume of PN 150 ml/kg/day. The rest of the volume may be given by oral route (if possible) or dextrose 10% if needed.

vanced aggressively as soon as possible. In some cases PN is available and there is experience, but an admixture unit in the hospital, with dedicated pharmacists for daily mixing of tailor-made PN solutions for individual infants, is unaffordable. A commercially prepared 3-in-1 lipid-amino-acid-glucose preparation for VLBW infants for short-term use (<3 weeks) is an affordable alternative (table 5). If PN is available, it is usually reserved for the infant with feeding intolerance or with a surgical condition such as bowel obstruction, NEC, spontaneous intestinal perforation, etc.

PN is initially administered through an umbilical venous line for a maximum of 7 days, and if still indicated, through a percutaneously inserted central line. The PN solution is administered over 24 h through a 1.2-μm filter and the administration tubing is changed every 24 h. Due to the high mineral content and osmolality of PN, administration through a peripheral line may result in tissue necrosis during the inadvertent leakage of PN fluid into the tissue. Stringent monitoring of the drip site is essential if this route of administration is used. Nursing staff should monitor the infusion site hourly for early signs of extravasation of PN fluid and thrombophlebitis. Early detection can minimize skin and tissue necrosis. Thrombophlebitis is usually avoided by changing the infusion site every 72 h and by sterilizing the skin thoroughly before insertion of the cannula.

Whether the PN is administered through an umbilical, central or peripheral line, no drugs or blood products should be administered through this line. The hub connection of the administration set remains the most important port of entry for bacteria and fungi during the administration of PN. The Clave® (ICU Medical, Inc., San Clemente, Calif., USA) needle-free connector and intravenous system provides a mechanically- and microbiologically-closed system for the administration of PN to protect the administration catheter from contamination that can lead to bloodstream infections. The Clave® systems may be unaffordable in resource-constrained countries. An affordable method of reducing hub infections during the administration of PN is to incorporate the catheter hub in the administration line with a polyvidone-iodine (betadine) connection shield [38]. A sterile 5 × 5 cm gauze square is soaked in betadine and wrapped around the hub connection and completely enclosed by waterproof Elastoplast® (Beiersdorf, Hamburg, Germany). It is replaced every 24 h along with the PN infusion set.

As the 3-in-1 PN solution is designed for short-term use, i.e. not more than 3 weeks, twice-weekly monitoring of electrolytes and weekly monitoring of liver function tests and a complete blood count are sufficient. The PN is advanced from 50% of the intravenous fluid intake needs on the first day of administration to the full volume the next day. The nutritional pathway for feeding a VLBW infant is presented in table 4.

Kangaroo Mother Care, Breastfeeding, and Preparing for Discharge

KMC facilities for the mothers of VLBW infants form an integral part of neonatal wards in developing countries [29]. Mothers of VLBW infants are immediately transferred to the KMC unit on discharge from the postnatal ward. The KMC unit is attached to the neonatal ward. This ensures that the mothers are available to provide colostrum and EBM from soon after birth and to assist with the care of their infants.

While the infant is still in the incubator and receiving intravenous feeding, the mother practices intermittent KMC lasting for a few hours per day and continues with regular breast milk expressing. Continuous KMC whereby the baby is in the skin-to-skin KMC position >20 h/day commences once the infant is gaining adequate weight, is off nasal continuous positive airway pressure, is stable and weighs at least 1,200 g. Although the infant is still being fed EBM by nasogastric tube, breastfeeding is now slowly introduced. The infants need to be woken to feed. Most premature infants attain maximal oral feeding by 35–37 weeks [39]. They are discharged while they are still developing their oral feeding skills, i.e. at weights of 1,600–1,800 g and a gestational age of approximately 34 weeks. As they are often not able to empty a breast and to obtain sufficient amounts of breast milk to meet their nutritional requirements they need top-up feeds. In hospital this is accomplished by additional nasogastric feeds of EBM. When the infant is fully established on the breast the nasogastric tube is removed. Nasogastric top-up feeding cannot be practiced at home but cup feeding can. There is ample time in the KMC unit for the mothers to be taught the correct method of cup feeding by the nursing staff. Immediately after the breastfeed the mother expresses milk from the partially emptied breast into a cup to ensure that the breast is fully emptied to maintain a good milk supply and she can give her baby a top-up feed by cup. Compared to a bottle and its teat, a cup is very easy to sterilize, even for mothers with no access to electricity or clean running water at home. While in hospital, an iron and vitamin-containing fortifier is added to the cup-fed PEBM. If no fortifier is available, a multivitamin and iron syrup, vitamin D, calcium, phosphate and vegetable oil are also administered.

Electrolyte levels including sodium, calcium, phosphate and hemoglobin levels are measured weekly once the infant is on exclusive breast milk feeding. Low serum sodium and phosphate levels are corrected by adding sodium chloride and phosphate to the feeds.

Inadequate protein intake during the early neonatal period in VLBW infants is associated with decreased head growth and poor long-term cognitive function [40]. Daily weight gain and weekly head growth should be plotted on a growth chart such as the Fenton Growth Chart for Premature Boys and Girls for the early identification of poor growth [41]. A daily weight gain of <12 g/kg/day and a head circumference at discharge <10th centile for gestational age have been associated with a poor neurodevelopmental outcome in ELBW infants [42].

Discharge

Infants are discharged home when they reach a gestational age of at least 35 weeks, a weight of 1,650–1,800 g, are gaining adequate weight, are fully breastfed and the mother is confident to care for her baby at home. Fortification is discontinued at discharge and a multivitamin and iron syrup is commenced which should be continued until at least 12 months of age (table 2). In malaria-endemic areas, screening for anemia is recommended and iron given if needed in the non-malaria (dry) season in conjunction with programs for diagnosis and treatment of malaria [14]. Feeding the infant formula milk and especially preterm formula has huge financial implications for the mother and is often associated with malnutrition due to incorrect reconstitution. It is critical that these infants are followed at clinics in their community and that their weight is meticulously monitored. Infants with poor weight gain are referred to a doctor. As VLBW infants are at a significant risk of a poor neurodevelopmental outcome, neurodevelopment assessments are of paramount importance. Nursing staff at the clinics should be trained to do basic assessments. Those infants with delayed milestones are referred to the hospital to be assessed by a doctor at 4–6 monthly intervals during the first year of life.

Nutritional Counselling Based on the Integrated Management of Childhood Illnesses (IMCI)

It is estimated that the energy needed from complementary foods during the ages 6–8, 9–11 and 12–23 months averages 270, 450 and 750 kcal/day, respectively [43]. Table 7 summarizes recommendations based on the IMCI to achieve this goal. The IMCI guidelines recommend the intake of foods that are rich in iron (e.g. meat, organ meats, chicken and dark-green vegetables); vitamin A (liver, mango, and sweet potato), zinc (meat, fish and legumes) and calcium (full-cream milk). Universal supplementation with iron, vitamin A and zinc is also a common practice in some developing countries. Micronutrient powders, also called sprinkles, containing iron, vitamin A, zinc and other vitamins and minerals can be sprinkled onto any semi-solid food at home; a recent meta-analysis concluded that home fortification of foods with sprinkles decreases anemia and iron deficiency in infants 6–23 months [44]. This strategy is recommended to improve iron status but no other micronutrient deficiencies [45]. However, there are still open questions with the use of sprinkles in terms of safety, in particularly the risk of enhancing infection risk, most appropriate conditions of use (daily vs. intermittent), and best mineral composition [46].

Summary of WHO Recommendations on Optimal Feeding of LBW Infants (Stable and >1 kg)

In 2011 the World Health Organization (WHO) convened a group of experts from the WHO regions to develop guidelines to improve the quality of care received by LBW infants in developing countries (WHO, 2011). These guidelines focused on the feeding of the clinically stable LBW infant and did not address the feeding of the

Table 7. Nutritional management at discharge based on IMCI

Age	IMCI recommendations
<6 months	For mother HIV–: – Exclusive breastfeed – Feed at least eight times in 24 h – Do not give other foods or fluids For mother HIV+: – Exclusive breastfeed (previous informed choice) or – If accessible, feasible, affordable, sustainable and safe: replacement feed exclusively (formula) (previous informed choice) – Stop breastfeeding completely at 6 months
6–12 months	For mother HIV–: – Breastfeed (previous informed choice) – Give three servings of nutritious complementary foods (malnourished infants may need 1 or 2 extra meals) – Always mix margarine, fat, oil, peanut butter or ground nuts with porridge – Mashed banana, beans, avocados, full cream milk, fruit and vegetables are other suitable complementary foods – Give egg, beans, lentils, meat, fish, chicken, locally available protein, full-cream milk, mashed fruit and vegetables For mother HIV+: – Do not breastfeed after 6 months – Formula feeds and complementary feeds as for mother who is HIV–

infant <1 kg. The recommendations were graded as: a) strong recommendation if there was confidence that the benefits clearly outweigh the harms; b) weak recommendation, when the benefits probably outweigh the harms, but there was uncertainty about the trade-offs. The main recommendations were:

- LBW infants should be fed mother's own milk (strong recommendation).
- If an infant cannot be fed mother's own milk, he or she should be fed donor human milk if safe banking facilities are available (strong situational recommendation).
- LBW infants who cannot be fed human milk should be fed standard infant formula; however, if they fail to gain weight they should be given preterm infant formula (weak situational recommendation).
- VLBW infants who fail to gain weight despite adequate breast milk feeding should be given human milk fortifiers (weak situational recommendation).
- VLBW infants should be given vitamin D supplements at a dose ranging from 400 to 1,000 IU until 6 months of age (weak recommendation). Note: we recommend to continue until 12 months of age [47].
- VLBW infants who are fed human milk (mother's own or donor) should be given daily calcium (120–140 mg/kg/day) and phosphorus (60–90 mg/kg/day)

supplementation during the first months of life (weak recommendation). Note: the benefit of calcium and phosphorus supplementation in terms of reducing metabolic bone disease is expected to be valued by providers and parents and the associated costs are low.

- VLBW infants fed human milk (mother's own or donor) should be given 2–4 mg/kg/day iron supplementation starting at 2 weeks of life until 6 months of age (weak recommendation). Note: we recommend to continue until 12 months of age [47].
- LBW infants should be put to the breast as soon as possible if stable (strong recommendation).
- VLBW infants should be given 10 ml/kg/day (trophic feeding) of enteral feeds, preferably EBM, starting day 1 of life, with the remaining fluid requirement met by intravenous fluids (weak situational recommendation). Note: our recommendation is to give 30 ml/kg/day if the infant is stable, in settings where intravenous fluids and other resources are limited. The infant should be carefully monitored and if signs of feeding intolerance appear, feeds should be stopped. Research is urgently needed to evaluate these recommendations.
- LBW should be exclusively breastfed until 6 months of age (strong recommendation).
- LBW infants who need to be fed by an alternative oral feeding method should be fed by cup (or palladai) or spoon (strong recommendation). Since cups are much easier to clean than bottles, feeding by cup could potentially reduce the risk of severe infections. Also, cup feeding is also associated with benefits in breastfeeding rates. On the other hand, one randomized controlled trial compared the effects of cup and bottle feeding on length of hospital stay in LBW infants. Infants in the cup-feeding group had a higher hospital stay (mean difference 10 days) [48]; this finding deserves further research.
- In VLBW infants, feed volumes can be increased by up to 30 ml/kg/day with careful monitoring for feed intolerance (weak recommendation).

Conclusions

Neonatal mortality is an important indicator of quality of neonatal care; most neonatal deaths occur in developing countries. Quality of neonatal care implies also a comprehensive approach which includes a continuum of care and optimal maternal and neonatal nutrition. Despite serious financial constraints in resource-limited countries, it is possible to provide adequate nutritional support to VLBW infants by using early and aggressive EBM feeding, breast milk fortification and selectively administer a 3-in-1 PN solution.

Preventing and caring for prematurity is an important part of the work that needs to be done to enhance newborn survival and health. The global Every Newborn action plan to be launched in 2014 hinges on this simple message: we can and must do better for the most vulnerable infants.

Practical Recommendations for VLBW Infants in Developing Countries

(1) Appropriate care practices and good nutrition including micronutrient supplementation to pregnant women may help decrease the incidence of LBW.

(2) Delayed cord clamping may improve the iron status of infants and decrease the need of blood transfusions and the incidence of NEC in VLBW infants.

(3) If parenteral nutrition is not feasible or affordable, enteral feeds should be started and advanced aggressively on day 1 of life for all stable babies and not be delayed beyond day 4 (if feeding is not contraindicated), for even the sickest infants (with careful monitoring of feeding tolerance). An intravenous solution with dextrose 10%, sodium, potassium, calcium and phosphate may be given to assure adequate volume and electrolyte administration.

(4) The use of large total daily feed volumes in smaller more frequent aliquots is helpful when high-density nutrient milk preparations are not available, to provide adequate nutrition at lower volumes.

(5) If fortifiers are not available, calcium and phosphate should be added to the feeding regime. If growth is suboptimal, cooking oil or vegetable coconut oil may be added.

(6) With a smaller budget, breast milk fortifier or preterm formula can be used for special groups like the VLBW infant and those with poor growth on maximal volumes of standard milk.

(7) Vitamins and iron should be provided to all infants born weighing <1.5 kg, especially those not receiving breast milk fortifiers.

Research Needs

(1) Define optimal micronutrient preparations and interventions for pregnant women.

(2) Improve and evaluate interventions to prevent LBW and ELBW.

(3) Assess skin to skin KMC advantages on specific outcomes.

(4) Perform comparative studies of cup feeding versus bottle feeding in low-resource settings.

(5) Define best 'comprehensive, aggressive and safe' practices to feed ELBW and LBW in low-resource countries and analyze long-term outcomes.

References

1 Lawn JE, Cousens S, Zupan J: Four million neonatal deaths: When? Where? Why? Lancet 2005;365:891–900.

2 Blencowe H, Cousens S: Addressing the challenge of neonatal mortality. Trop Med Int Health 2013;18:303–312.

3 Goldenberg RL, Culhane JF, Iams JD, Romero R: Epidemiology and causes of preterm birth. Lancet 2008;371:75–84.

4 Black RE, Victora CG, Walker SP, Bhutta ZA, Christian P, de Onis M, et al: Maternal and child undernutrition and overweight in low-income and middle-income countries. Lancet 2013;382:427–451.

5 Koletzko B, Brands B, Poston L, Godfrey K, Demmelmair H: Early programming of long-term health. Proc Nutr Soc 2012;71:371–378.

6 Admasu K, Haile-Mariam A, Bailey P: Indicators for availability, utilization, and quality of emergency obstetric care in Ethiopia, 2008. Int J Gynaecol Obstet 2011;115:101–105.

7 National Institute of Clinical Excellence: Weight Management Before, During and after Pregnancy. NICE Public Health Guidance 27. London, National Institute of Clinical Excellence, 2010.

8 Bhutta ZA, Das JK, Rizvi A, Gaffey MF, Walker N, Horton S, et al: Evidence-based interventions for improvement of maternal and child nutrition: what can be done and at what cost? Lancet 2013;382:452–477.

9 Victora CG, Adair L, Fall C, Hallal PC, Martorell R, Richter L, et al: Maternal and child undernutrition: consequences for adult health and human capital. Lancet 2008;371:340–357.

10 Symonds ME, Mendez MA, Meltzer HM, Koletzko B, Godfrey K, Forsyth S, et al: Early life nutritional programming of obesity: mother-child cohort studies. Ann Nutr Metab 2013;62:137–145.

11 Garofalo M, Abenhaim HA: Early versus delayed cord clamping in term and preterm births: a review. J Obstet Gynaecol Can 2012;34:525–531.

12 Van Rheenen P, De Moor L, Eschbach S, De Grooth H, Brabin B: Delayed cord clamping and haemoglobin levels in infancy: a randomised controlled trial in term babies. Trop Med Int Health 2007;12:603–616.

13 Hutton EK, Hassan ES: Late vs. early clamping of the umbilical cord in full-term neonates: systematic review and meta-analysis of controlled trials. JAMA 2007;297:1241–1252.

14 Prentice AM, Cox SE: Iron and malaria interactions: research needs from basic science to global policy. Adv Nutr 2012;3:583–591.

15 Sazawal S, Black RE, Ramsan M, Chwaya HM, Stoltzfus RJ, Dutta A, et al: Effects of routine prophylactic supplementation with iron and folic acid on admission to hospital and mortality in preschool children in a high malaria transmission setting: community-based, randomised, placebo-controlled trial. Lancet 2006;367:133–143.

16 Kumar V, Mohanty S, Kumar A, Misra RP, Santosham M, Awasthi S, et al: Effect of community-based behaviour change management on neonatal mortality in Shivgarh, Uttar Pradesh, India: a cluster-randomised controlled trial. Lancet 2008;372:1151–1162.

17 Baqui AH, El-Arifeen S, Darmstadt GL, Ahmed S, Williams EK, Seraji HR, et al: Effect of community-based newborn-care intervention package implemented through two service-delivery strategies in Sylhet district, Bangladesh: a cluster-randomised controlled trial. Lancet 2008;371:1936–1944.

18 Edmond KM, Zandoh C, Quigley MA, Amenga-Etego S, Owusu-Agyei S, Kirkwood BR: Delayed breastfeeding initiation increases risk of neonatal mortality. Pediatrics 2006;117:e380–e386.

19 Marriott BP, White A, Hadden L, Davies JC, Wallingford JC: World Health Organization (WHO) infant and young child feeding indicators: associations with growth measures in 14 low-income countries. Matern Child Nutr 2012;8:354–370.

20 Gartner LM, Morton J, Lawrence RA, Naylor AJ, O'Hare D, Schanler RJ, Eidelman AI; American Academy of Pediatrics Section on Breastfeeding: Breastfeeding and the use of human milk. Pediatrics 2005;115:496–506.

21 Agostoni C, Braegger C, Decsi T, Kolacek S, Koletzko B, et al: Breast-feeding: a commentary by the ESPGHAN Committee on Nutrition. J Pediatr Gastroenterol Nutr 2009;49:112–125.

22 Gupta A, Holla R, Dadhich JP, Suri S, Trejos M, Chanetsa J: The status of policy and programmes on infant and young child feeding in 40 countries. Health Policy Plan 2013;28:279–298.

23 Lizarazo-Medina JP, Ospina-Diaz JM, Ariza-Riano NE: The kangaroo mothers' programme: a simple and cost-effective alternative for protecting the premature newborn or low-birth-weight babies (in Spanish). Rev Salud Publica (Bogota) 2012;14(suppl 2):32–45.

24 Moore ER, Anderson GC, Bergman N, Dowswell T: Early skin-to-skin contact for mothers and their healthy newborn infants. Cochrane Database Syst Rev 2012;5:CD003519.

25 Rollins N, Meda N, Becquet R, Coutsoudis A, Humphrey J, Jeffrey B, et al: Preventing postnatal transmission of HIV-1 through breast-feeding: modifying infant feeding practices. J Acquir Immune Defic Syndr 2004;35:188–195.

26 Bhave S, Bavdekar A: Pediatric parenteral nutrition in India. Indian J Pediatr 1999;66(suppl):S141–S149.

27 Isaacs EB, Fischl BR, Quinn BT, Chong WK, Gadian DG, Lucas A: Impact of breast milk on intelligence quotient, brain size, and white matter development. Pediatr Res 2010;67:357–362.

28 Lucas A, Cole TJ: Breast milk and neonatal necrotising enterocolitis. Lancet 1990;336:1519–1523.

29 Hanson LA, Korotkova M, Haversen L, Mattsby-Baltzer I, Hahn-Zoric M, Silfverdal SA, et al: Breast-feeding, a complex support system for the offspring. Pediatr Int 2002;44:347–352.

30 Rodriguez NA, Meier PP, Groer MW, Zeller JM, Engstrom JL, Fogg L: A pilot study to determine the safety and feasibility of oropharyngeal administration of own mother's colostrum to extremely low-birth-weight infants. Adv Neonatal Care 2010;10:206–212.

31 Slutzah M, Codipilly CN, Potak D, Clark RM, Schanler RJ: Refrigerator storage of expressed human milk in the neonatal intensive care unit. J Pediatr 2010; 156:26–28.

32 Nwankwo MU, Offor E, Okolo AA, Omene JA: Bacterial growth in expressed breast-milk. Ann Trop Paediatr 1988;8:92–95.

33 Israel-Ballard K, Chantry C, Dewey K, Lonnerdal B, Sheppard H, Donovan R, et al: Viral, nutritional, and bacterial safety of flash-heated and Pretoria-pasteurized breast milk to prevent mother-to-child transmission of HIV in resource-poor countries: a pilot study. J Acquir Immune Defic Syndr 2005;40:175–181.

34 Besser M, Jackson DJ, Besser MJ, Goosen L: How long does flash-heated breast milk remain safe for a baby to drink at room temperature? J Trop Pediatr 2013;59:73–75.

35 Glynn L, Goosen L: Manual expression of breast milk. J Hum Lact 2005;21:184–185.

36 Kuschel CA, Harding JE: Multicomponent fortified human milk for promoting growth in preterm infants. Cochrane Database Syst Rev 2004;1:CD000343.

37 Charpak N, Ruiz JG: Breast milk composition in a cohort of pre-term infants' mothers followed in an ambulatory programme in Colombia. Acta Paediatr 2007;96:1755–1759.

38 Halpin DP, O'Byrne P, McEntee G, Hennessy TP, Stephens RB: Effect of a betadine connection shield on central venous catheter sepsis. Nutrition 1991;7: 33–34.

39 Jadcherla SR, Wang M, Vijayapal AS, Leuthner SR: Impact of prematurity and co-morbidities on feeding milestones in neonates: a retrospective study. J Perinatol 2010;30:201–208.

40 Poindexter BB, Langer JC, Dusick AM, Ehrenkranz RA: Early provision of parenteral amino acids in extremely low birth weight infants: relation to growth and neurodevelopmental outcome. J Pediatr 2006; 148:300–305.

41 Fenton TR, Kim JH: A systematic review and meta-analysis to revise the Fenton growth chart for preterm infants. BMC Pediatr 2013;13:1471–2431. http://www.biomedcentral.com/1471-2431/13/59. Access February 24th, 2014.

42 Ehrenkranz RA, Dusick AM, Vohr BR, Wright LL, Wrage LA, Poole WK: Growth in the neonatal intensive care unit influences neurodevelopmental and growth outcomes of extremely low birth weight infants. Pediatrics 2006;117:1253–1261.

43 Hendricks MK, Goeiman H, Dhansay A: Food-based dietary guidelines and nutrition interventions for children at primary healthcare facilities in South Africa. Matern Child Nutr 2007;3:251–258.

44 De-Regil LM, Suchdev PS, Vist GE, Walleser S, Pena-Rosas JP: Home fortification of foods with multiple micronutrient powders for health and nutrition in children under two years of age. Evid Based Child Health 2013;8:112–201.

45 Lazzerini M: Commentary on 'Home fortification of foods with multiple micronutrient powders for health and nutrition in children under two years of age'. Evid Based Child Health 2013;8:202–203.

46 Soofi S, Cousens S, Iqbal SP, Akhund T, Khan J, Ahmed I, et al: Effect of provision of daily zinc and iron with several micronutrients on growth and morbidity among young children in Pakistan: a cluster-randomised trial. Lancet 2013;382:29–40.

47 O'Connor DL, Unger S: Post-discharge nutrition of the breastfed preterm infant. Semin Fetal Neonatal Med 2013 (Epub ahead of print).

48 Collins CT, Ryan P, Crowther CA, McPhee AJ, Paterson S, Hiller JE: Effect of bottles, cups, and dummies on breast feeding in preterm infants: a randomised controlled trial. BMJ 2004;329:193–198.

49 Agostoni C, Buonocore G, Carnielli VP, De Curtis M, Darmaun D, Decsi T, et al: Enteral nutrient supply for preterm infants: commentary from the European Society of Paediatric Gastroenterology, Hepatology and Nutrition Committee on Nutrition. J Pediatr Gastroenterol Nutr 2010;50:85–91.

50 Blencowe H, Cousens S, Oestergaard MZ, Chou D, Moller AB, Narwal R, et al: National, regional, and worldwide estimates of preterm birth rates in the year 2010 with time trends since 1990 for selected countries: a systematic analysis and implications. Lancet 2012;379:2162–2172.

T. Murguia-Peniche, MD
Rollins School of Public Health
Hubert Department of Global Health, Emory University
Atlanta, GA 30322 (USA)
E-Mail tmdesierra@yahoo.com

Koletzko B, Poindexter B, Uauy R (eds): Nutritional Care of Preterm Infants: Scientific Basis and Practical Guidelines.
World Rev Nutr Diet. Basel, Karger, 2014, vol 110, pp 297–299 (DOI: 10.1159/000360195)

Recommended Nutrient Intake Levels for Stable, Fully Enterally Fed Very Low Birth Weight Infants

Berthold Koletzko[a] · Brenda Poindexter[b] · Ricardo Uauy[c]

[a]Dr. von Hauner Children's Hospital, University of Munich Medical Centre, Munich, Germany; [b]Riley Hospital for Children at Indiana University Health, Indianapolis, Ind., USA; [c]Department of Pediatrics, Catholic University, and Institute of Nutrition and Food Technology, University of Chile, Santiago de Chile, Chile

Abstract

Ranges of advisable nutrient intakes are presented for populations of fully enterally fed very low birth weight infants, based on current evidence and an intensive discussion with experts in July 2013. Recommended ranges of adequate nutrient intakes are expressed as amounts per kilogram body weight per day and also per 100 kcal energy intake. For many nutrients only limited evidence exists at present to precisely define quantitative ranges of adequate intakes. Future research may lead to better knowledge and modification of recommended intake values.   © 2014 S. Karger AG, Basel

Here we present our current recommendations for ranges of adequate daily nutrient intakes for populations of fully enterally fed, growing preterm infants with a birth weight up to 1,500 g (very low birth weight infants). These recommendations are based on the current knowledge as summarized in the various chapters of this book, as well as intensive discussions among the editors and authors held during a 2-day authors' meeting in July 2013 in Munich, Germany. Recommended nutrient intakes that are considered a reasonable goal to reach are presented as daily intakes per kilogram body weight (table 1). Recommended ranges of nutrient levels per 100 kcal energy intake have been calculated based on an energy supply of 110 kcal/kg/day considered the lower end of the range of adequate energy intakes. These recommended intakes are intended to meet the nutrient requirements of almost all medically stable and growing very low birth weight infants, although individual needs may differ according to gestational age, postconceptional age, birth weight, current weight, rates of weight gain, disease conditions, and other factors [1]. For comparative purposes, we also present the intake recommendations of the US Life Science Research Office, 2002

Table 1. Current recommendations of advisable nutrient intakes for fully enterally fed preterm very low birth weight infants per kilogram per day, and per 100 kcal energy intake, compared to the previous intake recommendations of the US Life Science Research Office (for formula-fed preterm infants only) [2, 3], of Tsang et al., 2005 [4], and of the European Society for Paediatric Gastroenterology, Hepatology and Nutrition (ESPGHAN), 2010 [5]

Nutrient	Current recommendation (per kg/day)	Current recommendation (per 100 kcal)	LSRO, 2002 (formula-fed infants only, per kg/day)	Tsang et al., 2005 (per kg/day)	ESPGHAN, 2010 (per kg/day)
Fluids	135–200	–	NS	150–200	135–200
Energy, kcal	110–130 (85–95 i.v.)	–	100–141	110–120	110–135
Protein, g	3.5–4.5	3.2–4.1	3.0–4.3	3.0–3.6	4.0–4.5 (<1 kg) 3.5–4.0 (1–1.8 kg)
Lipids, g	4.8–6.6	4.4–6	5.3–6.8		4.8–6.6 (<40% MCT)
Linoleic acid, mg	385–1,540	350–1,400	420–1,700	(4–15 E%)	385–1,540
α-Linolenic acid, mg	>55	>50	90–270	(1–4 E%)	>55
DHA, mg	(18–) 55–60	(16.4–) 50–55	NS	NS	12–30
EPA, mg	<20	<18	NS	NS	(<30% of DHA)
AA, mg	(18–) 35–45	(16.4–) 32–41	NS	NS	18–42
Carbohydrate, g	11.6–13.2	10.5–12	11.5–15.0 lactose 4.8–15.0	lactose: 3.8–11.8 oligomers: 0–8.4	11.6–13.2
Sodium, mg	69–115	63–105	46.8–75.6	0–23	69–115
Potassium, mg	78–195	71–177	72–192	0–39	66–132
Chloride, mg	105–177	95–161	72–192	0–35	105–177
Calcium, mg	120–200	109–182	148–222	120–230	120–140
Phosphate, mg	60–140	55–127	98–131	60–140	60–90
Magnesium, mg	8–15	7.3–13.6	8.2–20.4	7.9–15	8–15
Iron, mg	2–3	1.8–2.7	2–3.6	0–2	2–3
Zinc, mg	1.4–2.5	1.3–2.3	1.32–1.8	0.5–0.8	1.1–2.0
Copper, µg	100–230	90–210	120–300	120	100–132
Selenium, µg	5–10	4.5–9	2.2–6.0	1.3	5–10
Manganese, µg	1–15	0.9–13.6	7.6–30	0.75	<27.5
Fluoride, µg	1.5–60	1.4–55	NS	NS	1.5–60
Iodine, µg	10–55	9–50	7.2–42	11–27	11–55
Chromium, ng	30–2,250	27–2,045	NS	50	30–1,230
Molybdenum, µg	0.3–5	0.27–4.5	NS	0.3	0.3–5
Thiamin, µg	140–300	127–273	36–300	180–240	140–300
Riboflavin, µg	200–400	181–364	96–744	250–360	200–400
Niacin, mg	1–5.5	0.9–5	660–6,000	3.6–4.8	0.38–5.5
Pantothenic acid, mg	0.5–2.1	0.45–1.9	360–2,280	1.2–1.7	0.33–2.1
Pyridoxine, µg	50–300	45–273	36–300	150–210	45–300
Cobalamin, µg	0.1–0.8	0.09–0.73	0.096–0.84	0.3	0.1–077
Folic acid, µg	35–100	32–91	36–54	25–50	35–100
L-Ascorbic acid, mg	20–55	18–50	10–45	18–24	11–46
Biotin, µg	1.7–16.5	1.5–15	1.2–44.4	3.6–6	1.7–16.5
Vitamin A, µg RE	400–1,100	365–1,000	245–456	700	400–1,000
Vitamin D, IU	(400–1,000 per day, from milk + supplement)	100–350 from milk only	90–324	150–400	(800–1,000 per day) (100–350 per 100 kcal from milk only)
Vitamin E, mg α-TE	2.2–11	2–10	2.4–9.6	6–12	2.2–11
Vitamin K$_1$, µg	4.4–28	4–25	4.8–30	(300 bolus injection)	4.4–28
Nucleotides, mg	NS	NS	NS	NS	<5
Choline, mg	8–55	7.3–50	8.4–27.6	14.4–28	8–55
Inositol, mg	4.4–53	4–48	4.8–52.8	32–81	4.4–53

RE = Retinol equivalents; α-TE = α-tocopherol equivalents.

(for formula-fed preterm infants only) [2, 3], of Tsang et al., 2005 [4], and of the European Society for Paediatric Gastroenterology, Hepatology and Nutrition (ESPGHAN), 2010 [5].

We are aware that intakes outside of these recommended ranges may occur in infants fed human milk with added fortifiers or preterm infant formula, e.g. resulting from variation of nutrient contents in human or cow's milk, or from overages that occur to cover nutrient losses that may arise during handling and storage over a product's shelf life. The authors do not imply that nutrient contents below or above the ranges recommended here represent a risk for the target population.

These recommendations are based on a careful review of and discussion of current scientific knowledge and clinical experience by the expert group gathered in Munich on July 10–11, 2013. It is acknowledged that for many nutrients the available evidence on which the definition of an adequate intake range can be based is rather limited. The results of future research may result in redefining optimal nutrient intake levels and should lead to different desirable intake values for some nutrients in the future.

References

1 Uauy R, Koletzko B: Defining the nutritional needs of preterm infants; in Koletzko B, Poindexter B, Uauy R (eds): Nutritional Care of Preterm Infants. Basel, Karger, 2014, pp 4–10.

2 Klein CJ: Nutrient requirements for preterm infant formulas. J Nutr 2002;132(suppl 1):1395S–1577S.

3 Klein CJ, Heird WC: Summary and Comparison of Recommendations for Nutrient Contents of Low-Birth-Weight Infant Formulas. Princeton/NJ, Life Sciences Research Office, 2005.

4 Tsang R, Uauy R, Koletzko B, Zlotkin S: Nutrition of the Preterm Infant. Scientific Basis and Practical Application, ed 2. Cincinnati, Digital Educ Publ, 2005.

5 Agostoni C, Buonocore G, Carnielli VP, De Curtis M, Darmaun D, Decsi T, Domellof M, Embleton ND, Fusch C, et al; ESPGHAN Committee on Nutrition: Enteral nutrient supply for preterm infants: commentary from the European Society of Paediatric Gastroenterology, Hepatology and Nutrition Committee on Nutrition. J Pediatr Gastroenterol Nutr 2010;50:85–91.

Berthold Koletzko
Division of Metabolic and Nutritional Medicine
Dr. von Hauner Children's Hospital, University of Munich Medical Centre
Lindwurmstr. 4, DE -80337 Munich (Germany)
E-Mail Office.Koletzko@med.uni-muenchen.de

Koletzko B, Poindexter B, Uauy R (eds): Nutritional Care of Preterm Infants: Scientific Basis and Practical Guidelines.
World Rev Nutr Diet. Basel, Karger, 2014, vol 110, pp 300–305 (DOI: 10.1159/000360196)

Appendix

Appendix 1

Nutrient composition of preterm infant formulas and post-discharge formulas (PDFs)

	Mead Johnson Nutrition				Abbott		
	Enfamil® Premature 24	Enfamil® Premature 24 High Protein	Enfamil® Prematuros Premium†	Enfamil® Enfacare® Powder (post-discharge formula)	Similac® Special Care® 24 (SSC 24)	Similac® Special Care® 24 High Protein (SSC 24 HP)	Similac Expert Care® Neosure® (post-discharge formula)
Some markets where available	USA, Canada	USA, Mexico	Mexico, China	USA, Mexico	USA, Mexico, China	USA, Mexico, China	USA, Mexico, China
Energy per 100 ml, kcal	81	81	82	74	81.2	81.2	74.4
Energy per fl. oz, kcal	24	24	24	22	24	24	22
Energy, kcal	100	100	100	100	100	100	100
Protein, g	3	3.5	3	2.8	3	3.3	2.8
Carbohydrate, g	11	10.5	11	10.4	10.3	10	10.1
Lactose, g	4.5	4.2	4.5	6.8	5.15	5	5.05
Fat, g	5.1	5.1	5.1	5.3	5.43	5.43	5.5
MCT oil, % of fat	40%	40%		20%	50%	50%	25%
Linoleic acid, mg	810	810	810	860	700	700	750
α-Linolenic acid, mg	90	90	90	95			
Linoleic: linolenic, mg	9	9	9	9			
Arachidonic acid, mg	34	34	34	34	22	22	22
Docosahexaenoic acid, mg	17	17	17	17	14	14	14
ARA:DHA	2	2	2	2	1.57	1.57	1.57
Vitamin A, IU	1,250	1,250	1,250	450	1,250	1,250	350
Vitamin D, IU	240	240	240	70	150	150	70
Vitamin E, IU	6.3	6.3	6.3	4	4	4	3.6
Vitamin K, µg	8	9	8	8	12	12	11

Nestlé							Danone		
Gerber® Good Start® Premature 20	Gerber® Good Start® Premature 24	Gerber® Good Start® Premature 24 High Protein	Gerber® Good Start® Premature 30	Gerber® Good Start® Nourish (post-discharge formula)	SMA Gold Prem 1 24 Cal	SMA Gold Prem 2 Catch-up Formula (post-discharge formula)	Cow and Gate Nutri-prem 1	Cow and Gate Nutri-prem 2 (post-discharge formula)	Aptamil Preterm
USA	USA, Mexico	USA	USA	USA	USA, UK, China	USA, UK, Mexico, China	UK	UK	UK
68	81	81	101	74	82	73	80	75	80
20	24	24	30	22	24	22	24	22	24
100	100	100	100	100	100	100	100	100	100
3	3	3.6	3	2.8	2.7	2.6	3.3	2.7	3.3
10.5	10.5	9.7	10.5	10.5	10.2	10.3	10.5	9.9	10.5
5.25	5.25	4.85	5.25	6.3	5.1	7.8	5.8	7.8	5.8
5.2	5.2	5.2	5.2	5.2	5.4	5.4	4.9	5.3	4.9
40	40	40	40	20					
990	990	990	990	900	757	774			627
100	100	100	100	60	63	61			89.7
9.9	9.9	9.9	9.9	15	12	13.1	7	7.3	7
33	33	33	33	33	31	18	22	24.1	22
16.6	16.6	16.6	16.6	16.6	21	11	16.9	18.1	16.9
2.00	2	2	2	2	1.48	1.64	1.3	1.33	1.3
1,000	1,000	1,000	1,000	450	750	460	1,500	447	1,500
180	180	180	180	80	168	84	148	91.2	149.6
6	6	6	6	4	6	3.1	6.6	4.4	6.5
8	8	8	8	8	7.7	8.6	7.5	7.91	7.47

Appendix 1 Continued

	Mead Johnson Nutrition				Abbott		
	Enfamil® Premature 24	Enfamil® Premature 24 High Protein	Enfamil® Prematuros Premium†	Enfamil® Enfacare® Powder (post-discharge formula)	Similac® Special Care® 24 (SSC 24)	Similac® Special Care® 24 High Protein (SSC 24 HP)	Similac Expert Care® Neosure® (post-discharge formula)
Vitamin C, mg	20	20	15.9	16	37	37	15
Thiamin, µg	200	200	148	200	250	250	175
Riboflavin, µg	300	300	280	200	620	620	150
Pyridoxine, µg	150	150	150	60	250	250	100
Niacin, µg	4,000	4,000	2,800	1,000	5,000	5,000	1,950
Pantothenate, µg	1,200	1,200	1,200	850	1,900	1,900	800
Biotin, µg	4	4	4	5	37	37	9
Folate, µg	40	40	39	26	37	37	25
Vitamin B_{12}, µg	0.25	0.25	0.11	0.3	0.55	0.55	0.4
Sodium, mg	58	58	55	37	43	43	33
Potassium, mg	98	98	98	105	129	129	142
Chloride, mg	90	90	90	78	81	81	75
Calcium, mg	165	165	135	120	180	180	105
Phosphorus, mg	83	83	75	66	100	100	62
Magnesium, mg	9	9	9	8	12	12	9
Iron, mg	1.8 (0.5)	1.8	1.8	1.8	1.8	1.8	1.8
Zinc, mg	1.5	1.5	1.3	1	1.5	1.5	1.2
Copper, µg	120	120	110	120	250	250	120
Selenium, µg	2.8	2.8	3	2.8	1.8	1.8	2.3
Manganese, µg	6.3	6.3	6.5	15	12	12	10
Iodine, µg	25	25	25	21	6	6	15
Taurine, mg	6	6	3.9	6			
Carnitine, mg	2.4	2.4	2.4	2			
Inositol, mg	44	44	38	30	40	40	35
Choline, mg	20	20	20	24	10	10	16
Nucleotides, mg	4.2	4.2	4.2	4.2			

All values are in units per 100 kcal, unless stated otherwise.
All product forms are liquid, ready-to-use formulations, except where powder is indicated.
Missing values were either not specified, not available, or not applicable.
Values in parentheses indicate iron level in a non-iron fortified formulation.
All values are as reported in or calculated from publicly available sources as of August 2013.
Formulations included in this appendix are representative of major global manufacturers.
† Enfamil® Prematuros Premium is marketed in China and Mexico but label declarations are different between these countries due to different market requirements. The nutritional composition provided here matches the Mexico label.

Nestlé							Danone		
Gerber® Good Start® Premature 20	Gerber® Good Start® Premature 24	Gerber® Good Start® Premature 24 High Protein	Gerber® Good Start® Premature 30	Gerber® Good Start® Nourish (post-discharge formula)	SMA Gold Prem 1 24 Cal	SMA Gold Prem 2 Catch-up Formula (post-discharge formula)	Cow and Gate Nutri-prem 1	Cow and Gate Nutri-prem 2 (post-discharge formula)	Aptamil Preterm
30	30	30	30	20	18	15	21.2	16.1	21.2
200	200	200	200	150	170	150	170	120	170
300	300	300	300	200	240	220	250	200	250
200	200	200	200	100	150	110	150	110	150
4,000	4,000	4,000	4,000	1,500	2,900	1,400	3,990	2,400	3,990
1,400	1,400	1,400	1,400	1,000	1,300	550	1,100	800	1,100
5	5	5	5	3	2.9	2.9	4.36	4.02	4.36
45	45	45	45	25	35	20	43.6	26.8	43.6
0.25	0.25	0.25	0.25	0.25	0.23	0.3	0.3	0.3	0.3
55	55	55	55	35	53	37	87.2	37.6	87.2
120	120	120	120	105	90	97	102	104	102
85	85	85	85	74	82	79	94.5	70.1	94.5
164	164	164	164	120	124	100	117	117	117
85	85	85	85	65	74	58	77.4	63	77.4
10	10	10	10	10	10	9	10	9.37	10
1.8	1.8	1.8	1.8	1.8	1.7	1.7	1.99	1.61	1.99
1.3	1.3	1.3	1.3	1.2	1	1	1.37	1.21	1.37
150	150	150	150	120	110	85	99.1	80.2	99.1
2	2	2	2	2.9	2.1	2.1	5.61	2.28	5.61
7	7	7	7	7	5.8	6.8	12.5	13.4	12.5
35	35	35	35	20	12	14	32.7	26.8	32.7
10	10	10	10	10	6.9	6.9	6.85	6.6	6.9
2.6	2.6	2.6	2.6	2.6	3.2	1.5	2.2	1.2	2.2
35	35	35	35	30	37	35	29.9	29.5	29.9
15	15	15	15	24	18	18	21.2	17.4	21.2
4.6	4.6	4.6	4.6	4.6	not added	3.9	3.99	4.3	3.99

Appendix 2

Nutrient composition of human milk fortifiers

	Preterm Human Milk Estimate	Amount added to 100 ml milk				Mixed as directed†				Amount per 100 kcal* mixed as directed†			
		Mead Johnson Enfamil® Human Milk Fortifier Acidified Liquid	Abbott Similac® Human Milk Fortifier Powder	Danone Cow and Gate Nutriprem Breast Milk Fortifier Powder	Nestlé SMA Breast Milk Fortifier Powder	Mead Johnson Enfamil® Human Milk Fortifier Acidified Liquid (4 vials + 100 ml)	Abbott Similac® Human Milk Fortifier Powder (4 packets + 100 ml)	Danone Cow and Gate Nutriprem Breast Milk Fortifier (2 sachets + 100 ml)	Nestlé SMA Breast Milk Fortifier Preterm (2 sachets + 100 ml)	Mead Johnson Enfamil® Human Milk Fortifier Acidified Liquid*	Abbott Similac® Human Milk Fortifier Powder	Danone Cow and Gate Nutriprem Breast Milk Fortifier*	Nestlé SMA Breast Milk Fortifier Preterm*
Markets where available	N/A	USA, Mexico	USA, Mexico, China	UK	UK	USA, Mexico	USA, Mexico, China	UK	UK	USA, Mexico	USA, Mexico, China	UK	UK
Energy, kcal	67	30	14	16	14.6	97	79	80	84.6	100	100	100	100
Protein, g	1.62[a]	2.2	1	1.2	1	3.8	2.35	2.6	2.8	4	2.97	3.25	3.3
Carbohydrate, g	7.3[a]	<1.2	1.8	2.8	2.4	7.9	8.2	9.6	9.4	8.1	10.4	12	11.1
Lactose, g	7.3	none added		0.02		7.3		6.92		7.5		8.65	
Fat, g	3.5[a]	2.3	0.36	0	0.16	5.8	4.14	3.5	4.16	6	5.24	4.38	4.92
MCT oil, %	not relevant												
Linoleic acid, mg	480[b]	230				710				730			
α-Linolenic acid, mg	30[b]	28				58				60			
Linoleic: linolenic, mg	16	8.2				12.2				12.2			
Arachidonic acid, mg	16.5[c]	20				37				38			
Docosahexaenoic acid, mg	11.2[c]	12				23				24			
ARA:DHA	1.47	1.67				1.6				1.6			
Vitamin A, IU	48[d]	1,160	620	773	450	1,210	983	1,050	>900	1,250	1,245	1,313	>1,064
Vitamin D, IU	8[e]	188	120	200	304	200	119	207	>304	210	150	259	>359
Vitamin E, IU	0.39[d]	5.6	3.2	1.94	4.5	6	4.2	4.24	>4.5	6.2	5.3	5.3	5.32
Vitamin K, µg	2[f]	5.7	8.3	6.4	11	7.7	8.3	7.23	>11	7.9	10	9.04	>13
Vitamin C, mg	4.4[d]	15.2	25	12	40	20	34.8	16.52	>40	21	44	20.7	>47.3
Thiamin, µg	8.9[g]	184	233	132	220	193	247	142	230	200	313	178	272
Riboflavin, µg	27[g]	260	417	174	260	290	453	203	290	300	574	254	343
Pyridoxine, µg	6.2[g]	140	211	112	260	146	220	121	270	151	278	151	319
Niacin, µg	210[g]	3,700	3,570	2,400	3,600	3,900	3,623	2,490	3,810	4,000	4,587	3,113	4,504
Pantothenate, µg	230[g]	920	1,500	758	900	1,150	1,636	997	1,130	1,190	2,072	1,246	1,336
Biotin, µg	0.54[g]	3.4	26	2.6	1.5	3.9	25.7	2.86	2.5	4	32.6	3.58	2.96
Folate, µg	3.1[g]	31	23	30	30	34	25.6	35.11	33.1	35	32	43.9	39.1
Vitamin B_{12}, µg	0.02[g]	0.64	0.64	0.2	0.3	0.66	0.67	0.23	0.32	0.68	0.85	0.29	0.38
Sodium, mg	28[a]	27	15	36	18	55	39	63.5	48	57	49	79.4	56.7
Potassium, mg	50[a]	45	63	24	28	95	117	72.6	88	98	148	90.8	104
Chloride, mg	58[a]	28	38	26	17	86	91	80.3	76	89	115	100	89.8
Calcium, mg	25[a]	116	117	66	90	141	138	91.4	112	145	175	114	132
Phosphorus, mg	14.5[a]	63	67	38	46	78	78	52.2	60	80	98	65.3	70.9
Magnesium, mg	3.3[h]	1.84	7	5	3	5.1	9.8	8.13	5.5	5.3	12.4	10.2	6.5
Iron, mg	0.09[i]	1.76	0.35	0		1.85	0.46	–		1.91	0.6		
Zinc, mg	0.37[j]	0.96	1	0.6	0.26	1.33	1.31	0.9	0.66	1.37	1.65	1.13	0.78

Appendix 2 Continued

	Preterm Human Milk Estimate	Amount added to 100 ml milk				Mixed as directed[†]				Amount per 100 kcal* mixed as directed[†]			
		Mead Johnson Enfamil® Human Milk Fortifier Acidified Liquid	Abbott Similac® Human Milk Fortifier Powder	Danone Cow and Gate Nutriprem Breast Milk Fortifier Powder	Nestlé SMA Breast Milk Fortifier Powder	Mead Johnson Enfamil® Human Milk Fortifier Acidified Liquid (4 vials + 100 ml)	Abbott Similac® Human Milk Fortifier Powder (4 packets + 100 ml)	Danone Cow and Gate Nutriprem Breast Milk Fortifier (2 sachets + 100 ml)	Nestlé SMA Breast Milk Fortifier Preterm (2 sachets + 100 ml)	Mead Johnson Enfamil® Human Milk Fortifier Acidified Liquid*	Abbott Similac® Human Milk Fortifier Powder	Danone Cow and Gate Nutriprem Breast Milk Fortifier*	Nestlé SMA Breast Milk Fortifier Preterm*
Copper, µg	38[d]	60	170	36		98	228	75		101	289	93.8	
Selenium, µg	2.4[l]		0.5	1.8				4		2.5	2.4	5	
Manganese, µg	0.36[k]	10	7.2	8.2	4.6	10.4	7.6	8.54	>4.6	10.7	10	10.7	>5.44
Iodine, µg	17.8[f]			11			10	27.8		18.4	13	34.8	
Taurine, mg	4[m]												
Carnitine, mg	0.7[m]												
Inositol, mg			4				18				22.9		
Choline, mg			2				11				14		

Missing values were either not specified, not available, or not applicable.

Formulations included in this appendix are representative of major global manufacturers.

* Values are calculated based on the caloric value per 100 ml milk as provided by the product labels and may vary between individuals.

[†] Formulas within these sections should not be directly compared as each manufacturer may use different values for the nutrient composition of preterm human milk.

All values are as reported in or calculated from publicly available sources as of August 2013.

[a] Gross SJ: N Engl J Med 1983;308:237–241 (postpartum week 3) – protein, fat, carbohydrate, Ca, P, Na, K, Cl.

[b] Jensen RG: Prog Lipid Res 1996;35:53–92 (gestational age 21–36 weeks, postpartum day 42).

[c] Brenna JT, et al: Am J Clin Nutr 2007;85:1457–1464.

[d] Adapted from Moran JR, et al: J Pediatr Gastroenterol Nutr 1983;2:629–634 (21-day sample).

[e] Atkinson SA, et al: Nutr Res 1987;7:1005–1011 (14–21 days).

[f] Vitamin and Mineral Requirements in Preterm Infants; Tsang RC (ed). New York, Dekker, 1985.

[g] Ford JE, et al: Arch Dis Child 1983;58:367–372 (16–196 days).

[h] Adapted from Atkinson SA, et al: Early Hum Dev 1980;4:5–14 (first 4 weeks).

[i] Adapted from Mendelson RA, et al: Early Hum Dev 1982;6:145–151 (28–30 days).

[j] Adapted from Ehrenkranz RA: Pediatr Res 1984;18:195A, abstr 597 (28-day sample).

[k] Personal communication concerning Atkinson SA, et al: FASEB J 1989;3:A1246, abstr 5930 (2–4 weeks).

[l] Nutritional Needs of the Preterm Infant; Tsang RC, Lucas A, Uauy R, Zlotkin S (eds). Baltimore, Williams & Wilkins, 1993.

[m] Committee on Nutrition, American Academy of Pediatrics: Pediatric Nutrition Handbook, ed 2; Forbes GB, Woodruff CW (eds). Elk Grove Village/IL, American Academy of Pediatrics, 1985.

Author Index

Subject Index

carbohydrates and lung function studies in neonates 242
gross intake 65
neurodevelopment role 194
parenteral nutrition 182
protein-energy metabolism
    energy costs
        growth 71
        nitrogen balance impact of intake 72, 73
        protein and tissue synthesis 71, 72
    overview 70, 71
    recommendations
        intake 77, 78
        research 78
    requirements
        factors affecting
            age 67, 68
            body size 70
            clinical conditions 70
            metabolic factors 69
            physical activity 68, 69
            temperature of environment 69
        fetus 65–67
        preterm infants 67
Enteral nutrition, *see also specific nutrients*
    administration 206, 207
    developing countries 283
    human milk, *see also* Human milk
        benefits 202, 203
        donor human milk 203, 204
        fortification 204, 205
    infant formula 205
    initiation 185, 186, 205
    logistics 209
    minimal enteral feeding 206, 210
    overview 201, 202
    recommendations 209–211, 297–299
    tolerance 208
Estimated average requirement (EAR), definition 7
Evidence-based medicine (EBM)
    application of evidence 45, 46
    best evidence finding 40–42
    critical appraisal 42–45
    grading criteria 46
    overview of steps 39, 40
    question formulation 40
Extracellular fluid (ECF)
    overview 100
    regulation 101–103

Fat, *see* Lipids
Feeding guidelines, benefits of standardized guidelines 21, 22
Feeding tube, *see* Enteral nutrition
Folate
    functions and requirements 160–162
    heat, light, and freezing effects 153
    neurodevelopment role 193, 197
Fortification, *see* Human milk

Galactose, intake and utilization 76
Gestational age (GA)
    determination 12, 13
    nutritional needs by week 269
Glucose
    intake and utilization 74, 75
    neurodevelopment role 193
GRADE system 46
Growth curves
    birth weight-derived intrauterine growth curves 12–15
    fetal weight-derived growth curves 16
    postnatal growth curves 17
Growth failure, *see* Postnatal growth failure
Gut microbiota, *see* Intestinal microbiota

Hospital discharge
    developing countries 290, 291
    feeding practices for preterm infants
        formula 268–270, 300–303
        guidelines 266, 267
        overview 264, 265
        recommendations 274, 275
    monitoring after discharge 272, 273
    nutritional deficiencies 270, 272
    nutritional status at discharge 265, 266
    postnatal growth failure monitoring after hospital discharge 236, 237
    prospects for study 273
    vitamin D requirements of preterm infants 147, 148
Human immunodeficiency virus (HIV), transmission through milk 282–294
Human milk
    bioactive compounds 215–217
    composition 219, 220, 235, 236
    developing countries and expressed breast milk
        administration 285, 286
        fortification 285, 286
        precautions 282–285

Magnetic resonance imaging (MRI), brain volume measurement 21
Mammalian target of rapamycin (mTOR), neurodevelopment role 195, 198
Manganese
    functions and requirements 130–133
    recommendations 133
Mannose, intake and utilization 77
Medium-chain triglycerides (MCTs)
    formula composition 85
    parenteral administration 95
Mendelian randomization 37, 38
Meta-analysis
    definition 28, 30
    individual patient data 33
    multiple-treatments meta-analysis 33, 34
Methylxanthine, preterm infant studies 113
Microbiota, *see* Intestinal microbiota
Minimal enteral feeding (MEF) 206, 210
Molybdenum
    functions and requirements 135, 136
    recommendations 136
MOOSE, reporting standards 39
Multiple-treatments meta-analysis (MTM) 33, 34
Myristic acid, breast milk 84

Necrotizing enterocolitis (NEC)
    antibiotic effects 171
    carbohydrate intake studies 76
    clinical signs 255, 256
    diversity of microbes 171, 255
    epidemiology 202
    indomethacin risks 260
    laboratory evaluation 256, 257
    medical management 257, 258
    microbe-induced inflammation 260
    milk protection 216, 217, 259
    outcomes and complications 260
    pathogenesis 253–255
    prebiotic studies 173
    prevention 258, 259
    probiotic studies 172, 173, 260
    prospects for study 261
    radiography 257
    transfusion association 259, 260
    ultrasound 257
Neurodevelopment
    brain volume measurement 21
    docosahexaenoic acid benefits 5, 19

growth factors 198
nutrients in critical period
    energy 194
    lipids 194, 195
    minerals 195–197
    overview 193, 194
    protein 195
    vitamins 197, 198
overview of nutrition interactions 190–193
plasticity and vulnerability of neonatal brain 192
Niacin
    functions and requirements 159, 161, 162
    heat, light, and freezing effects 153
Nitrogen balance, impact of intake
    minerals 73
    protein-energy 72, 73
Nutritional needs
    definition 6, 7
    enteral 7
    individual 7

Osteopenia of prematurity, etiology 140

Palmitic acid, breast milk 84
Pantothenic acid
    functions and requirements 160–162
    heat, light, and freezing effects 153
Parenteral nutrition, *see also specific nutrients*
    developing countries 287, 288
    indications and benefits 178, 179
    initiation and enteral nutrition transition 185, 186
    overview 177, 178
    practical aspects 181, 183
    prospects for study 186
    quality assurance and good practice 184, 185
    risks 179, 180
    solutions 182, 183
    standardization 184
Pasteurization, expressed breast milk 285
Patent ductus arteriosus (PDA), clinical trials of fluid and sodium intake 100, 108–110
Peripherally inserted central catheter (PICC), parenteral nutrition risks 179, 180
Phosphorous
    enteral requirements 142–144
    hospital-discharged infants 270
    lung function studies in neonates 246

milk fortification in developing
   countries 286
perinatal homeostasis 141
Polyunsaturated fatty acids (PUFAs), *see also*
   specific fatty acids
digestion and absorption 87, 88
enteral administration
   practical aspects 91–93
   timing and amount 88–91
fetal accretion and metabolism 85–87
lung function studies in neonates 244–246
neurodevelopment role 193–195
parenteral administration
   practical aspects 94–96
   timing and amount 93, 94
Population reference intake (PRI),
   definition 7, 8
Postnatal growth failure
consequences 230, 231
definition of growth faltering 231, 232
early nutritional support in prevention
   goals 232
   intravenous amino acids 233, 234
   optimization 233
   prescribed versus actual intake
      234, 235
   protein optimization 235
incidence 229
monitoring after hospital discharge 236,
   237
neurodevelopment studies 194, 195, 231
risk factors 230
Potassium
conditions of excess and deficiency 114
input, factors affecting 105
output, factors affecting 105, 106
postnatal adaptation of fluid and electrolyte
   homeostasis in preterm infants
   clinical trials
      phase I 108–110
      phase II and III 111, 112
      respiratory distress syndrome 108
      stabilization with problems 112, 113
      stabilization without problems 112
   phases 106, 107
Potential renal solute load (PRSL) 105, 107
Prebiotics
necrotizing enterocolitis studies 173
overview 173, 174
Primary peritoneal drainage (PPD),
   necrotizing enterocolitis management 258

PRISMA, reporting standards 39
Probiotics
monitoring 173
necrotizing enterocolitis studies 172, 173,
   260
overview 172
Protein, *see also* Amino acids
digestion and absorption 53, 54
early nutritional support optimization 235
enteral nutrition
   practical aspects 60
   preterm infant requirements 57, 58
fortifiers 221, 222
human milk composition 219, 220, 235,
   236
lung function studies in neonates 243, 244
metabolism and distribution 52, 53
neurodevelopment role 193, 195
overview 50
parenteral nutrition 181
protein-energy metabolism
   energy costs
      growth 71
      nitrogen balance impact of intake
         72, 73
      protein and tissue synthesis 71, 72
   overview 70, 71
quality in formula and human milk
   58–60
Pyridoxine
enteral feeding 163
functions and requirements 159–162
heat, light, and freezing effects 153
neurodevelopment role 193

Randomized control trial (RCT)
overview 34
rapid critical appraisal 42, 43
Recommended daily allowance (RDA),
   definition 7, 8
Reference nutrient intake (RNI), definition
   7, 8
Respiratory distress syndrome (RDS), clinical
   trials of fluid and sodium intake 108, 109
Riboflavin
enteral feeding 163, 164
functions and requirements 159, 161, 162
heat, light, and freezing effects 153

Selenium
enteral nutrition 136